The Clinical Field

ITS USE IN NURSING EDUCATION

Dorothy E. Reilly, R.N., Ed.D., F.A.A.N.
Professor of Nursing
College of Nursing
Wayne State University
Detroit, Michigan

Marilyn H. Oermann, R.N., Ph.D.
Associate Professor of Nursing
College of Nursing
Wayne State University
Detroit, Michigan

APPLETON-CENTURY-CROFTS/Norwalk, Connecticut

To our mentors whose wisdom and caring influenced our careers.

0-8385-1127-9

Notice: The authors and publisher of this volume have taken care that the
information and recommendations contained herein are accurate
and compatible with the standards generally accepted at the time of publication.

Copyright © 1985 by Appleton-Century-Crofts
A Publishing Division of Prentice-Hall, Inc.

85 86 87 88 89 / 10 9 8 7 6 5 4 3 2 1

Prentice-Hall of Australia, Pty. Ltd., Sydney
Prentice-Hall Canada, Inc.
Prentice-Hall Hispanoamericana, S.A., Mexico
Prentice-Hall of India Private Limited, New Delhi
Prentice-Hall International (UK) Limited, London
Prentice-Hall of Japan, Inc., Tokyo
Prentice-Hall of Southeast Asia (Pte.) Ltd., Singapore
Whitehall Books Ltd., Wellington, New Zealand
Editora Prentice-Hall do Brasil Ltda., Rio de Janeiro

Library of Congress Cataloging in Publication Data

Reilly, Dorothy E.
  The clinical field.

  Includes index.
  1. Nursing—Study and teaching. 2. Medicine,
Clinical—Study and teaching. I. Oermann, Marilyn H.
II. Title. [DNLM: 1. Education, Nursing.
2. Preceptorship. WY 18 R362c]
RT73.R43 1985   610.73'07'11   85-11234
ISBN 0-8385-1127-9

Design: Lynn Luchetti

PRINTED IN THE UNITED STATES OF AMERICA

Contents

Meaning of Professional Practice/1; Theories of
Practice/2; Purposes of Clinical Practice in an
Educational Program/4; Nursing as a Practice
Discipline/7; Theory of Practice in
Nursing/9; Clinical Practice Setting: Laboratory or
Field/10; Historical Perspective of Clinical Practice
in Nursing Education/12

Rationale for a Conceptual Framework of the
Teaching–Learning Process/17; Learning Concept
Rooted in Human Science Theory/18; Concept of
Learning/20; Concept of Teaching/29; The
Dynamic: Teaching and Learning/35; Relevance of
Conceptual Framework of the Teaching–Learning
Process to Teaching in the Clinical Field/36

A Concept of Nursing Process/41; Derivation of the
Nursing Process/42; Nature of Nursing
Process/43; Nursing Process—Nursing
Frameworks/56; Teaching the Nursing Process in
the Clinical Field/57

10. Clinical Evaluation.. 297

Concept of Evaluation/298; Nature of Clinical
Evaluation Process/301; Relationship of Clinical
Evaluation to Objectives/303; Methods of
Evaluating Clinical Practice/305; Use of Multiple
Strategies for Clinical Evaluation/321; Evaluation
Protocol for Unit on Chronic Pain/322

11. Grading of Clinical Field Experience................. 331

Meaning of Grades/331; Uses for
Grades/334; Types of Grading Systems/335; Issues
on Grading Clinical Performance/338; Grading
Systems for Clinical Practice Experience/340

12. A Future Perspective: The Clinical Field............. 351

The Information Society/352; Prospective Payment:
Impact on Health Care Settings/359; The Use of
the Clinical Field in the Future/368; Effect of
Change on Purposes for Use of Clinical
Field for Preparation of Practitioners/372

Index... 381

Foreword

It is interesting that the first major text on clinical education appears a little less than a hundred years after Annabelle McCrae was employed as the first teacher of nursing. Dorothy Reilly and Marilyn Oermann, Professors of Nursing at Wayne State University, are pathfinders. They have written a theoretical text about the realities of teaching clinical disciplines. The chapters in this book discuss cognitive, psychomotor and affective clinical learning, the placement of clinical practice within the curriculum, clinical evaluation and grading and the use of the nursing process and conceptual frameworks in a clinical milieu. The senior author, Dorothy Reilly, is well-recognized in educational circles and has written definitively about the structural elements of nursing education. In this new text she makes a conceptual leap and charts a course along an unexplored terrain, the clinical education of the professional.

How many of us have wondered about the quality of our clinical teaching? Frequently these concerns are expressed by arguments about appropriate faculty/student ratios, percentage of course grades to be given for clinical work, and the appropriate length of each clinical experience. *The Clinical Field: Its Use in Nursing Education* provides a comprehensive overview against which we can measure our teaching practices and evaluate the usefulness of traditional concepts and methodologies. It will help seasoned and new teachers to raise questions about their world views and their methods of instruction. The act of bringing teachers to self-examination, requires that we submit our theories in use and theories of practice to quantitative and qualitative analysis.

This text is not a how-to-do-it book. Rather it is a thoughtful reflection on professional practice and the forms of education which develop clinical acumen and judgment. Read it.

Sister Rosemary Donley, Ph.D., R.N.
Dean, Catholic University of America
School of Nursing
February 12, 1985

Preface

The clinical field is an opportunity. Its rich and diverse resources present an ever increasing challenge to nursing educators. How should it be used to maximize its potential within nursing education programs toward the goal of preparation of nurses for practice? Oftentimes, when one element in a program is in constant usage, there is a tendency to ignore the need for a periodic scrutiny of its role thus resulting in a general acceptance of present practices. A somewhat routinized usage occurs with little acknowledgement of the changes, both internally and externally, which demand new considerations.

In this book, we have explored the clinical field component of nursing education programs within the context of present and emerging trends in nursing, health care and education and have offered proposals for its usage. The book is of particular significance to educators in schools of nursing and in-service departments in health care agencies and to graduate students preparing for the teaching role. Its value extends further to those faculty in other health care disciplines who incorporate clinical field practice in their educational programs.

The use of the clinical field is viewed in its total spectrum—its purpose, structure and the processes entailed within its boundaries. Philosophical, theoretical and practical perspectives constitute the framework for the presentations in each chapter.

The theoretical framework of clinical practice in Chapter 1 is derived from that of Argyris and Schön which extends the notion of field practice in a professional program beyond the generally accepted purpose of providing the opportunity to apply theory to practice with real clients. Their emphasis on the competencies of the professional person capable of responsible practice in a rapidly changing society serves as a theme throughout the book in terms of the purposes to be achieved and the teaching practices demanded within the clinical field.

A conceptual framework of the teaching–learning process in Chapter 2 provides the basis for proposals of learning activities, teaching methodologies and evaluation strategies offered throughout the book.

Because nursing process is the methodology of practice, it receives special emphasis in Chapter 3 relative to the competencies required and the teaching processes which are appropriate. Special acknowledgement is extended to five of nursing's noted theorists for their contribution to this chapter. Each theorist, Imogene King, Betty Neuman, Dorothea Orem, Martha Rogers and Sister Callista Roy, most generously critiqued the concept of nursing process depicted for her theory and made the appropriate modifications in the text. Their contribution to this book is most remarkable for it enables us to demonstrate the similarities and differences among the theorists in their approach to nursing process.

The clinical field as a milieu for learning nursing practice is presented in Chapter 4, followed in Chapter 5 by a description of the multiple teaching and learning strategies available for use in the clinical setting to meet varied objectives.

The next three chapters, 6, 7, 8, are allocated to a substantive discussion of the teaching of each of the three domains of learning: cognitive, psychomotor and affective. It is recognized that all three domains are interrelated in most learning, but the three are treated in this book as discrete entities in recognition of the fact that there are specific behavioral outcomes for each and that teachers use specific teaching and evaluation methods when emphasizing each one.

In Chapter 9, a unit on instruction demonstrates the approach to planning a curriculum component which uses both clinical and classroom activities. The teaching and learning activities are prescribed in accord with the objectives of the unit. The following two chapters, 10 and 11, draw upon this chapter to present concepts and processes of evaluation and grading of clinical practice learning in the field.

The final chapter, 12, includes a projection for the future usage of the clinical field in nursing education with particular reference to current major changes occurring in the health care system; technology entrenchment, and newer patterns of reimbursement for hospital care which seek to address the limitations in the monies for health care.

Many individuals have made contributions to us during the writing of this book; our students who helped us in the formulation of many ideas; our faculty colleagues at the College of Nursing, Wayne State University: Geraldine Flaherty, Judith Floyd, Marjorie Isenberg, Norma McHugh, Kathleen Monahan, Barbara Pieper, Fern Sturgis, and Ann Whall, who responded with their wise and astute criticisms when called upon for specific parts of the book; our very skillful, knowledgeable and patient typist, Julia Ploshehanski, who prepared the final manuscript; and David Oermann, who was a sustaining supporter during the entire enterprise.

We are most indebted to our friend and professional colleague, Maria Phaneuf, who served as a continuous expert reviewer and critic during the evolution of the book. Her breadth of vision, knowledge of nursing and matters pertinent to health care, and her literary expertise greatly influence the text in terms of both substance and effect.

We are grateful for the opportunity to present this book to our associates in nursing education.

D.E.R.
M.H.O.

1

A Theoretical Perspective of Clinical Practice

Professionals practice. This statement determines the entire spectrum of professional education: substance, methodology, setting, and future directions. It is therefore clear that professional education must provide for a practice component where the student learns to think and act like the professional in the specific discipline. Its practice component differentiates a professional discipline from an academic discipline. Donaldson and Crowley (1978) note the distinction between the two disciplines. "Academic disciplines emphasize knowing and the theories are descriptive. Professional disciplines are directed toward practical aims and thus generate prescriptive as well as descriptive theories" (p. 115).

MEANING OF PROFESSIONAL PRACTICE

Professionals in a society serve in an area important to that society and through possession of expertise in a specific domain of knowledge serve in behalf of particular needs of designated clients. The practice of professionals in service fields comprises clinical judgments derived from theories, laws, knowledge, principles, and some intuition; the use of specialized skills; and the acceptance of the client as an autonomous being with own inherent rights. Practice is defined as a deliberately planned sequence of action carried out by highly skilled individuals in response to particularized needs of clients.

Practice, so described, suggests that a professional makes a commitment of service to a particular clientele and that this commitment requires a lifetime career. An additional component to the service element is its legitimization granted by society to members of the profession as long as those members perform their tasks for the good of society. Society in some ways declares ownership of the professional; for the right to practice can be withdrawn whenever society deems that its needs are not being served in accord with accepted standards.

Two notions are significant. One is that the professional possesses a unique body of knowledge and skills used in service to clients in a community; the other is that this service represents a lifelong career commitment. A professional's practice occurs in juxtaposition with the practice of other professionals within a larger society, which itself is in a constant state of flux as it responds to multiple currents in the world of ideas and actions. The body of knowledge and skills that the professional brings to practice in that society can be no more static than the events occurring in society at large at any given time. Client systems may change, client problems may change, the expectations of service may change, indeed, the nature of the professional's knowledge and skills may be markedly altered over a career span. The role of the professional is subject to change as society becomes more knowledgeable and more differentiated relative to the services it demands.

The education of the professional requires more than the use of current knowledge and skills within a delineated practice mode. Preparation for practice addresses skills in learning to learn, initiating or responding to change, and maintaining a realistic perspective of one's practice within the framework of ideas and events of society at any point in time. Society's tendency toward differentiation of services means that no one professional's area of practice is "turf bound"; thus skills of interdisciplinary collaboration in addressing client needs are required. Practice must be viewed continuously within spatial and temporal dimensions.

THEORIES OF PRACTICE

The charge to educators of professionals is to prepare practitioners who not only possess the requisite knowledge and skills inherent in their practice, but who also have the ability to evolve their own theory of practice, which is congruent with the expectations of the discipline as it interfaces with society. Such a practitioner does not limit the perception of his or her own actions to the ability to meet client needs, but also sees the opportunity these actions provide for reflection on their meaning, significance, and potential for generating new knowledge for future practice.

Argyris and Schön (1974) define a theory of action as it pertains to the activities of an individual in practice: "A theory of action is a theory of deliberative human behavior which is for the agent a theory of control, but which, when attributed to that agent serves to explain or predict behavior" (p. 6). Within the scope of practice, the activity selected by the practitioner to meet a particular client need is defined by the practitioner in terms of a specific knowledge referent. The consistency with which the individual uses an action in practice for a specifically determined purpose results in that person's identification with the act and the nature of the practice in use. The scope of theories of action with any one profession's practice is extensive because of the complexity of client needs and the environment in which the practice occurs.

Does a theory of practice exist? What are the dimensions? Argyris and Schön (1974) support the notion of a theory of practice with the following definition:

> A theory of practice, then, consists of a set of interrelated theories of action that specify for the situations of practice, the actions that will under relevant assumptions yield intended consequences. Theories of practice usually contain theories of intervention, that is theories of action aimed at enhancing effectiveness; these may be differentiated according to roles in which intervention is attempted. (p. 6)

A discipline's theory of practice incorporates theories relevant to the nature of the services it renders, theories of communication and interaction relating to the mode of interaction of the participants, and social and political theories which provide knowledge of the dynamics of structures within which the practice occurs. The profession identifies the theories of action pertinent to its practice and then assumes responsibility for assuring that its practitioners are competent in their use.

The inclusion of practice in a profession implies activity: a "doing," an experiencing. It is more than engaging in an intellectual process relative to theories of action. It means participation in activities which lead to competent use of these theories of action. Practice entails thoughtful consideration of a setting where students have the opportunity to develop skill in use of the theories. Schein (1972) refers to practice as putting the students in a position where they deal with *real* problems. Thus, the nature of the practice setting is determined by the opportunities it provides for students to apply the theories of action with real clinical problems. The emphasis of the reality dimension on the *clinical problem* rather than the setting is significant. Too often the practice setting is described as the real world when in reality it may be the opposite in terms of career practice goals of many students. Furthermore, because of specialization in health care, many settings are a distortion of the real world; for example, an acute children's hospital in a medical center is not the real world to learn about the health care needs of children, for most children's health care is delivered in ambulatory settings.

PURPOSES OF CLINICAL PRACTICE IN AN EDUCATIONAL PROGRAM

Clinical practice provides the opportunity for students to become skillful in the use of theories of action. This statement is a technical perspective whereby one learns the skills necessary to address client problems. A traditionalist might support this perspective as the sole purpose, but teachers of professional students need to recognize that clinical practice experience provides many other learnings essential for competent professional practice. Clinical practice is envisioned as more than the opportunity to put theory learned in the classroom into practice. Benner (1983) notes that "theory offers what can be made explicit and formalized, but clinical practice is always more complex and presents many more realities than can be captured by theory alone" (p. 36). Faculty who conceptualize clinical practice from a narrow perspective limit the opportunities for growth in other dimensions which the individual needs to function with confidence in an evolving society and profession.

Learning How to Learn
The professional is an eternal learner throughout the duration of the professional career. Expansions in the frontier of knowledge and the changing expectations of society continuously influence the nature of practice. The student in the profession needs to develop learning skills which facilitate inquiry, pursuit of ideas, concentration, integration, and evaluation. Security in the known as the basis for making clinical decisions is not self-serving. Since this knowledge serves others, responsibility for maintenance of current knowledge is a high priority for a professional practitioner.

Clinical practice provides a fertile experience in learning how to learn. The reality of problems guarantees students will encounter variations in "normal" responses that challenge them to seek alternative knowledge and skills for resolution. The multidisciplinary encounters in most clinical practice sites expose the learner to differing approaches to similar problems. The student is challenged to examine and to try new modalities of care. The faculty is challenged to accept risk-taking behavior. This behavior is not chance behavior, but a carefully thought out plan of action in which possible consequences have been noted but the actual outcome remains uncertain. Calculated risk means consideration of risks ranging from reasonable anticipated best outcomes of the action to the potentially worse outcomes of the action for all participants. This process of risk analysis is problem-solving behavior using divergent thinking, a critical element in learning how to learn.

The encouragement of the student for calculated risk-taking in meeting client needs fosters a lifelong learner open to new ideas and

experiences. The demand for "tried and true" practice stifles learning potential and fosters the development of a practitioner restricted
to "what is" and reticent to deal with new ideas.

Handling Ambiguity

Professional practice is concerned with the known and the unknown. Some aspects of practice are convergent (one action is possible) since their rationale is supported by theory. Other components
of practice are divergent (multiple actions are possible), since no one
theory provides the support for a response. Schein (1972) speaks of
the important component of a professional program as "training for
uncertainty." He describes the characteristic skills as, "maintenance of one's self-confidence even when one does not have a clear
answer to the problem; willingness to take responsibility for key
decisions that may rest on only partial information, and willingness
to make decisions under conditions of high risk" (p. 45). Clinical
practice must provide the student with both convergent and divergent components of professional practice. Too often the convergent
component receives priority while divergent thinking, which demands dealing with ambiguities and risk taking, is often avoided.
The critical question: "What else is possible?" when students suggest an action will help them move from a dualistic approach to a
relativistic one.

Skill in handling ambiguity is also a function of the student's
ability to deal with role conflict encountered when in the clinical
field. Hursh and Borzak (1982) report on this matter in the report of
the study of the role of field work in cognitive development. They
state, ". . . the student fluctuated between pleasures of giving, relating, helping, doing on the one hand and taking, learning, objec-
tifying, analyzing on the other" (p. 69). Students faced with such a
dilemma need to come to a resolution by identifying the common
denominators of both the student and caregiver roles. Viewing the
situation from both perspectives calls upon problem-solving skill. A
reconciliation of these roles is posed by Hursh and Borzak (1982):

> (a) modifying role of the student toward that of scholar, i.e., one who as
> an adult is interested in learning things in systematic ways, and (b)
> emphasizing in the role such capacities as a systematic (rather than
> hunch based) problem solving, informed (rather than speculative) deci-
> sion making, effective communication and periodic distancing in order
> to maintain objectivity and allow for careful observation of events
> (rather than subjective identification with them). (p. 75)

Think Like Professionals

Practice enables the student to develop the process of thinking most
appropriate to the profession. Professional knowledge includes the
abstract and the concrete. Professionals approach their practice

from a problem-solving perspective rather than a task-oriented perspective. The problem-solving approach which incorporates skill in divergent thinking enables the learner to pose questions whose resolution will contribute to the development of a theory of practice for the individual.

Professionals are expected to think about their practice within the broader context of the society in which it occurs. Although some professionals have developed tunnel vision about their practice, whereupon the focus is confined to the sphere of their own individual activities, an informed public is demanding that all professionals address their practice within social demands and expectations. The practice component of a professional program contributes significantly to the socialization of the student into the professional role and its concomitant values of social consciousness, ethical and moral accountability, and responsibility to society.

Develop Personal Causation

Argyris and Schön (1974) suggest another important outcome of clinical practice learning: the acceptance of the notion of personal causation, the commitment to be responsible for one's own actions. Societal permission for professionals to practice implies that it will hold each professional accountable for all actions relative to practice. The clinical practice experience enables the student to minister to real clients in the management of real problems inherent in their practice. As students, clinical assignments are relegated on the basis of the knowledge and skills possessed at any particular time. Practice enables the student to develop competency to a designated level under the supervision of a faculty or preceptor. Even within this early structured process, the student learns to be accountable for preparation for the learning experience and recording the results according to established protocol. The notion of personal causation learning requires a deliberative process, which is developmental in nature. It must be a positive learning experience, not one of threat, which adds the element of fear to the learning experience.

In summary, clinical practice experience serves a multipurpose role in the education of professionals. It provides experience necessary for the learner to develop knowledge, skills, and values inherent in the theories of action accepted by the profession and necessary for the individual to be self-confident, responsive to society's expectations, and a continuous learner in pursuit of new knowledge that will have an impact on practice. The nature of the contributions of clinical practice experience calls for it to be an integral part of the total curriculum, not an added experience in the final term of studies. The competencies to be achieved are developmental and, thus, must be provided for in increasing complexity in a sequential pattern of experience throughout the total program.

NURSING AS A PRACTICE DISCIPLINE

Is nursing a practice discipline? Nursing research is posing questions as to the nature of a nursing science and its practice element. It is acknowledged that nursing professionals possess expertise in specific areas of knowledge which is used in behalf of particular needs of designated clients. Its practice represents clinical judgments derived from theories, laws, knowledge, principles, and some intuition; the use of specialized skills; and the acceptance of the client as an autonomous being with own inherent rights. This description reflects nursing's compatibility with the description of practice noted earlier in the chapter.

Clinical practice may be conceptualized as the medium through which the nurse uses a particular constellation of abilities based on selected theories of action to meet health needs of clients. It is a dynamic comprised of cognitive, psychomotor, and affective behaviors. It is a synthesis of all of these behaviors into a holistic framework called nursing process, the methodology of the practice. It is problem oriented; it involves decision making; it calls for the best of fit between scientifically determined assessed data and intervention strategies reflecting the appropriate theories of action.

Conceptualization of the phenomenon of nursing is being subjected to much research from various perspectives. Definitions of nursing are varied, often reflecting the particular perceptions of the different researchers. Donaldson and Crowley (1978) analyzed nursing literature and arrived at three generalizations which form the core of a nursing discipline:

1. Concern with the principles and laws that govern the life processes and optimum functioning of human beings—sick or well.
2. Concern with the patterning of human behavior in interaction with the environment in critical life situations.
3. Concern with the processes by which positive changes in health status are affected. (p. 113)

Fawcett (1984) describes a metaparadigm on nursing which incorporates the four major concepts generally accepted by nursing theorists: *recipient* of care (individual, family, group, community, society); the *environment*, encompassing relevant inanimate and animate surroundings; *health*, referring to wellness or illness; and *nursing actions*, which include all activities of members of the profession.

Two definitions proposed by nursing authorities are most appropriate to the discussion of the clinical practice component of nursing. The Social Policy Statement of the American Nurses Association (1980) supporting the language in the New York State Practice Act states: "Nursing is the diagnosis and treatment of human responses to actual or potential health problems" (p. 9). Schlotfeldt

(1981) provides the following definition: "Nursing is assessing and enhancing the general health status, health assets, and potential of human beings" (p. 298). These definitions convey the notion of goal-directed services within a defined scope of practice.

Nursing, like other professions, has various categories of practitioners whose level of mastery of knowledge and skill is delineated by the nature of their preparation for entry into the field. Many approaches to differentiating the practice of each of these categories have been proposed with little success in outcome. Delineation is important if the use of the clinical practice experience is to be maximized. Since all groups are involved in making clinical decisions, the nature of the decisions each group makes could serve as the critical criterion for defining boundaries of practice. Relevant to these decisions are the types and depths of interventions for which the nurse will be held accountable and for which learning experiences in the clinical field must be designed.

Practical nursing programs address those clinical decisions that relate to the overt needs of clients' daily living activities. Since these activities are incorporated in the nursing process, practical nurses would be expected to use the process under the direction of the registered nurse. In addition to developing competencies in their own areas of practice, practical nurses would learn those skills essential for a supportive role to the registered nurse.

Programs for associate and diploma students address clinical decisions relating to the overt and covert needs of the client in those areas of care where prescriptive nursing measures are already described for nursing management. Nursing process is developed to a level of mastery with decision making directed toward a differential selection of the appropriate prescriptive management protocol for any given situation.

Programs in baccalaureate nursing address clinical decisions involving overt and covert needs of clients, not only where prescriptive nursing exists, but also where nursing decisions entail developing new modes of nursing management based on analysis of nursing and supportive theories. Nursing process relates to the known and unknown with the nurse having the ability to develop hypotheses that can be tested on the basis of suitable theories of action.

Graduate programs address clinical decision-making involving multivariate or highly specialized client problems which entail the known and unknown. A research posture is in order as the graduate practitioner uses the nursing process to meet specialized client needs. Theories of action are tested and synthesized into a theory of use for each practitioner.

Whatever the level of practice, all categories of nurses providing nursing care to clients have specific skills to perform and a body of knowledge which must be translated into action. The depth and breadth of the practice and the dimensions of accountability are described by the expectations of practice.

THEORY OF PRACTICE IN NURSING

Nursing theory development proceeds on multiple fronts at this time in nursing history, and the processes involved are duly recorded in the nursing literature (Fawcett, 1984; Kim, 1983; Newman, 1979). A framework particularly useful for the discussion of the clinical practice component of nursing education programs is the theory of practice defined by Argyris and Schön (1974). Elements of the theory include:

1. A set of interrelated theories of action that specify for the situations of practice actions that will, under relevant assumptions, yield intended consequences.
2. Theories of intervention are composed of theories of action aimed at enhancing effectiveness. These may be differentiated according to roles in which intervention is attempted. (p. 6)

Theories of Action

Nursing is an intervention activity for the health of individuals in interaction with their environment during all stages of life in any state of health or illness. Nursing represents multiple theories of action as it seeks to answer to the health-related responses of the clients. The nature of nursing lends itself to three classifications of theories of action, namely, people-centered, health, and nature of practice milieu.

People-centered Theories of Action
Interpersonal interaction
Intrapersonal interaction
Communication
Interviewing
Teaching
Counseling
Group process
Systems
Change

Health Theories of Action
Health promotion
Health maintenance
Disease/illness prevention
Disease/illness intervention
Human systems functioning
Observation

Therapeutic intervention
Mobility
Environmental management

Nature of Practice Milieu Theories of Action
Decision making
Collaboration
Leadership
Power and influence
Conflict resolution
Organizational behavior
    Agency
    Community
    Profession

The relationship of these theories to the practice of nursing in terms of their expression in practice requires much research. Argyris and Schön (1974) differentiate between *espoused theory,* that which is at least tacitly acknowledged and to which the individual gives allegiance when asked, and *theory in use,* that which the individual actually uses as a guide for action. The latter is based upon assumptions about self, others, the situation and connections among action, consequence, and situation. The position of Benner (1983) that there is a lack of knowledge of what occurs over time in actual nursing practice is consistent with Argyris and Schön's position that professions lack knowledge about theory in use. Benner states:

> Knowledge development in an applied discipline consists of extending practical knowledge (know-how) through theory-based scientific investigations and through the charting of existing "know-how" developed through clinical experience in the practice of the discipline. (p. 3)

The nurse uses and examines these theories of action on a selective basis as they pertain to a role or function at any particular time. The unique constellation of theories of action developed into theories of intervention and used in a consistent manner becomes the individual's theory of practice.

CLINICAL PRACTICE SETTING: LABORATORY OR FIELD

The clinical setting in which students develop the competencies essential for professional practice is often referred to as a laboratory. Webster's dictionary states that a laboratory is a place equipped for experimental study in science or for testing and analysis. It provides a broader interpretation which identifies the laboratory as a place where there is opportunity for experimentation, observation, or practice in a field of study. Absent from the definition is the word *experiencing*. Experiencing implies the notion of involvement in a process; i.e., the nursing student is experiencing the practice of nursing, not remaining outside the learning event as often occurs in science laboratories.

The word laboratory often conjures up an image of a controlled unipurpose environment in which the object of learning is isolated and all of the energy of the learner is directed toward the learning event. Distractions are generally eliminated, the learning activity is assured, and a reasonable time frame can be determined. However, in an activity-oriented, multipurpose environment, control of the object of learning is uncertain, distractions are indigenous, and time is less easily controlled. The energy of the learner must be shared between the need to address the learning object and self-management within the demands precipitated by the situation. In the laboratory, the practice of interviewing can be focused and controlled. In a clinical setting the practice of interviewing may be influenced by the changing health status of the client, demands on the client from others in the setting, and concurrent diverse activities which may be occurring in the setting at any one particular time.

Labels have significance in conveying meaning and in establishing a mind set. Because the word laboratory may conjure up an image of controlled learning experience primarily focused on the manipulation of objects and the cognitive processes necessary for interpretation, another word is needed to convey a concept of selective learning within a dynamic environment. Many professional disciplines refer to a *practice field* rather than to a *practice laboratory*. Field suggests a gestalt, a locus of operations where multiple goal-directed activities are taking place concurrently. Faculty may not control the field but can select the learning activity from the field and delineate its boundaries. However, the control is not absolute and faculty must be prepared to accommodate uncontrollable events and to maximize serendipitous learning events which may arise.

A comparison of the characteristics of the laboratory and the field concept is depicted in Table 1.

The notion of a field practice instead of laboratory practice is more compatible with the purposes of clinical practice described earlier in the chapter. A faculty who perceives the setting as a field will approach the environment from a broader vision of its potential for developing various professional competencies than will faculty who sees the setting as a laboratory with sharply defined goals for learning. Most nursing programs do have a laboratory which reflects the described characteristics and is often referred to as a learning resource laboratory where students can practice in a con-

TABLE 1. CHARACTERISTICS OF LABORATORY AND FIELD

Laboratory	Field
Predictable environment	Nonpredictable environment
Unipurpose	Multipurpose
Learning experience controlled	Learning experience selected

Learning activity
  manipulation of object
	Learning activity
	  experiencing

Learner energy focused	Learner energy shared
Distractions limited	Distractions indigenous
Time determined	Time uncertain

trolled environment. Maximizing that setting as a true laboratory for initial practice, faculty can use the field setting for reality practice, analysis, and synthesis.

HISTORICAL PERSPECTIVE OF CLINICAL PRACTICE IN NURSING EDUCATION

Christy (1980) reminds us that clinical practice has always been a function of nursing education, although the role has experienced varied interpretations. Florence Nightingale posited an educational value to clinical practice in the program she established at St. Thomas Hospital. Her emphasis on autonomy for the school from the hospital demanded three requisites, namely:

- It must be an independent educational institution.
- It must have its own independent funds.
- It must have its own board of trustees.

Such a position enabled the school to pursue its educational mission and develop a systematic approach to the theoretical and practice components of the program. The Nightingale system saw the beginning of the unification model in the appointment of a matron responsible to the hospital for care of the patients and to the school for the education of the students. This position reflected Nightingale's belief in the interrelationship of nursing education and service.

Practice in the wards was conducted in an apprenticeship mode under the tutelage of ward sisters, paid by the hospital with an increment for teaching. Teaching emphasis was placed on helping pupils develop skills in *how* to observe, *what* to observe, *how* to think, and *what* to think. Methods included ward teaching, case study, and use of procedure sheets in medical-surgical settings and later in the community. Clinical practice sites in the hospital were selected on the basis of their relevance to the educational program, not in terms of patient care needs.

Although the Nightingale system of nursing education was adopted by three hospitals in the United States in 1873 (The Connecticut Training School, The Boston Training School, and The Bellevue School), the educational value inherent in the system was soon diminished as hospitals realized the potential for nursing schools to provide pupils to meet the need for care of the sick. Roberts (1954) reports that by the end of the first decade in the twentieth century, nursing schools increased from 437 to 1129. Most of these schools were started for economic, not educational reasons, and the primary mode of education was trial-and-error in the ward setting.

This period is often noted as the time of apprenticeship learning in nursing education, but it was not, for there was no one under whom students could serve as apprentices. Instruction in the hospital was by fellow students, seniors, or ward aides, although in a random fashion, doctors did some lecturing and bedside instruction. The first position of instructor to nurses, as noted by Roberts (1954), was the appointment of Jane Delano in the University of Pennsylvania School of Nursing in 1890. In 1885, Isabel McIsaac, principal of the Illinois Training School for Nurses, and a superlative teacher, is believed to be first to institute instruction in nursing procedures. However, by 1910, only one-half of the schools of nursing employed instructors.

The change in emphasis of the nursing school from one of education to one of care of the sick had a profound impact on the development of the clinical field as a learning environment. Services to patients superseded the learning needs of the students, and the notion of time in the clinical setting as constituting "work" persisted long after nursing education became more goal directed and structured into a regular educational pattern. The Goldmark Report in 1928 and the Grading School Committee Report in 1934 noted the inequities in nursing programs, particularly in relation to the overuse of clinical practice to the detriment of any theoretical learning. Assignments to clinical areas were based on patient care needs, not learner needs, and instruction occurred after patient demands were met. This practice continued even though collegiate education programs were developing.

The entrance of federal funding into nursing education through the Cadet Corps was a major impetus in changing the role of the clinical field. Criteria for a school of nursing receiving funds required upgrading of many schools and moneys were made available for the employment of faculty. The directions charted by this government program were compatible with such efforts by nursing leaders to develop truly educational programs in nursing. This movement was further supported by the G.I. Bill after World War II, which enabled many nurses to attend institutions of higher learning for advanced study and degrees. The return of many of these prepared nurses as faculty, knowledgeable about many of the science disciplines supporting nursing, enabled nursing education to find its theoretical base and seek a complimentary relationship between learning in the classroom and the clinical setting. The advent of the control of nursing programs by universities, colleges, and community colleges and the development of accreditation standards and processes directed clinical practice in nursing programs toward the Nightingale model where practice sites are chosen in accord with learner needs and instruction is provided by prepared nurses designated as faculty.

As often happens when a control system is changed, the new order takes over in totality without a careful analysis of the resources developed under the previous control mechanism. The movement from nursing service responsibility for teaching in the clinical setting to the school's responsibility through its own faculty ignored the rich potential that skilled nurses in practice have to contribute to students' learning. The current trend is toward the use of these skilled nurses in a preceptor role in the clinical setting, reflecting the possibility for a true apprenticeship experience for students and new graduates entering the field.

The clinical field continues to be a significant environment for learning nursing practice, although its potential is still not realized. Its contribution beyond applying classroom learned theory to practice in the care of the patient needs to be identified, planned for, and institutionalized in the educational program.

SUMMARY

Clinical practice is a function of all educational programs preparing professional practitioners, especially in the service fields. To meet the particular type of clinical judgments and specialized skills demanded of such practitioners in a dynamic society, clinical practice provides more than the opportunity to develop the ability to use professional knowledge and skills within a circumscribed practice mode. It facilitates the ability of the student to learn how to learn, handle ambiguity, think like professionals, develop a notion of personal causation, and evolve one's own theory of practice.

Nursing, a practice discipline, encompasses theories of action related to its people-centered mission, concern with matters of health/illness, and the nature of its process within the practice milieu. The theories to be developed and their degree of development are a function of the category of nursing practitioner. The setting in which the learning occurs may be perceived as a field rather than a laboratory to accommodate its dynamic nature, the reality of the client situations and the potential it has to address the multipurpose expectations of clinical practice within an educational program.

Clinical practice has always been a function of nursing. Its historical development evidenced a deviation from its educational commitment to meet the economic expectations of hospitals for nursing care of patients. Through the efforts of nursing leaders, the input of federal funding for nursing programs, the advanced preparation of faculty, and the development of nursing schools within institutions of higher learning, clinical practice is once more viewed as an educational experience in concert with theory and as an integral part of a systematically developed curriculum.

REFERENCES

Argyris, C., & Schön, D. (1974). *Theory in practice: Increasing professional effectiveness.* San Francisco: Jossey-Bass.

Benner, P. (1983). *From novice to expert.* Menlo Park, Calif.: Addison-Wesley.

Christy, T. (1980). Clinical practice as a function of nursing education. *Nursing Outlook, 28,* 493–97.

Donaldson, S., & Crowley, D. (1978). The discipline of nursing. *Nursing Outlook, 26,* 113–20.

Fawcett, J. (1984). *Analysis and evaluation of conceptual models of nursing.* Philadelphia: F. A. Davis.

Hursh, B., & Borzak, L. (1982). Toward cognitive development through field studies. *Journal of Higher Education, 50,* 63–77.

Kim, H. (1983). *The nature of theoretical thinking in nursing.* Norwalk, Conn.: Appleton-Century-Crofts.

Newman, M. (1979). *Theory development in nursing.* Philadelphia: F. A. Davis.

Nursing: A social policy statement. (1980). Kansas City, Mo.: American Nurses Association.

Roberts, M. (1954). *American nursing history and interpretation.* New York: MacMillan.

Schein, E. H. (1972). *Professional education: Some new directions.* New York: McGraw-Hill.

Schlotfeldt, R. (1981). Nursing in the future. *Nursing Outlook, 29,* 295–301.

BIBLIOGRAPHY

Baron, R. J. (1981). Bridging clinical distance: An emphathetic rediscovery of the known. *Journal of Medical Philosophy, 6,* 5–23.

Brown, J. S., Tanner, C. A., & Padrick, K. (1984). Nursing search for scientific knowledge, *Nursing Research, 33,* 26–32.

Carnegie Commission on Higher Education. (1971). *Higher education and the nation's health.* New York: McGraw-Hill.

Donahue, M. P. (1983). Isabel Maitland Stewart's philosophy of education. *Nursing Research, 32,* 140–46.

Ellis, R. (1982). Conceptual issues in nursing. *Nursing Outlook, 30,* 406–10.

Entry into professional practice: Proceedings of National Conference. (1978). Kansas City, Mo.: American Nurses Association.

Greene, J. A. (1979), Science, nursing and nursing science: A conceptual analysis. *Advances in Nursing Science, 2,* 57–64.

Johnson, D. E. (1983). *Physicians in the making: Personal, academic and socioeconomic characteristics of medical students from 1950–2000.* San Francisco: Jossey-Bass.

Kernan, T., Aiken, L., & Cluff, L. E. (Eds.). (1981). *Nurses and doctors: Their education and practice.* Cambridge, Mo.: Oelgeschlager, Gunn and Hain.

Mayhew, L. B. (1971). *Changing practices in education for the professions.* Atlanta: So. Regional Education Board.

McGlothin, W. J. (1960). *Patterns of professional education.* New York: G. P. Putnam,

Nightingale, F. (1859). *Notes on nursing: What it is and what it is not.* London: Harrison & Sons.

Olsen, E. M. (1983). Baccalaureate student's perception of factors assisting knowledge application in the clinical laboratory. *Journal of Nursing Education, 22,* 18–21.

Reed, S. (1984). Commentary on models of basic nursing education. *Nursing & Health Care, 5,* 263–67.

Stewart, I. M. (1943). *The education of nurses.* New York: Macmillan.

Styles, M. (1982). *Nursing toward a new endowment.* St. Louis: C. V. Mosby.

2

Conceptual Framework of the Teaching–Learning Process

The clinical setting is a dynamic multipurpose environment in which the various goals of clinical practice in a professional curriculum can be attained. The teacher enters the setting to teach. How does the teacher perceive this action? How does the teacher perceive the learning action in which students are engaged? Each teacher must ponder these questions and arrive at his or her own answers, for the answers will influence significantly the direction of the educational process.

RATIONALE FOR A CONCEPTUAL FRAMEWORK OF THE TEACHING–LEARNING PROCESS

A conceptual framework of the teaching–learning process, representative of a synthesis of compatible beliefs about the nature of both the teaching and learning processes, serves as the basis for all decisions relative to the learning of clinical practice competencies. The framework is descriptive rather than prescriptive. It provides the source for decisions relative to the selection of learning objectives for practice sessions in relation to the total program, the choice of learning experience and teaching strategies, and the determination of expectations in the performance of students and teachers. It is particularly important in assisting both students and teachers to maintain a reality perspective of the learning process so that the learner model, not the practitioner model, provides a referent for performance evaluation. Marshall (1973) addresses the need for a teacher to have "a logically consistent framework through which the evaluative process may be fruitfully viewed" (p. 10). He suggests the need for each teacher to be sure of his or her own goals, values, and criteria so that "they are anchored in something deeper than the convenience of the moment or a simple hunch with which to evaluate progress and the success of the effort" (p. 10).

Instructional decisions must have a rationale supported by theory and fundamental values that reflect the integrity and worth of each student. Teachers need an explicit philosophy of the educational process and must function from a firmly established and supported concept of teaching and learning.

LEARNING CONCEPT ROOTED IN HUMAN SCIENCE THEORY

A conceptual framework of the teaching–learning process is rooted in theory. The teacher has numerous theories of learning, some descriptive and some prescriptive, from which to select and develop a unique concept of learning. The notion of the learning process may be based on one theory or it may be eclectic, derived from compatible elements from several theories. No predictive theory of instruction has been developed, but various descriptions of the process are found in the literature. The teacher must be certain that there is congruence between the concepts of the learning process and the teaching process if the total dynamic is to be developed for use in the clinical field.

The purpose of clinical practice in a nursing program as described suggests a learning theory that addresses cognitive, developmental, and humanistic processes. Nursing is a cognitive activity. Although its practice entails numerous psychomotor and affective skills, the underlying activities are problem-solving and decision-making skills relative to clinical judgments. Its charge to act within an ambiguous, ever-changing society demands that its practitioners be skillful in learning to learn and continually relate nursing practice to developing events at any point in time.

The nature of the learning process appropriate for a teacher in a clinical setting is derived from theorists who perceive learning from a human science perspective rather than one of natural science. Theorists subscribing to a human science view of learning are those associated with gestalt/cognitive field theory, development theory, and humanism theory. These theorists are often referred to as phenomenologists because of their approach to the study of mental activities from a meaningful holistic framework rather than the analysis of each part of the activity. The fundamental difference between those who approach learning from a natural science perspective and those who approach learning from a human science perspective is rooted in their basic beliefs about the nature of man. The human science view of man is the most compatible with the nature of nursing and the processes by which learners achieve practice competencies.

Milhollan and Forisha (1972) differentiate man as perceived by these two groups of theorists.

> The behaviorist orientation considers man to be a passive organism governed by stimuli supplied by the external environment. Man can be manipulated, that is, his behavior controlled through proper control of environmental stimuli. Furthermore the laws that govern man are primarily the same as the universal laws that govern all natural phenomena. Therefore, the scientific method, as evolved by the physical sciences, is appropriate as well for the study of the human organism.
>
> The phenomenological orientation considers man to be the source of all acts. Man is essentially free to make choices in each situation. The focal point of this freedom is human consciousness. Behavior is, thus, only the observable expression and consequences of an essentially private internal world of being. Therefore, only a science of man which begins with experiences . . . as it is immediately given in this world of being can ever be adequate for a study of the human organism. (p. 13)

Dubos (1981) differentiates between the capacity of man from that of animals. He states, "whereas animal life is a prisoner of biological evolution which is essentially *irreversible,* human life has the wonderful freedom of social evolution which is rapidly reversible and creative" (p. 6).

The phenomenologic perspective sees man as a purposive, goal-directed individual in constant interaction with the environment. Cognitive abilities enable the individual to seek meaning in and order to all experiences. Mental capacities enable the person to be curious, creative, imaginative, and free to make choices. These abilities reflect characteristics of individual uniqueness, human consciousness, complexity, and unpredictability. The possession of mental processes of thinking and discrimination enable one to be both a generator and a transmitter of knowledge.

Each individual, although involved in the events occurring in the environment, lives in a very private, subjective world of feelings, emotions, and perceptions. Thoughts and behavior arise from this inner world and the individual seeks to maintain balance between both the inner and outer worlds. Therefore, any study of man must occur within the context of a human world of meaning and values where the individual demonstrates an active mind and free will.

A concept of learning based on the phenomenologic view of man recognizes the uniqueness of the individual and the mental capacities that enable a person to (1) grasp meaning from experiences in a creative way; (2) make choices and decisions based upon thoughtful deliberations; and (3) be the source of one's own responses to events in both the internal and external environment. This concept accepts the notion that learning behavior is often an internal process which may be inferred from behavior change rather than be primarily dependent upon observation as professed by supporters of learning as studied by a natural science.

The acknowledgment of the individual as an open system in simultaneous mutual interaction with the environment is more compatible with a learning concept fundamental to the instructional process directed toward cognitive, feeling, and action inherent practice, than the more mechanistic, environmentally controlled notion of the individual as a closed system espoused in the behaviorist theory of learning.

The emphasis on the notion of learning from a holistic perspective is congruent with the involvement of the whole person in learning the phenomenon of practice within the field setting. The selection of cognitive theory as the nucleus of the framework differentiates the preparation for nursing practice as an educational experience rather than a training one. Chickering (1976) makes a distinction between the two processes: "Training starts with the task and conforms a person to it; education starts with the learner and uses tasks in service of increased differentiation and integration" (p. 82).

CONCEPT OF LEARNING

Learning and Experience

Learning is a process by which behavior is changed as a result of experience. Hergenhahn (1982, p. 4) sees learning as a process that mediates behavior and acts as the intervening variable between certain experience and behavior change. He diagrams the process as follows:

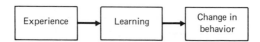

Some individuals conceptualize learning as outcome and state that learning *is* a change in behavior as a result of experience. It is the learning process that is critical to this presentation and the outcome is perceived as "what is learned."

The notion of experience in any concept of learning is critical, for it differentiates change in behavior which may be the result of maturation or alteration in structure or function in any component of the individual's being. Dewey, the master theorist in the domain of experience as it relates to theory and its role in the learning process, cautions us that all experience is not equally educational. Stressing the need for quality experience, Dewey (1963) states:

> The central problem in education based in experience is to select the kind of present experiences that live fruitfully and creatively in subse-

quent experiences. The essence of experience for learning is its meaningfulness to the educational goals of the learner and its ability to
prepare the individual for deeper and more complex experiences in the
future. (pp. 26–27)

Dewey (1963) provides two criteria to discriminate between ed-
ucative and miseducative experiences:

1. *Continuity of experience*: every experience both takes something
   from those which have gone before and modifies in some way the
   qualities of those that come after. Continuity means continued
   growth.
2. *Interaction*: consigns equal rights to both factors in experience—
   objective and internal conditions. An experience is always what it is
   because of a transaction taking place between an individual and
   what, at the time, constitutes own environment. (pp. 33–34)

Piaget (Hergenhahn, 1982) supports Dewey's notion of the role
of experience in growth in referring to the need for "experiences to
be moderately challenging in order to stimulate cognitive growth"
(p. 291). As stated by Dewey, a meaningful educational experience
is one through which the knowledge and skills gained are able to be
effective in managing comparable situations which follow. It is the
connectiveness of experience that is the essential criterion in any
planning for learning.

Steinaker and Bell (1979) conceptualize the process of experience as an involvement of the total person: a living through activity.
They propose a hierarchy of behavior which connotes various progressive stages the learner goes through in meeting the goal of
learning from the experience. The categories are:

1. Exposure: consciousness of the experience
2. Participation: decision on basis of data already received to
                    become physically a part of the experi-
                    ence
3. Identification: union of learner with what is to be learned
                    in an organizational, emotional, and in-
                    tellectual context for purposes of achiev-
                    ing objectives.
4. Reinforcement: experience incorporated and fitting into
                    other aspects of a person's life.
5. Dissemination: experience extends inwardly and outward-
                    ly with the learner in more control than
                    previously.

This structural format for viewing experience in the teaching
and learning situation serves to guide the teacher toward appropriate activities which facilitate the learner's progress. Experiential
learning is the essence of clinical practice and as such must be

conceptualized thoughtfully within the total teaching–learning framework used by the teacher.

Learning and Perception
The concept of the individual as an open-ended system in continuous, simultaneous interaction with the internal and external environment suggests that there is in each person's environment a perceptual field or life-space, which is unique. This life-space is the internal environment which contains the cognitive structures, feelings, and potentials of the individual. Learning involves the interaction between both the inner and outer world so that new learnings can be incorporated within the life-space.

Human science theorists recognize the perceptual field phenomenon but approach the learning process from different perspectives. Gestalt and cognitive field theorists relate learning to perception and consider learning to be a reorganization of the perceptual field. The notion of the reorganization process suggests that the human has the ability to organize in a meaningful way the events and experiences that are accepted into the field. The perceptual field is more than the sum of its parts, for the process of organization establishes meaning which is not inherent in any of the elements. The process by which sensory data are organized into meaningful patterns is attributed by field theorists to brain function, genetically determined, so that there is a state of isomorphism between psychological experience and processes that exist in the brain. The perceptual field is a dynamic, continually changing, interrelated system of elements, with each element affecting every other element as well as the total field.

The stimulus to learning occurs when an individual is confronted with a problem and a state of cognitive disequilibrium results until there is a resolution. The origin of the problem may arise from factors in the outer environment or from problems of inner needs often related to self-actualization. The law of Pragnaz (Hergenhahn, 1982) states that "cognitive balance is more satisfying than cognitive disequilibrium" (p. 256). Therefore, the learner seeks a resolution of the state of disequilibrium through a problem-solving process aimed at bringing order to the field.

Problem solving requires the interpretation and analysis of the meaning of the problem so as to gain appropriate insights for problem solution. Insight development requires change in perception of the problem. Three processes are involved in changing perceptions:

Grouping: categorization of facts
Recentering: focus on an aspect
Reorganizing: from insight and figure background, focus on something that was in the background

Wertheimer, in his book, *Productive Thinking,* (1945, p. 190) used the Gauss problem to explain this phenomenon:

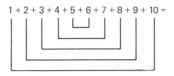

At first view, the problem appears to be a series of discrete numbers. A further analysis of the problem results in a different perspective of the problem.

Grouping: numbers can be categorized into multiples of 11
Recentering: 11 as the figure in the background
Reorganizing: 5 multiples of 11: solution $= 11 \times 5 = 55$.

The change in the perception of the problem enabled the problem solver to gain insight into its meaning and, thus, solve the problem. The problem supports the notion that the solution of a problem lies within the problem (multiples of 11 were already present).

Insight, as noted by Gestalt and cognitive field theorists, is a deliberative approach to problem solving whereby the inner relations or basic principles are sought instead of using trial and error. Insightful learning may involve a total pattern or a partial feel for the pattern. Hergenhahn (1982) cites four characteristics of insightful learning:

1. Transition from pre-solution to a solution is sudden and complete.
2. Performance based upon solutions gained by insight is usually smooth and free of errors.
3. Solution of a problem gained by insight is retained for a considerable length of time.
4. Principles gained by insight are easily applied to other problems; a process of transposition. (p. 26)

Once the new insight is gained it forms a new cognitive structure and causes a reorganization of the perceptual field. Learning, then, is not an additive process, but rather an integrative one.

Piaget (Hergenhahn, 1982) considers schema, the potential to act in a certain way, as an element in cognitive structures. He identifies two circumstances under which these schemata change:

1. *Assimilation*: the process of responding to the environment in accordance with one's own cognitive structures and the physical environment.
2. *Accommodation*: the process by which cognitive structures are modified—the major mechanism for intellectual growth. (pp. 283–284)

Vinacke (1952) sees the relationship between formation of cognitive structures and concept formation:

> Concept formation involves processes of perception and learning by means of which the individual develops an organized and coherent relation to the external world. The consequences of these processes is the establishment of concepts, cognitive structures, which link the individual's present perceptions and learning to previous experience. (p. 98)

Concepts, as such, facilitate the efficient use of experience through the identification and classification of objects and the use of symbolic responses which are known.

Bruner (1963) considers the act of learning as involving three almost simultaneous processes:

1. Acquisition of new information: refinement of previous knowledge.
2. Transformation: way of dealing with information to go beyond it.
3. Evaluation: check on pertinence and adequacy of knowledge to task at hand. Judgment of knowledge's plausibility. (pp. 92–93)

Carl Rogers (1983) supports the notion of learning through insight, a process by which perceptual relationships in the field are identified. He particularly emphasizes the learning behavior that affects the component of the field which relates to the "self," the particular meanings and values which are identified with self-actualization. His phenomenologic perspective of learning is presented as: "Significant learning combines the logical *and* the intuitive, the intellect *and* the feelings, the concept *and* the experience, the idea *and* the meaning" (p. 20).

Learning as conceptualized by these theorists is a holistic process involving perceptions, meanings, principles, and relationships resulting in new cognitive structures which are incorporated in the perceptual field. New learnings are accepted when related to present content of the perceptual field and result in a reorganization of the field. Its paradigm is stimulus-organism-response (S → O → R), which notes the role of the organism, (individual) in interpreting the stimulus and determining the response.

Learning and Thinking

The fundamental process in cognitive learning is reflective thinking, that which occurs in an experience when an organism meets, recognizes, and solves a problem. Wertheimer (1945) differentiates productive thinking from blind, habitual, mechanical thinking when he says, "Productive thinking consists in envisaging, realizing structural features and structural requirements; proceeding in accordance with and determined by these requirements" (p. 190). Reflective thinking fosters divergent thinking, the derivation of more than one solution to a problem. Divergent thinking is a creative process, essential for effective problem solving; it is productive thinking. Convergent thinking, derivation of only one solution, is reproductive thinking, often resulting from rote or memorization.

Although the analytic process in productive thinking is stressed, Bruner (1963) is concerned that intuitive thinking, the process of arriving at plausible but tentative formulation without going through the analytic process, is neglected in educational practices. He says: "The shrewd guess, the fertile hypothesis, the courageous leap to a tentative conclusion—these are the most valuable coin of the thinker at work, whatever the line of work" (p. 13). Carl Rogers concurs with Bruner on this point and recognizes the significance of intuitive thinking in problem solving. Intuitive thinking, although not based on a rational thinking process, is not an irrational process, for it depends upon the existence of previous experience in the perceptual field which can be applicable to solving the new problem.

Transfer of Learning
Compatible with the beliefs of the theorists relative to significance of the development of insight through perception change and the search for meaning and order in the new learning task, transfer of that learning is dependent upon the understanding of the meaning of the task. Bruner (1963) sees a relationship between the nature of the learning and the transfer. "Massive general transfer can be achieved by appropriate learning, even to the degree that learning properly under conditions (optimum) leads one to learn how to learn" (pp. 6–7). He emphasizes that learning the structure of a subject, the understanding of it in a way that permits many other things to be related to it meaningfully, is the "center of the problem of transfer."

Cognitive theorists relate transfer of learning to the significance of perceptions in noting similarities in situations, i.e., meanings, generalizations, concepts, or insights gained in previous learning experiences. Transfer is not simply related to mastery of facts and techniques and their applicability to the new situation. The transfer requires that the individual grasp the nature of the phenomenon to be transferred so that its applicability can be determined.

Learning and Knowledge
A concept of learning must not only incorporate the process but must also consider the scope of learning and the meaning of knowledge. Perry (1970) addresses the intellectual and ethical development of students relative to the nature of knowledge, truth, values, and the meaning of commitment. His schema, representing four general categories (dualism, multiplicity, relativism and commitment), describes the development of students from a "simplistic cat-

egorical view of the world to a realization of contingent nature of knowledge, relative values, and affirmation of own commitment" (pp. 57–58).

This schema addresses the ability of students to deal with knowledge outside the perspective of absolutism. It is the discriminating use of knowledge and the potential for seeing various meanings of knowledge in a broader context that leads the learner to creative, reflective thinking in problem solving. The dualistic thinker is a convergent thinker unable to relate to a world of uncertainty.

Whitehead (1967) is also concerned about what individuals do with knowledge when he refers to "'inert ideas,' those ideas merely received into the mind without being utilized or tested or thrown into fresh combinations" (p. 1). Both Dewey and Whitehead see knowledge as the greatest freedom. Whitehead (1967) relates knowledge to "wisdom which concerns handling of knowledge, its selection for the determination of relevant issues, its employment to add value to an immediate experience" (p. 32).

Learning and Processing of Information

In addition to the cognitive process of learning, two factors concerning the handling of information are significant to teaching clinical practice skills. One factor refers to the cognitive style of the learner and the other relates to cultural patterns of learning accepted by various groups.

Recent research is suggesting that there are different cognitive styles that relate to the way individuals process information. Cognitive style is not related to intelligence, skill performance, or cognitive performance or the *what* of learning, but rather, it addresses the process of data handling, i.e., the *how* of learning, namely perceiving, thinking, problem solving, and interactions with others. Cognitive style is a habitual mode of information processing which, as heretofore supported in research, is not amenable to major change.

Messick (1976) clarifies the difference between ability and cognitive styles by presenting the characteristics of each. Table 2 is extracted from his discussion.

The work of Witkin, Moor, Goodenough, and Cox (1977) is directed toward two different styles of habitual information processing and interacting: field independence and field dependence. Table 3 identifies the characteristics of individuals representing the two different cognitive styles.

This classification and the defined characteristics are helpful in understanding a process by which some learners handle information in their learning behavior pattern. The field independent–field dependent classification is one of several ways of approaching this important dimension of learning.

TABLE 2. COMPARISON OF CHARACTERISTICS OF COGNITIVE STYLE AND ABILITY

Cognitive Style	Ability
1. Addresses question of *how*	1. Addresses question of *what*
2. Measurement of characteristic modes in terms of typical performance—emphasis on process	2. Measurement of capacities in terms of maximal performance—emphasis on level of accomplishment
3. Bipolar—dynamic gestalt pits one syndrome or complex of interacting characteristics against contrasting complex at opposite end of pole	3. Unipolar—the top is significant
4. Range from one extreme to another. Each end has different implication for education	4. Range from zero to higher denotes greater facility
5. Value differentiated—each pole has adaptive value in different circumstances	5. Value directional—more is better
6. Neither end is more adaptive—it is a function of the situation	6. The higher the value, the more adaptive
7. Cuts across all domains	7. Usually delineates a basic dimension underlying a fairly limited area specific to a particular domain of content or function
8. Roots in study of perception and personality—close ties with laboratory or clinic	8. Measurement—roots in mental test theory in schools

The second factor that influences learning behavior is the influence of culture on learning. Cultural determinants are significant in any concept of learning, for they denote the structure of knowledge, its meaning and relationships, and the process by which members of a culture learn. Hall (1961) sees learning as an adaptive mechanism used by the culture as an agent of acculturation of its members as well as a mechanism for its continuance. Since people in various cultures learn to learn differently, a pattern not readily alterable, responses to learning situations will also vary. Differences occur in temporal and spatial dimensions as well as content and meaning. American culture values active involvement (the "doing," during the learning experience), rewards rapidity in grasping the learning task, and accepts the notion of pressure as an ingredient of the learning process. Other cultures may value the skill of memory or rote learning and reward correct learning regardless of the time needed so that the time pressure is not a factor.

Hall proposes three models of learning: formal, informal, and technical. Formal learning, the result of precept or admonition, establishes patterns by mistakes. It is a dualistic approach, emphasizing right/wrong or yes/no, and is suffused with emotion. Informal

TABLE 3. CHARACTERISTICS OF DIFFERENT COGNITIVE STYLES

Field-Independent	Field-Dependent
1. Perception of figures more or less separate from surrounding field	1. Perception dominated by perceptual field
2. Able to dissemble a salient element from background	2. Difficulty in dissembling elements because of global view of the field
3. High in cognitive restructuring skills	3. Low in cognitive restructuring skills
4. Impersonal orientation—low in social skills	4. Social orientation—high in social skills
5. Preference—domains featuring analysis of items within the field	5. Preference—domains featuring interpersonal relationships and day-to-day work with people
6. High in analytic and differentiation skills	6. Low in analytic and differentiation skills
7. Hypothesis testing approach in concept formation	7. Spectator approach in concept formation—trial and error
8. Adept at learning material with natural science content	8. Adept at learning and memorizing material with social content
9. Intrinsic motivation for learning	9. Extrinsic motivation for learning—social group
10. Unstructured inner-directed environment	10. Structured outer-directed environment
11. Capacity to be self-referent for self-definition	11. Rely on external referent, particularly by authority, for self-definition
12. Autonomous	12. Low in personal autonomy
13. Low response to personal criticism	13. High response to criticism, positive or negative
14. Performs best when own strategies developed	14. Needs more explicit instruction and more exact definition of performance outcome

learning occurs as a result of identification with a model, often an "out of awareness" phenomenon. The learner asks no questions but follows the behavior pattern of the model. Technical learning results from the transmission of information, often after a mistake has been made. In contrast to the normal learning pattern, the learner in this pattern is supported and receives clarification and correction in a facilitative tone.

Because anthropology is concerned with the meanings of knowledge and behavior from a societal perspective, it is concerned with the influence of a group's perception or response to a learning event. Mead (1955) recognizes the difference in what a society accepts as proper reward or praise behavior, its notion of dualism and competition, and the content it deems to be acceptable in a teaching situation.

Crick (1982) raises questions about the notion of an anthropology of knowledge which would address meanings, cognitive knowledge, and how different cultures think. He notes that if the aim of anthropology is to make social life intelligible and knowledgeable, it can be assumed that knowledge must be seen in a social context. Accepting the notion of an early development in the domain of anthropology of knowledge, Crick raises questions that anthropology must answer. These questions are: Does language represent knowledge, or is there a linguistic language and a cultural language? How are ritual and knowledge related? How are knowledge and power related in a society? As the anthropology of knowledge is explored and articulated, the impact of culture in influencing meanings and learning styles will become even more significant to a framework of the learning phenomenon. Cultural influence on learning cannot be ignored.

CONCEPT OF TEACHING

Relationship to Concept of Learning

The concept of learning presented as relevant to teaching in the clinical field includes significant ideas that influence the process of teaching, for the two processes must be interrelated. Learning is an individual process; it is active, experiential; it is holistic, involving the total being and the environment. It emphasizes meanings, principles and relationships among phenomena, and it is concerned with perception, insight, and cognitive structure formation. It is an integrative process through which new learnings are incorporated into a perceptual field, thus causing a reorganization of the field; and it provides for transfer of knowledge or skill when there is relevance in meaning between previous experience and the new one. Learning is often precipitated by cognitive disequilibrium requiring problem solving based on reflective thinking for solution, although sometimes intuitive thinking is effective. The learning style is influenced by the cognitive style of the learner and the cultural pattern of learning adopted by the learner's referent group. Learning is perceived from a cognitive perspective because knowledge and its use is basic to all other domains of learning inherent in professional practice.

What process of teaching is most compatible with the above description of learning? It is certain that the notion of teaching as "telling" through which information is dispensed is not appropriate. Teaching is the facilitation of learning, which involves a sharing and mutual experience of learning on the part of both teacher and learner. It is a sharing of the perceptual field of both participants toward a goal-directed encounter with new experiences.

Teaching seeks to assist students in developing a sense of excitement, curiosity, and discovery about the world. It asks for involvement of the learner, not passivity, and provides the supportive environment required. It provides for experience in problem solving and accommodates reflective and intuitive thinking. It assists students in the pursuit of new knowledge and the skills in utilizing that knowledge in practice. It includes the total learner in the experience, guarding against overemphasis on one domain, such as cognitive, to the exclusion of other domains, particularly the affective domain, which provides the value base for use of new knowledges and skills.

Teaching: An Intervention Process

Teaching, like other service professions, is a helping field which addresses the growth and developmental needs of individuals. It is a diagnostic and intervention process similar in structure to the nursing process. A comparison of these two processes is shown in Table 4.

The diagnostic process in teaching involves assessment of the individual's resources and limitations to enter into the task as well as the nature of the learning required for its attainment. Bloom (1980) states that educational research is moving from a study of the characteristics of teachers and students to direct observation of learning taking place in the interactions between students and teachers. The teaching process is the focus of the research. Bloom, Hastings, and Madaus (1971), using John Carroll's Model of School Learning, developed a mastery of learning model based on Carroll's premise that "if students are normally distributed with respect to aptitude, but the kind and quality of instruction and learning time allowed are made characteristic to needs of each learner, the majority of students will achieve mastery of the subject" (p. 46). The five variables in this model can be used most effectively in diagnosing learner needs as a basis for planning instruction. The five variables are:

1. Aptitude for particular kinds of learning: the time required to attain mastery of the learning task.
2. Quality of instruction: the degree to which the presentation, explanation, and ordering of elements of the task to be learned approach the optimum for a given learner.
3. Ability to understand instruction: the ability of the learner to understand the nature of the task to be learned and the procedures to be followed in the learning.
4. Perseverance: the time the learner is willing to spend in the learning.
5. Time allowed for learning: time allowed for learning to take place.

TABLE 4. COMPARISON OF NURSING PROCESS AND TEACHING PROCESS

Nursing	Teaching
Goal: Change in behavior—coping with health/illness	*Goal:* Change in behavior—new learning

Assessment:
Client needs—health
Nature of problem
  Health deficiency
  Health maintenance
  Health promotion
Priority based on nursing diagnosis
	Assessment:
	Client needs—learning
	Nature of problem
	  Learning deficiency
	  Learning continuance
	  Learning promotion
	Priority based on diagnosis of learning needs

Planning: Determine short- and long-term goals with client Establish pertinent objectives Select intervention strategies to meet objectives	*Planning:* Determine short- and long-term goals with student Establish pertinent objectives Select intervention strategies to meet objectives
Intervention: Supplemental Supportive Curative Educational	*Intervention:* Supplemental Supportive Alternate pacing Alternate experience
Evaluation: Outcome—goals of health status Process—means by which outcome was obtained	*Evaluation:* Performance—goals of learning Process—means by which learning experience outcome was obtained

Bloom (1982, p. 11) is now involved in his current research, which addresses a causal system of relations between selected variables and selected learning outcomes. The diagram which explains the system is:

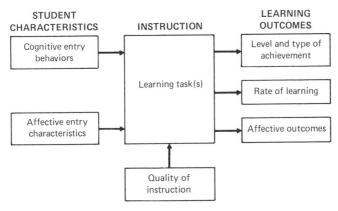

32

THE CLINICAL FIELD: ITS USE IN NURSING EDUCATION

The following variables are designated: cognitive entry behaviors, affective entry behaviors, and quality of instruction. Entry behaviors are derived from the history of the learner's experiences at the time of entry into the task and related to the demands of the new task. The quality of instruction variable addresses the elements in the mastery of learning concept. The emphasis in the model is on the identification of alterable variables, those which can be manipulated, and the causal processes by which they can be altered. Bloom (1980) presents four alterable variables relevant to this discussion:

1. Available time vs. time on task: time on task refers to the active learning time that students are engaged in learning; not time available. This appraisal of time provides both a qualitative and quantitative dimension.
2. Intelligence and cognitive entry characteristics: intelligence and aptitude are generally stable, but abilities, knowledge, or skills (essential prerequisites for a particular learning task) have a high relation to achievement and are alterable since they can be addressed in the educational process.
3. Summative vs. formative tests: formative tests are used to provide feedback to help students correct errors in learning with additional time to reach standards of achievement. Summative tests are used for grading at the conclusion of a learning experience.
4. Teachers vs. teaching: the quality of teaching, not the quality of the teacher, is the focus of present research (pp. 382–85).

Three characteristics of teaching as proposed by Bloom (1982) are:

(a) cues—instruction of what is to be learned as well as directions as to what the learner is to do in the learning process
(b) reinforcement—extent to which the learner is rewarded or reinforced in learning
(c) participation—extent to which the student actively participates or engages in learning (pp. 115–22).

This focus on alterable variables provides a diagnostic framework for determining both teacher and learner behavior in the teaching–learning process and the significance of the outcome.

Intervention addresses strategies for assisting the learner to achieve educational goals. The expediting or retarding of the pace of learning may be relevant for the learner with temporal needs for grasping the meaning of new learnings. Use of resources (teacher as well as library, field, or outside experts) is an important teaching strategy. Modifications in or use of alternative teaching methodologies compatible with the goals of the learning task are useful in broadening the experience of some students or helping to clarify new learnings for other students.

Witkin, Moore, Goodenough, and Cox (1977) suggest teaching strategies that are appropriate to different types of cognitive styles of learning. Field-dependent learners, with their inclination toward global perceptions of the field and domains that feature interpersonal relations, respond best to teaching methods that entail group interaction with responsibility shared by the teachers and students. Because they do not readily use a hypothesis testing approach to problem solving and concept formation, they require more specific instruction and more exact definition of performance expectation. They are dependent upon salient cues for learning, and because of their use of the social group as a self-referral, they are more responsive to criticism of their performance, whether positive or negative.

The field-independent learners seek teaching strategies that stimulate analytic skills, and they prefer lecture and discovery methods. Their predilection for examining elements in a field and the interrelationships support a hypothesis testing approach to problem solving and concept formation. They rely less on structure or cue saliency. With an internalized frame of reference and self-defined goals, they are minimally affected by criticism of their performance.

In the process of accommodating learning expectations and teaching strategies to meet the various needs of students, Bruner (1963) cautions us about the tendency in teaching groups of students to "unequalize" learning expectations. He states:

> The pursuit of excellence must not be limited to the gifted student. But the idea that teaching should be aimed at the average student in order to provide something for everyone is an equally inadequate formula. The quest is to devise material which will challenge the superior student, while not destroying the confidence and will to learn of those who are less fortunate. (p. 70)

Teaching and the Teacher

In the dynamic phenomenon of teaching and learning, it is the teacher who must assume the primary responsibility for the quality of the learning environment relative to the prevailing climate, availability of resources, and process of goal-directed learning. The climate is supportive to learning; it reflects caring about and liking students; it is generated by the teacher's enthusiasm for teaching; it accepts the involvement of the total learner in the process, regardless of the nature of the learning task.

The teacher recognizes variability in learner response to the learning task, sometimes due to differences in aptitude, preference, experience, or motivation relative to task achievement. Although motivation lies within the province of the learner, the teacher seeks to help the learner find meaning and relevance to the new experience. The teacher recognizes the role that biases, prejudices, and fear of change or self-encounter play in preventing the learner from entering new experiences which result in new insights and behavior change, and develops strategies that will assist the learner in becoming open.

The teacher identifies the potential of each student and encourages, through sharing, the evolution of a sense of self. Nouwen (1971) describes a sharing which contributes to the growth of both the faculty and student:

> Students grow during those moments in which they discover they have offered something new to teachers without making them feel threatened, but rather, thankful. And teachers could be much better teachers if students were willing to draw the best out of them and show their acceptance by thankfulness and creative work. Too many people cling to their own talents and leave them untouched because they are afraid there is nobody who is really interested. (p. 17)

The climate is a humanistic one which is authentic, supportive, and caring. However, the charge for learning to occur requires that it be stimulating, provocative, and disciplined in the pursuit of new learnings. Sensitivity and caring about learner needs does not mean lessening of acceptable performance; it means consideration of strategies directed toward helping the learner attain the desired goals. It means enhancing the learner's perspective so that learning does not become viewed as a personal possession, but rather it becomes a way of relating to the world at large, that is, the student's world and the outside world are an integral part of learning.

Eble (1972, p. 37) in his research on teachers, has identified qualities of the effective teacher:

1. Discipline   without rigidity
2. Generosity   of spirit, outlook, give student chance to succeed
3. Energy   performing aspect, mental energy of mind
4. Variety   styles: delivery, mood, format, timing, pace
5. Use of illustrations   clarification, relevance
6. Enthusiasm   for teaching and subject matter
7. Clarity and organization   teacher's performance, know many things, curiosity of world, see relationships
8. Honesty   responding to conscience, resisting temptation, admitting error
9. Sense of proportion   willingness to enter into mutual experience

The teacher is a vital link in the teaching–learning dynamic. Expertise in subject matter and teaching are basic requirements, but they must be accompanied by the human qualities that make the total experience stimulating, developmental, and fulfilling for both the teacher and the learner. It is the teacher, through the use of a theoretically based concept of the teacher–learning process, that sets the tone and provides for smooth functioning of the total endeavor.

THE DYNAMIC: TEACHING AND LEARNING

Teaching and learning, two discrete processes, can be interrelated so as to form a gestalt that reflects a dynamic process. Congruency in the fundamental constructs of each provides a consistent pattern which unites the two processes. The dynamic which has been presented is eclectic, reflecting concepts and theories of theorists who view learning from the perspective of human science rather than natural science. It is an interactional phenomenon whereby the fields of the participants, teacher, and learner intersect and are open to new experiences. Total beings are involved in this interaction and learning occurs in all three domains: cognitive, affective, and psychomotor. The dynamic requires giving and receiving by both parties as each pursues the continuous search for knowledge, self-identity, and living within the reality of one's own existence.

In a professional field, the participants in the process are not equal, for the field requires a distinct repertoire of skill and knowledge for its practice. The "knower" (the teacher) guides the "uninformed" (the student) through the learning process in pursuit of the requisite competencies for practice. Because of the continuous introduction of the "new" into the realm of practice, the teacher often becomes a learner when engaged in the dynamic and the learner may become the teacher as his or her own experiences elucidate practice behavior and provide data which contribute to the development of new insights. The total process, then, reflects the goals, experiences, and values of the participants at any point in time.

Learning can occur without teaching. Teaching can occur without learning as a result. In the educational field, however, the two ought to be interactive in accord with specifically defined goals appropriate to the parties involved. When the gestalt is perceived, there is greater attention to the congruency of the two processes, so that the outcome can be achieved with greater efficiency and the evaluation can be concerned with both the outcome (learning) in terms of desired goals and the process (teaching) by which it was guided.

RELEVANCE OF CONCEPTUAL FRAMEWORK OF THE TEACHING–LEARNING PROCESS TO TEACHING IN THE CLINICAL FIELD

As stated earlier, each teacher develops his or her own conceptual framework which can be operationalized in all decisions pertinent to curriculum matters. The framework presented represents concepts and theories deemed relevant to the educational experience that occurs in the clinical practice component of a nursing program. The framework recognizes that the three domains of learning; i.e., cognitive, affective, and psychomotor, occur within the clinical setting, but it also emphasizes the cognitive processes of learning as the principal element. This choice was made because nursing involves cognitive skills in all dimensions of its practice; clinical judgments inherent in its problem-solving process of care and the delivery of care; choice in the selection and use of intervention strategies and their alternatives necessitated by individual response; and moral reasoning essential for determining actions in a complex field of practice. Nurses "do," but behind all actions are cognitive processes, even though some are primarily carried out as habit—an automatic response which results from previous cognitive experience.

A framework which supports problem solving and experiential learning is particularly relevant to teaching nursing practice competencies in a clinical setting, since they are the two processes that dominate the experience. The problem-solving activity is not only essential for individualizing client care, but it is also a means by which the learner develops skill in discrimination when ambiguous choices are encountered, broadens perspectives so that alternative responses or actions are evident in practice, and helps in learning how to learn so that a questioning posture may be established, thus enabling continuous evaluation of new and continuing practice modes.

Experiential learning is essential in a practice discipline and provides opportunities for problem-solving practice with real clients and problems in the setting, hands-on experience in ministrations of care, and moral or ethical decision making relative to client, setting, or self. The knowledge of field-independent and field-dependent cognitive styles of processing information is particularly relevant here. Nursing is a people-oriented field and the practice setting provides the opportunity to work with people. The environment is well-suited to the field-dependent individual, but what can the teacher expect from the field-independent learner? Are nurses primarily field-dependent? Quinland and Blatt (1973) did a study of nurses in terms of cognitive style and found that high-achiever psychiatric nurses were field dependent while high-achiever surgical nurses were field independent. Psychiatric nurses' mode of practice is personal interaction; surgical nurses (particularly those in the operating room) work with much instrumentation selected from the operating field.

Nursing today requires the cognitive skills of analysis and hypothesis testing (field independent) and personal interaction skills (field dependent). Both types of behaviors are goals of clinical practice. How do we accommodate the predilections of each group and yet require both cognitive and social skill? The recognition of the cognitive style phenomenon enables teachers to foster the preferences of each type of learner and devise strategies for developing the opposite skill so that achievement can be attained.

Theorists who emphasize problem solving and experiencing as teaching modalities highlight the role of perception, insight, and general principles in the transfer of learning. The stress on meanings and the connections between previous experience and new learning highlight the importance in developing the understanding which underlies all nursing actions and not the "doing" of the action itself.

Teaching in the clinical field according to this teaching–learning concept is concerned with a learning climate that supports the activities of the learners in a situation where the learner is most vulnerable. Diagnostic and intervention components of teaching facilitate both teaching and learning activities. Consideration is given to providing sufficient time for problem solving and the carrying out of nursing ministrations; supporting creative proposals made by the learner and accepting the potential of mistakes as an inherent part of any learning experience. The learner is not a practitioner; yet, in the clinical field where experienced practitioners are engaged in their respective activities, expectations of acceptable performances by the learner are often judged on the basis of what is observed in practice.

Opportunities to use knowledge under various circumstances foster the ability to transfer learnings by finding new meanings and relationships. The accumulation of learning culminates in a repertoire of related knowledge which comprises the basis of nursing practice.

SUMMARY

Knowledge, skill, and value commitment are the outcomes of clinical practice experience. All can be achieved in the practice setting if the teacher has a theoretically based conceptual framework of the teaching–learning process used in making all decisions relative to goals of the experience, diagnosing learner needs, selection of learning and teaching strategies, management of learner responses during the experience, and use of self as a facilitator. The framework, proposed as appropriate for teaching in the clinical field, is derived from cognitive field theory and the ideas of others who perceive learning from a human science point of view.

Cognitive field theory, which stresses reflective divergent thinking in problem solving and decision making, is the focus because cognition is a critical competency in nursing. The role of perception, insight, meanings, relationships, and principles in learning and the transfer of learning is the essence of learning. Dewey's theory of experiential learning provides criteria for determining the educational value of the clinical experience. Bruner's stress on the importance of teaching the structure of knowledge (its meaningfulness and its relatedness) suggests the approach to teaching nursing's body of knowledge; Carl Roger's concern about the role of education in moving people toward self-actualization provides the stimulus to support the growth and development of the person who is to be the nurse. Perry's thesis about the need for education to move individuals from dualistic thinking to relativistic thinking and commitment challenges nursing teachers to enable students to deal with the uncertainties of a field which is an inexact science. Witkin's work on the significance of cognitive style in learning behavior provides another basis for understanding learner needs and responses in the clinical practice site while Hall's and Mead's theses about cultural influences on the learning process provide new insight into a dimension of learning which has had little emphasis heretofore.

Teaching is a facilitative, supportive process; it is humanistic, but demanding of acceptable performance on the part of the teacher and the learner, which is compatible with an articulated concept of learning. It is a diagnostic and intervention process. Bloom's contribution to the teaching field in the development of the mastery of learning mode and the present research into teaching with a focus on alterable variables has major implications for the teacher or students engaged in multiple learning tasks in a multipurpose environment.

Teaching and learning is a dynamic which is mutually interactive and needs to be viewed as such by the teacher in the clinical setting. This perspective enables learners and teachers to engage in a sharing experience which highlights problem solving and experiential learning, is appropriate for meeting the multiple goals of clinical practice in the nursing program, and forms the basis for the learners eventual development of their own theory of practice.

REFERENCES

Bloom, B. S. (1980). The new directions in educational research: Alterable variables. *Phi Delta Kappa, 61*, 382–85.
Bloom, B. S. (1982). *Human characteristics and school learning*. New York: McGraw-Hill.

Bloom, B. S., Hastings, J. T., & Madaus, G. P. (1971). *Handbook on formative and summative evaluation of student learning*. New York: McGraw-Hill.

Bruner, J. S. (1963). *The process of education*. New York: Vintage Books.

Chickering, A. W. (1976). The double bind of field dependence/independence in program alternatives for educational development. In S. Messick & Associates, *Individuality in learning*. San Francisco: Jossey-Bass.

Crick, M. (1982). Anthropology of knowledge. *Annual Review of Anthropology, 11*, 287–313.

Dewey, J. (1963). *Experience in education*. New York: Collier Books.

Dubos, R. (1981). *Celebrations of life*. New York: McGraw-Hill.

Eble, K. E. (1972). *Professors as teachers*. San Francisco: Jossey-Bass.

Hall, E. (1961). *Silent language*. New York: Premier Books.

Hergenhahn, B. R. (1982). *An introduction to theories of learning* (2nd ed.). Englewood Cliffs, N.J.: Prentice-Hall.

Marshall, J. P. (1973). *The teacher and his philosophy*. Lincoln, Neb.: Professional Publications Inc.

Mead, M. (1955). *Cultural patterns and technical change*. New York: Menton.

Messick, S. (1976). Personality competencies in cognition and creativity. In S. Messick & Associates, *Individuality in learning*. San Francisco: Jossey-Bass.

Milhollan, F., & Forisha, B. (1972). *From Skinner to Rogers*. Lincoln, Neb.: Professional Publications Inc.

Nouwen, H. (1971). *Creative ministry*. New York: Doubleday.

Perry, W. G., Jr. (1970). *Forms of intellectual and ethical development in the college years*. New York: Holt, Rinehart & Winston.

Quinland, D. W., & Blatt, S. J. (1973). Field articulation and performance under stress: Differential prediction in surgical and psychiatric nursing training. *Journal of Consulting and Clinical Psychology, 39*, 517.

Rogers, C. (1983). *Freedom to learn in the 80's*. Columbus, Ohio: Chas. E. Merrill.

Steinaker, N. B., & Bell, M. R. (1979). *The experiential taxonomy: A new approach to teaching and learning*. New York: Academic Press.

Vinacke, W. E. (1952). *The psychology of thinking*. New York: McGraw-Hill.

Wertheimer, M. (1945). *Productive thinking*. New York: Harper.

Whitehead, A. N. (1967). *The aims of education*. New York: Free Press.

Witkin, H. A., Moore, C. A., Goodenough, D. R., & Cox, P. W. (1977). Field-dependent and field-independent cognitive styles and their educational implications. *Review of Educational Research, 47*, 1–64.

BIBLIOGRAPHY

Bandura, A. (1977). *Social learning theory*. Englewood Cliffs, N.J.: Prentice-Hall.

Bass, J. (1977). The motivation to teach. *Journal of Higher Education, 48*, 243–48.

Bevis, E. O. (1982). *Curriculum building in nursing* (3rd ed.). St. Louis: C. V. Mosby.

Bigge, M. L. (1982). *Learning theories for teachers* (4th ed.). New York: Harper & Row.

Bruner, J. S. (1966). *Toward a theory of instruction*. Cambridge, Mass: Belknap Press of Harvard University Press.

Chickering, A. W. (1969). *Education and identity*. San Francisco: Jossey-Bass.

Cooper, L. N. (1980). Sources and limits of human intellect. *Daedalus, 109* (2), 1–17.

Cross, K. P. (1981). *Adults as learners*. San Francisco: Jossey-Bass.

Duck, L. (1981). *Teaching with charisma*. Boston: Allyn & Bacon.

Hammock, F. M. (1982). Education for nursing: Problems and prospects. *New York Educational Quarterly, 13*(2), 8–14.

Hilgard, E. R., & Bower, G. H. (1975). *Theories of learning* (4th ed). Englewood Cliffs, N.J.: Prentice-Hall.

Hullfish, H. G., & Smith, P. G. (1961). *Reflective thinking: The method of education*. New York: Dodd, Mead.

Intellect and imagination: The limits and presuppositions of intellect. *Daedalus*, 1980, *109*(2).

James, W. (1962). *Talks to teachers*. New York: Dover.

Kitchner, K. S. (1983). Educational goals and reflective thinking. *Educational Forum, 47*(5), 75–79.

Kneeler, G. R. (1965). *Introduction to philosophy of education*. New York: Wiley.

Knowles, M. & Associates. (1984). *Andrology in action: Applying modern principles of adult learning*. San Francisco: Jossey-Bass.

Kramer, M., Tegan, E., & Knowler, J. (1970). Effect of presets on creative problem solving. *Nursing Research, 19*, 303–11.

May, R. (1953). *Man's search for himself*. New York: Dell.

Merrit, S. L. (1983). Learning style preferences of baccalaureate nursing students. *Nursing Research, 32*, 367–72.

Nuernberger, P. (1984). Mastering the creative process. *The Futurist, 18*(4), 30–32.

O'Shea, H. S. (1981). Role orientation and role strain of clinical nurse faculty in baccalaureate programs. *Nursing Research, 31*, 306–10.

Parnes, S. J. (1984). Learning creative behavior. *The Futurist, 18*(4), 30–32.

Piaget, J. (1966). *Psychology of intelligence*. Totowa, N.J.: Little-Adams.

Smith, C. E. (1978). Planning, implementing, and evaluating learning experiences for adults. *Nurse Educator, 3*(4), 31–36.

Tarnow, K. G. (1979). Working with adult learners. *Nurse Educator, 5*(2), 34–40.

Valiga, T. M. (1983). Cognitive development: A critical component of baccalaureate nursing education, *Image, 15*(4), 115–23.

Wolfgard, M. E., & Dowling, W. D. (1981). Differences in motivation of adult and younger undergraduates. *Journal of Higher Education, 52*, 640–48.

3

Nursing Process:
A Practice Modality

The term *nursing process* is very much in the literature in the eighties. However, this inclusiveness does not necessarily imply that it is accepted as an integral part of practice or, indeed, even understood by many nurses practicing in the field in spite of the literature which addresses the nature of the process and its use in meeting clients' health-care needs. Nursing process is the *methodology* of nursing practice. As such, it is learned in the clinical field through continuous practice. The concern of this book is the teaching of the process in the clinical setting, for nursing has many excellent authorities, such as Yura and Walsh (1983), Marriner (1983), Mayers (1983), Griffith and Christensen (1982) and Carnevali (1983), who address the process from the theoretical and practice perspective.

A CONCEPT OF NURSING PROCESS

Nursing process is a systematic series of sequential, but interrelated interdependent nursing actions with the ultimate goal of meeting a client's health need to the level of optimum wellness for that client. The client may be an individual, family, or community. The nursing process is primarily a cognitive activity, although the actions inherent in the process represent all three domains: cognitive, psychomotor, affective. According to Reilly (1980), the process involves:

1. Intellectual operations, such as problem solving, concept formalization, inference reasoning, judgment, and decision making, and the application of a synthesis of theories, ideas, and concepts.
2. Value judgments based on the respect of the dignity and worth of human beings.
3. Psychomotor skills, both for assessment and intervention. (p. 153)

The potential variability of nursing activities, ranging from simple to complex, which are inherent in the process, provide the nurse with a framework for individualizing client nursing care in terms of implicit and explicit needs determined by both the nurse and the client. The process order, defined by its four steps (assessment, planning, implementation, and evaluation), facilitates a systematic approach to addressing real needs of clients. As with any process, it is a dynamic series of activities directed toward change.

DERIVATION OF THE NURSING PROCESS

Florence Nightingale delineated nursing actions from physician actions, particularly in the realm of environmental and supportive measures to ease the discomfort and to facilitate the recovery of the patient. However, in the early years of nursing, most nursing and physician activities were palliative, for there was a limited knowledge base for intervening in the course of the disease. Patient care was shared by the two disciplines. With the advent of the germ theory and other scientific developments, an increasing array of intervention activities became available. Physician education moved into the university setting to receive the benefits of the knowledge gleaned from the developing scientific community. Nursing education, however, remained in the hospital setting, continuing to emphasize palliative and environmental measures, with little impact from the scientific revolution that was occurring.

The separation of physician and nurse became increasingly more marked as scientific knowledge altered the delivery of care to the patient. Physicians could now intervene in the disease process, and because of the nurse's lack of scientific knowledge, the nurse began to see the patient through the "physician's eyes," and a pattern of nursing care developed which was composed primarily of delegated tasks. Nurses tended to patients in terms of designated medical intervention.

The movement of nurses into institutions of higher learning, especially after World War II which brought about the G.I. Bill, enabled nurses to obtain the critical biologic, behavioral scientific knowledge and began the evolution of a patient care modality in which nurses saw the patient through "their own eyes." This evolutionary movement has now reached the point where nursing research is addressing nursing's own science.

Nursing process has been one result of this evolutionary movement. The "seeing of the patient through one's own eyes" demanded a system of relating these observations to a method of nursing intervention in the patient's health problem. Yura and Walsh (1983) note that prior to the 1960s, the term nursing process was seldom seen in the nursing literature, although references to a process inherent in nursing practice was reported by Peplau (1952), Hall (1955), Johnson (1959) and in the early sixties by Orlando (1961) and Wiedenbach (1964). Nursing process is now acknowledged as the phenomenon of nursing practice, especially since nursing theorists have incorporated the process into their theory development. In the eighties, precision in identifying nursing diagnoses, the last phase of the assessment process, has become the concern of nursing researchers and practitioners, for it is the nursing diagnosis that directs all actions of the nurse toward meeting client needs.

Chinn and Jacobs (1983) see that the nursing process "has developed from a skeleton description of actions that were intended to replace rule-oriented and principle-oriented approaches to nursing with a more detailed description of the components of thought and action that constitute effective practice" (p. 29). Nursing practice viewed from the "nurse's eyes" now requires a more deliberative, thoughtful systematic activity that reflects judgment and creativity.

The evolution of nursing process as a systematic method has been influenced by the advent of systems theory, which addresses whole phenomena and the dynamic interaction of its parts toward a clearly defined goal. The nature of wholeness is acknowledged in the nursing process, as all phenomena acting upon an individual in the health–illness spectrum is of concern to the nurse throughout the total process. Nursing process, defined as a sequential series of operations toward the goal attainment of optimal health for a particular client, reflects the nature of any system that synthesizes the actions of each part into a unified, goal-directed function.

NATURE OF NURSING PROCESS

Nursing process is a series of sequential interrelated steps in a goal-directed delivery of nursing care; yet the sequence is not inviolate, and there can be movement among the different steps. Various proposals have been made for the desired number of steps in the process, but there is general agreement that four steps comprise the essence of the process. The four steps and their operations are:

1. Assessment	Problem recognition
	Data gathering
	Data analysis
	Nursing diagnosis
2. Planning	Desired goal setting
	Priority setting
	Selection of intervention measures
3. Implementation	Carrying out of nursing actions
	Formative evaluation of actions
	Change as indicated
4. Evaluation	Relationship of outcome to defined goals
	Consistency of actions in process steps with predetermined criteria and standards of care

> Influence of structural variables on outcome and
> process (environment, agency policies and pro-
> cedures, staffing in relation to quality and
> quantity)

These operations are reflected in the American Nurses Association
(ANA) Standards of Nursing Care, which serves as a valuable resource in process evaluation.

The ordering of the steps in the nursing process is comparable
to that in the problem-solving process, but there are other significant processes involved. It is the development of these processes and
their synthesis into a unified whole of action for delivering nursing
care that is of concern to the teacher in the clinical field, since it is in
this setting that actual delivery of care occurs. An examination of
the various operations in the total process and each of the steps
signals the charge to the nursing instructor.

Assessment

Assessment is an interactive process involving the nurse, client,
family, and significant others in defining the health problem(s) to be
addressed. Skills in all three domains are involved. Cognitive skills
in problem solving, concept formation, inference reasoning, critical
thinking, decision making, and judgment are used. Psychomotor
skills which determine anatomic and physiologic functioning status
provide critical data. Skills in valuing individual's rights to self-
personhood and to be a participant in the assessment process as a
primary source, when possible, are essential if data supplied are to
meet the criterion of reality.

There are four parts to this step; problem recognition, data
gathering, data analysis, and nursing diagnosis. The term nursing
diagnosis is here referred to as the use of categories in naming the
health problem, but in reality all steps in the assessment process
can be recognized as the *process* of nursing diagnosis.

Problem Recognition. This action is a function of the nurse's
knowledge by which the nurse recognizes an implicit or explicit
potential health problem which requires delineation of nursing actions. The stimulus may arise from the client, significant others,
nurse, or other caregivers.

Data Gathering. Reflective of a holistic perspective of nursing,
data are gathered on major matters related to clients' health. Client
responses to occurring phenomena provide cues to the client's health
status in relation to assets and deficits for handling the health problem and to the potential level of wellness if needs are met. Perception is a critical factor here, for data must reflect the client's or

significant other's perception of events that are occurring as well as those of the caregivers. Knowledge of the anticipated pattern in relation to the suspected health problem direct the nurse in data gathering, but data must be within the context of other knowledge, which also influences client responses. Such knowledge includes cultural, social, interpersonal, and systems and patterns of communication. Gordon (1982) suggests important cues for data gathering which contribute to the nursing diagnosis:

1. Change in a client's usual pattern that is unexplained by expected norms of growth and development. (Change may be either positive or negative).
2. Deviation from an appropriate population norm.
3. Behavior that is nonproductive in the whole-person context.
4. That which indicates pattern development. (p. 137)

Cognitive skills of observation, communication, perception, and interviewing in concert with physical assessment skills provide the means for obtaining data. Basic to these skills is the nurse's repertoire of knowledge for appropriate retrieval.

Data Analysis. Cognitive functioning is the critical process in this activity, for more is involved than interpreting each discrete item of data on the basis of biologic or behavioral science principle. Analysis calls for information-processing strategies that depict the relationship among data, discriminate data cues suggestive of a real or potential problem from those that are reflective of wellness, and provide a basis for designating health problem(s) for which a course of action is to be prescribed. Clinical knowledge recall, perceptual skills for seeing relationships among cues in the data field, and inferential reasoning are the significant intellectual operations during this stage. Gordon (1982) notes the significance of inference in the process which she describes as "the ability to make judgments on the basis of information and to go beyond information to predict or explain" (p. 13). The judgment the nurse makes at this juncture to attest the relationship among data cues enables the nurse to cluster discrete data cues with common properties into cue sets or groups. Gordon suggests three possible errors in data clustering:

1. Premature clustering—inadequate data support.
2. Incorrect clustering—inadequate knowledge of critical signs and symptoms.
3. Failure to or delay in synthesizing—leads to error of omission. (p. 220)

The clustering activity prepares the way for the final activity in the assessment step of the process. This activity is the identification of the nursing diagnosis.

Nursing Diagnosis. At the point at which the cue sets are identified, a concept of the health problem is ready to be stated and a nursing diagnosis made. Gordon defines nursing diagnosis as "an actual or potential health problem amenable to nursing therapy" (p. 7). Aspinall (1976) conceives nursing diagnosis as "a process of clinical inference from observed changes in a patient's physical or psychological condition; if it is arrived at accurately and intelligently, it will lead to possible causes of symptomatology" (p. 434). Guzzetta and Forsyth (1979) state that "the process of nursing diagnosis involves the placing of a patient in a diagnostic category for the purpose of identifying and directing nursing management" (p. 28).

The concept attainment reflected in the diagnostic category represents a clinical judgment, a decision on the part of the nurse which was derived from all activities in the assessment process. It is, however, a probabilistic statement, for clinical data are subject to differing perceptual interpretation on the part of the client and caregiver. Reliable and valid data arise from rigorous scientific investigation, Kritek (1979) supports this notion when she refers to the difficulty nurses have in their commitment to the value of holistic nursing by "the state of the knowledge regarding complex judgments, the interaction of diverse human variables and the process of decision making" (p. 75).

The categorization of health problems into nursing diagnoses is the most significant component of the nursing process, for it provides the focus for determining goals of care, the derivation of an appropriate realistic plan of care, the selection and use of pertinent nursing actions of intervention, and the evaluative judgments pertinent to the client's progress toward goal attainment. In other words, all therapeutic activities of the nurse involving the client arise from nursing diagnosis. It is a problem statement; not one of need or a way of meeting the need. It is important to emphasize that the diagnostic process and the resultant categorization are functions of nursing and its domains of practice and do not involve the diagnostic process of other health caregivers. A diagnosis of ineffective breathing patterns is a nursing diagnosis; a diagnosis of emphysema is a medical diagnosis.

The statement of a nursing diagnosis includes two major concerns: the substance of the statement and the classification system for selecting a diagnosis. Gordon (1982, p. 89) proposes three essential components in a statement of a nursing diagnosis, which she refers to as PES format:

P—*Health Problem* or health state of client stated in clear, concise words.

E—*Etiologic Factors:* the probable factors causing or maintaining the client's health problem; behaviors of client, factors in the environment, interaction of both.

S—*Defining signs and symptoms:* a cluster of critical defining signs and symptoms which permit discrimination among health problems. It is a subcategory of the diagnostic category.

In the 1980s the process of categorization of nursing diagnosis is an activity engaging many nurses at both the theoretical and empirical levels. This activity is a critical one, for any science must have a classification system which serves as a communication avenue among its practitioners and directs the activities of the group. In nursing it is an outgrowth of nurses seeing "the patient through one's own eyes." A classification is an important component of a nursing science.

Abdellah's 21 nursing problems (1960), McCain's schema of assessment in 13 problem areas (1965), and Henderson's 14 basic needs (1966), were early movements toward giving nursing its unique focus, different from that designated by the medical profession. In 1973, the First National Conference in Classification of Nursing Diagnosis was held in an attempt to define nursing's own classification system. Five other conferences were held since that date resulting in a listing of 51 diagnoses ready for clinical testing (Kim, McFarland & McLane, 1984), (Table 5).

The first conference approached the task from an inductive methodology, which involves proceeding from the particular to the general. Nurses in practice described client health problems with which they were concerned during the course of their practice as a participant observer or through recall of previous experiences. Other nurse scholars, such as Campbell (1978) also used nurses in practice in their pursuit of nursing diagnoses labels.

By the third conference in 1978, a need for a conceptual framework was recognized, for there was no system by which data could be organized and classified. The use of a conceptual framework signifies a deductive approach, the movement from the general to the particular. It is apparent that both deductive and inductive methodologies will be used in the search for a classification system.

The pursuit of a classification system for nursing diagnosis is an ongoing activity in the eighties. Jones (1979) suggests five steps in the process of developing a taxonomy of nursing diagnosis:

1. Defining nursing (so defined as "caring which assists person, family, community in coping with their response to actual or potential threat to health").
2. Identification of parameters of nursing assessment (data base).
3. Selection of terminology to describe nursing problems.
4. Definition of these terms.
5. Development of a system of classification. (p. 67)

TABLE 5. LIST OF APPROVED NURSING DIAGNOSES AT FIFTH NATIONAL CONFERENCE

Activity intolerance
Activity intolerance potential
Activity clearance, ineffective
Anxiety
Bowel elimination, alteration in: constipation
Bowel elimination, alteration in: diarrhea
Bowel elimination, alteration in: incontinence
Breathing pattern, ineffective
Cardiac output, alteration in: decreased
Comfort, alteration in: pain
Communication, impaired: verbal
Coping, family: potential for growth
Coping, ineffective family: compromised
Coping, ineffective family: disabling
Coping, ineffective individual
Diversional activity, deficit
Family process, alteration in
Fear
Fluid volume alteration in: excess
Fluid volume deficit, actual
Fluid volume deficit, potential
Gas exchange, impaired
Grieving, anticipatory
Grieving, dysfunctional
Health maintenance, alteration in
Home maintenance management, impaired
Injury, potential for: (poisoning, potential for: suffocation, potential for: trauma, potential for)
Knowledge deficit (specify)
Mobility impaired, physical
Noncompliance (specify)
Nutrition, alteration in: less than body requirements
Nutrition, alteration in: more than body requirements
Nutrition, alteration in: potential for more than body requirements
Oral mucous membrane, alteration in
Parenting, alteration in: actual
Parenting, alteration in: potential
Powerlessness
Rape trauma syndrome
Self-care deficit: feeding, bathing/hygiene, dressing/grooming, toileting
Self-concept, disturbance in: body image, self-esteem, role performance, personal identity
Sensory-perceptual alteration: visual, auditory, kinesthetic, gustatory, tactile, olfactory
Sexual dysfunction
Skin integrity, impairment of: actual
Skin integrity, impairment of: potential
Sleep pattern disturbance
Social isolation
Spiritual distress (distress of the human spirit)
Thought processes, alteration in
Tissue perfusion, alteration in: cerebral, cardiopulmonary, renal, gastrointestinal, peripheral
Urinary elimination, alteration in patterns
Violence, potential for: self-directed or directed at others

(From Kim, M. J., McFarland, G. K., & McLane, A. M. Classification of nursing diagnosis: Proceedings of the fifth national conference, 1984, with permission.)

Whatever system is eventually developed, it is essential that diagnoses are clear, concise statements acceptable to and understood by practitioners as well as investigators. Once categories are identified, they need to be validated; i.e., reliable indicators for each category must be determined before the classification can be standardized and incorporated into a nursing diagnosis taxonomy.

Search for nursing theory is proceeding on many fronts in the eighties, all of which have an impact on the nature of the classification system. Although classifications arise from specific knowledge, values, and philosophies, in nursing there are diverse philosophies reflected in the notions of nursing as a science and practice discipline by the various theorists. The concepts of nursing diagnosis held by King, Neuman, Orem, Rogers and Roy are noted later in this chapter in Table 6; each suggests a different perspective and approach to problem solution. Can a classification system be developed that is understood by all nurses, yet accommodate to differing philosophies of nursing?

The notion of patterning as a function of nursing assessment appears in the nursing literature relative to nursing diagnosis. In an effort to address the diversity in perspective of nursing theorists yet recognizing the need for some unity in nursing practice for standardizing the assessment process, Gordon (1982) has proposed a typology of assessment areas, functional health patterns common to all clients. This typology attempts to provide unification of structural areas while leaving the approach to assessment and analysis of data to the domain of each of the theorists.

The 11 functional health patterns proposed by Gordon (Note 1) are:

1. *Health-perception–health-management pattern.* Describes client's perceived pattern of health and well-being and how health is managed.
2. *Nutritional-metabolic pattern.* Describes pattern of food and fluid consumption relative to metabolic need and pattern indicators of local nutrient supply.
3. *Elimination pattern.* Describes patterns of excretory function (bowel, bladder, and skin).
4. *Activity-exercise pattern.* Describes pattern of exercise, activity, leisure, and recreation.
5. *Cognitive-perceptual pattern.* Describes sensory-perceptual and cognitive pattern.
6. *Sleep-rest pattern.* Describes patterns of sleep, rest, and relaxation.
7. *Self-perception–self-concept pattern.* Describes self-concept pattern and perceptions of self (e.g., body comfort, body image, feeling state).
8. *Role-relationship pattern.* Describes pattern of role engagements and relationships.
9. *Sexuality-reproductive pattern.* Describes client's patterns of satis-

faction and dissatisfaction with sexuality pattern; reproductive patterns.
10. *Coping-stress-tolerance pattern.* Describes general coping patterns and effectiveness of the pattern in terms of stress tolerance.
11. *Value-belief pattern.* Describes patterns of values, beliefs (including spiritual), or goals that guide choices or decisions. (p. 81)

Suffice to say, nursing diagnosis is a critical component of the nursing process. The standardization of the classification system is the province of nurse theorists, researchers, and practitioners, a task urgently needed if nursing practice is to have a scientifically determined, goal-directed, orderly process for meeting health care needs of clients. Knowledge has advanced sufficiently at this time to enable nurses to accept the notion of nursing diagnosis and to develop practice modes in accordance with this notion, while still realizing that there is a probabilistic dimension to nursing diagnosis.

Planning

Nursing diagnosis sets the stage for the second step of the nursing process: the design for nursing care which addresses the client's health problem. Nursing literature includes much recent discussion concerning this step in the process by such authorities as Mayers (1983), Yura and Walsh (1983), Marriner (1983), Carnevali (1983), Bower (1982), and Carpenito (1983). Of particular concern in this book is the identification of the critical elements in this step that are significant to the teacher in the clinical field. Planning is an intellectual and ethical operation involving decision making, critical thinking, and value choice making. It calls upon the nurse to activate the problem statement into a process by which the solution is pursued. Bower (1982) notes three ethical issues which are of concern to nurses in planning care:

1. What is best for the client in order for maximum benefits to occur.
2. Whether the client's rights were protected when decisions were made about the plan.
3. Whether there has been justice in the way materials, resources, and time have been allocated to the client. (p. 134)

Goal Setting. The use of nursing diagnosis, a reflection of a clustering of signs and symptoms, rather than the use of each sign and symptom as a discrete item, enables the nurse to direct nursing actions in a holistic manner toward resolution of the total problem. The nursing diagnosis directs the nurse in the determination of goals, the desired outcome of care. These goals refer to the desired level of wellness/health status appropriate for the client and describe a state, condition, or behavior. The goals specified must be congruent with the goals of other caregivers for the concern is a unified approach in the management of the total needs of the client.

Goals are designated as either short-term or long-term, for the time variable is an important dimension. Short-term goals are noted in times of urgency or as interim steps toward a goal requiring a greater time span for achievement. Long-term goals recognize the health problem as an episodic event in the life activities of the client whose management greatly influences the quality of the total life span. Immediate short-term resolution is not an end in itself but must be viewed within the context of the client's total existence.

Participation of the client or significant others in the assessment process continues in this step of the nursing process, as goals must be mutually met by all concerned. It is imperative that both the caregiver and the client have the same perception of the desired goals so that there is a complementary and supportive interaction in problem resolution. Goal setting is a function of the nurse's knowledge and the client's acceptance.

Priority Setting. Often, multiple diagnoses are developed for an individual client and the nurse is called upon to determine a priority among the various goals since all goals cannot, or in all probability should not, be addressed at the same time. This process entails the establishment of a preferential order of goals which provides direction for nursing actions. Priority setting entails skills in decision making and judgment, drawing upon the nurse's repertoire of knowledge and the ensuing nursing action required.

Bower (1982) suggests three criteria for determining a hierarchy of importance of problems for priority setting:

1. Those which threaten the life, dignity, and integrity of the individual, family, or community.
2. Those which threaten to change destructively the individual, family, or community.
3. Those which affect the normal developmental growth of the individual, family, or community. (pp. 22–23)

In addition to the criteria stated above which relate to the nature of the health problem, other factors may be considered in establishing priorities. In some instances, the treatments the client receives may have a high priority because of their impact on promoting or maintaining the integrity of the individual's functioning. Treatments may be those prescribed by nurses or by other caregivers, such as physicians or specialty therapists. The relationship of nursing actions to those of other caregivers must be considered in any priority setting for there must be coordination of all actions involving the client. Factors such as availability of time for goal attainment, resources (finances, facilities, services, people) essential for therapeutic management, and the social, cultural, psychologic and spiritual meanings of events are important in the ordering of goals in those instances where the criterion of urgency does not apply. Priority setting requires skill in discriminating among various goals so that planning for care is congruent with the needs of the client and proceeds according to the range of intensity of these needs.

Selection of Intervention Strategies. The designation of a goal signals the need to determine strategies by which the nurse can intervene for purposes of resolving or ameliorating disturbances in response patterns and lead a client to the desired state of health as specified in the goals. As with the other parts of the planning process, the client or significant others are participants in the decisions.

Intervention modalities are directed toward the etiology factor, which is noted in the statement of the nursing diagnosis. Some selections are the result of convergent thinking, since therapeutic measures have been specifically identified as prescriptions for particular types of responses. However, in many situations, nursing prescriptions are not readily available and the need for divergent thinking resulting in creative management strategies is paramount. The nurse needs to be prepared to consider alternatives for intervention and should be willing to be a risk taker when proposing new strategies whose outcome is uncertain. A careful examination of the potential consequences of the action enables the nurse to anticipate the degree of risk involved and reach the decision as to whether or not to proceed with the action.

Although nursing does have some prescriptive actions for certain diagnoses which can be incorporated in a plan of care, many times even the prescription has to be evaluated in terms of its appropriateness to a particular client. Gordon (1982) suggests six areas of information that are essential in individualizing interventions for a particular client:

1. Personal client factors—unique characteristics.
2. Client's perception—particularly any misconceptions related to etiology.
3. Current level of compensation—resources, strengths.
4. Problem magnitude and urgency—type and timing of nursing actions.
5. Extended effects—influence on other areas of client's life.
6. Cost-benefit factors—financial, social and psychologic. (pp. 244–245)

Individualization in the selection of nursing intervention actions calls upon, once more, the nurse's ability to be creative in the selection of alternatives, each of which has the capability to address the health problem.

Nursing practice includes a repertoire of intervention modalities available to the nurse. Three different forms of nursing action are proposed by the Nursing Theories Conference Group (1980):

1. Assuming responsibility for a person until he or she is able to be responsible for self.
2. Changing (manipulating) environment to facilitate health.
3. Helping person toward some goal. (p. 216)

Therapeutic communication skills of listening, observing, interacting, and transacting with clients are important methods by which the nurses use themselves in the process of care. Teaching is a communication skill which is a significant intervention strategy, ranging from information sharing to assisting the client in developing new patterns of functioning. Teaching is a function of nursing, and its substance for any particular client is derived from the assessment process, inclusive of the diagnostic statement, which delineates the knowledge status of the client. Teaching, selected for a care plan, addresses knowledges the client needs to cope with a real or potential disturbed health state and to partake in one's own care during the illness episode and that which is essential for promoting or maintaining an optimum level of wellness.

The development of a protocol for teaching a client is the prerogative of nurse functioning in accord with the stated nursing standards. Nurses who rely on physician approval for the plan and its implementation view teaching as a delegated function rather than a nursing function. Protocols for teaching clients in a health care setting need to be reviewed and approved by a nursing board, not a medical board, as happens in some settings. Teaching methods selected for the plan relate to the goals to be achieved, the ability and resources of the learner, and the nature of the material to be learned.

Psychomotor skills represent many intervention strategies, which may be either for restorative or supportive purposes. Their selection is determined by the problem to be addressed, and their actions may be carried out solely by the nurse, solely by the client, or by both. The range of skill involved varies from the simple to the complex, which calls upon more than one psychomotor skill for the total operation. The selection of the appropriate skill is a judgment decision on the part of the nurse; however, the client is afforded the opportunity to be a part of the decision-making process and to be fully informed as to the procedure and what is entailed in the skill.

The American Nurses Association Social Policy Statement (1980) indicates that the aims of nursing actions are to ameliorate, improve, or correct conditions to which those practices are directed to prevent illness and promote health. The planning for all actions recognizes the integrity of the individual as a total phenomenon.

The selection of intervention strategies may be prescriptive or it may be exploratory requiring validation. Regardless of the derivation of the strategy, the nurse must be able to predict the probability that such a measure will be effective in meeting the desired outcome of care. The prediction is a function of the nurse's knowledge about nursing actions and their relationship to various health–illness phenomena.

Implementation

This is the action step of the process and represents the implementation of the nursing plan. It demands not only skill in performance of the activities, but the process of perception and observation in the continuous appraisal of the actions as they occur. It requires critiquing skills as actions are viewed in terms of goals to be achieved and the original data base on which they were based. Nursing judgments are made and decisions are often arrived at to modify actions or to obtain other types of data when there is a suggestion that the client is not being moved toward the desired goal. Judgments are also made about the interrelationship of nursing interventions and those of other caregivers who are also ministering to the client. The interventions of all concerned must be complimentary and directed toward the desired health status goal.

Nursing textbooks contain detailed information of various intervention modalities which nurses use for designated purposes. It is sufficient here to acknowledge that this phase includes the "doing" for, about, or with the client and the use of feedback to ascertain the effectiveness of the "doing" or the need for alternative approaches when intervention is not achieving the desired result.

Evaluation

The fourth step in the nursing process, evaluation, is concerned with the quality dimension of care. It answers such questions as: Were client outcomes achieved? If not, why not? How was the process executed? What events in the setting influenced positively or negatively the outcome and the process? Answers to these questions rely upon professional judgment based on skills of perception, analysis, and knowledge retrieval.

Most references to this step in the process include the evaluation of process and outcome. Little emphasis is placed on the role assumed by characteristics of and events in the setting in influencing both process and outcome. Donabedian (1969) refers to three components in assessing the quality of health care: structure in which health care occurs, process of care, and the outcomes of care.

Outcome, the health characteristics, behavior, and states, which were specified as goals following the diagnostic process, are the foci of the nurse's evaluation efforts in terms of the effectiveness of care. They are assumed to be the result of interventions, although such a causal relationship is difficult to ascertain because of the inexactness of predictability. The outcomes are client centered; i.e., what happened to the client; not caregiver centered in terms of the quality of the performance.

Process is another focus of evaluation of the nursing process. Phaneuf (1976) describes the actions involved:

> Evaluation of process of care entails appraisal of all major or minor steps taken in the care of the patient with attention to the nature of the rationale for, and the sequence of the steps and the degree to which they help the patient reach specified and attainable therapeutic goals. (p. 21)

Evaluation questions address the comprehensiveness and accuracy of the assessment, the precision of the inferences and resulting diagnosis, the relevance of the goals of care to the stated diagnosis, the appropriateness of the plan components, and the effectiveness of the implementation activities.

The American Nurse's Association Standards of Nursing Care provides a framework for this activity, for the standards are described from a nursing process perspective. Generic standards and specialty standards are available. The nursing audit is another means for evaluating the process of care.

Structural variables are significant in their impact on both process and outcome, yet they are seldom incorporated in the evaluation protocol of direct care. They are more likely to appear in quality assurance programs of a total health care delivery service. The beliefs, values, policies, and procedures of an agency; the quantity and quality of the staff of nursing and other caregivers and support services; the availability of resources needed for care; the financial resources of the institution; the interpersonal interaction patterns; and the management style with particular emphasis on locus of decision making all influence the ability of the nurse to carry out the nursing process. An evaluation of care without consideration of the role played by some of the variables mentioned above can often produce spurious results.

Evaluation is a critical step in the nursing process. At this stage, it is a summative evaluation, a declaration of *what is* in contrast to formative evaluation which is ongoing in the previous steps, particularly in implementation, which states *what is and what can be.* Appraisal of client outcome in relation to the total effect and the structural variables' influences on the process and its outcome constitutes an effective framework for professional judgment as to the quality of nursing care.

Data dealing with outcome collected at this time are valuable resources for determining the effectiveness of nursing's impact in the health care delivery system. Compilation of outcome data and their interpretation related to cost factors, decrease in recidivism, and effective use of time and resources would be most influential in portraying the real significance of the nurse as a health care provider.

NURSING PROCESS—NURSING FRAMEWORKS

Earlier, the nursing process was identified as the methodology of nursing, the means by which the delivery of nursing care is administered to clients. The substance of that delivery system is determined by the framework of nursing beliefs accepted by an individual nurse, a nursing service, or a school of nursing. lt is the belief about nursing that gives direction to the activities inherent in the nursing process. It is generally accepted that professionals go to the theory base of their discipline to obtain the basis for curriculum and program development, research, and practice. The very fact that the discipline exists provides the source of authority for its practitioners (Reilly, 1975).

Nursing is in pursuit of its own science as various theorists in nursing propose their philosophic notions of nursing and the relevant elements and their relationships which characterize the practice. Some theorists have operationalized their beliefs into a pattern of practice, while others have described their theory in abstract terms. Nursing literature is replete with data which describe the various frameworks of nursing, the ongoing research related to each, and the critiques, both positive and negative. All frameworks are abstractions, but some are postulated as theories, while others are referred to as conceptual representations. Reilly (1975) differentiates between these two frameworks:

> A conceptual model (framework) provides a perspective, a way of looking at nursing. It is a representation of reality since it is derived from and pertains to reality, but it *does not constitute* reality. A theoretical model (framework), on the other hand, *does constitute* reality since it has a scientifically accepted base. (p. 567)

Some nursing educational programs and nursing care settings have adopted a particular nursing theorist's framework or have developed an eclectic framework reflective of components from several theories, nursing and other disciplines. All such frameworks acknowledge the nursing process as the means by which nursing care is delivered to clients. In situations where no nursing framework exists, nursing process may or may not be the accepted mode.

Fawcett (1984) recognizes the role of conceptual models of nursing as a guideline for all aspects of practice. She concludes: "the model tells the clinician what to look at when interacting with clients and how to interpret observations. It also tells the clinician how to plan interventions in a general manner and provides beginning criteria for evaluation of interventions and outcomes" (p. 27).

Gordon (1982) emphasizes the significance of a nursing model "because nursing diagnosis cannot be done without a *nursing model* that provides clear guidelines for the collection of clinical information. It is the model that delineates the data to be assessed, their rationale and the resultant nursing diagnosis" (p. 28). It is because at this time there is not one nursing theory or nursing science that Gordon proposes the use of functional health patterns, described earlier as a framework for assessment, so that there may be some consistency in the type of data collected. The meaning and interpretation of data remain within the realm of the nursing framework chosen by the individual nurse or the agency.

Table 6 depicts the nature of nursing process within the concept of nursing as described by five theorists. The theorists selected are not meant to be inclusive of all nursing theories, but are selected because they are at this time generally recognized in the nursing community and they reflect different levels of theory development. Their inclusion in this chapter is an attempt to emphasize that nursing process is not a suitable conceptual framework, as perceived in some schools of nursing and health care settings, but is in reality the means of operationalizing nursing as conceptualized in a framework.

TEACHING THE NURSING PROCESS IN THE CLINICAL FIELD

Because the nursing process is a practice model, its teaching for competency can only be obtained in a practice field where students care for real clients with real or potential health problems. Attainment of competency requires a progression of experiences reflecting increasing complexity over a period of time which, although variable in accord with individual differences, is sufficient for development to occur.

A Holistic Process

The teaching of the nursing process must respect its holistic nature: four steps, discrete in themselves, but interrelated into a total phenomenon. It is the interrelationship among the steps that provides the essence of the process. Although, as noted earlier, each step has its own goal, purpose and specialized tasks, its significance in patient care is only in terms of its relationship to the goals, purposes and tasks of the other steps. Data obtained in assessment are of little value if they are not formulated into a plan of care which denotes intervention strategies which are implemented and evaluated. Likewise, a technically developed plan of care, not based on

TABLE 6. NURSING PROCESS ACCORDING TO FIVE NURSING THEORISTS

	King	Neuman
Definition of Nursing	Nursing is a helping profession involving a process of action, reaction, interaction and transaction whereby nurse and client share their perceptions in the nursing situation through: purposeful communication, identify specific goals, problems, or concerns; explore means to achieve a goal; agree to means to the goal; and both move toward goal attainment.	Nursing is a unique profession concerned with all variables affecting a client(s)' response to stressors. Nursing actions are appropriate to the total needs of the client on his/her own wellness/illness continuum toward providing client/client system stability.
Goal of Nursing	Promote health: i.e., help individuals and groups attain, maintain, and restore health and if not possible, help individuals die with dignity.	Promote client/client system integrity through retention, attainment, and/or maintenance of an optimal functional level for the client.
Concept of Nursing Process	Nursing is a process of human interaction leading to goal attainment. It is a process of action, reaction, interaction, and	Nursing process is systemized into the following three categories: *Nursing diagnosis—* Accomplished by

(*Continued on page 60*)

TABLE 6. (*Continued*)

Orem	Rogers	Roy
Nursing is a human service whose concern is the individual's need for self-care action and the provision and management of it on a continuous basis in order to sustain life and health, recover from disease or injury and to cope with their effects. Conditions that validate the existence of requirement for nursing as an adult are the absence of ability to maintain continuously that amount and quality of self-care which is therapeutic in sustaining life and health, in recovery from disease or injury or in coping with their effects. In children, the condition is the ability of parent (or guardian) to maintain continuously for the child, the amount and quality of care that is therapeutic.	Nursing is a science and an art. A science is defined as an organized body of abstract knowledge arrived at by scientific research and logical analysis. The art of nursing is the imaginative and creative use of this knowledge in human service. The practice of nursing is the use of the body of abstract knowledge in service to people. A science of unitary human beings basic to nursing requires a new world view and a conceptual system specific to nursing's phenomenon of concern. People and their environments are perceived as irreducible energy fields integral with one another and continuously creative in their evolution. It is postulated that people have the capacity to participate knowingly and probabilistically in the process of change.	Nursing is a scientific way of providing care for the ill or potentially ill person which acts through nursing process to promote adaptation in each of the four modes of adaptation in situations of health and illness.
Dependent upon the particular self-care demand and degree of self-care agency, goals are to (1) protect or promote the individual's capabilities for rendering care to self, (2) meet the person's self-care demand, (3) promote the capabilities of the dependent care agent for rendering care to patient.	Maintenance and promotion of maximum well-being within the potential of individuals and groups through utilization of descriptive, explanatory, and predictive principles deriving from the conceptual system. Nurses are concerned with all people whoever they are and whether they may be deemed well or sick.	Promotion of a person's adaptation in physiologic needs, self-concept, role function, and relations of interdependence in situations of health and illness.
Consciously selected activities directed by the nurse toward accomplishing nursing goals within a health care	The utilization of the science of unitary human beings in continuously innovative ways through evaluative and interventive	A problem-solving approach required by client-centered goal of nursing and the need to verify the service the

(*Continued on page 61*)

TABLE 6. (*Continued*)

	King	Neuman
Concept of Nursing Process (*cont.*)	transaction where nurse/patient share mutually set goals and move toward goal attainment. Nursing process is the standard method used in most nursing situations which has identified some of the essential functions of the nurse: assessment of patient's health, formulation of a plan on the basis of information gathered, implementation of a plan of care, and evaluation of its effectiveness.	acquisition of an appropriate data base and synthesis of theory for determining variance from wellness from which hypothetical interventions can be made to reach the desired client/client system stability or wellness level. *Nursing Goals*—Arrived at by data analysis, data related to theory and client negotiations for prescriptive change which form the bases for nursing intervention strategies and are postulated to retain, attain and/or maintain client/client system stability. *Nursing Outcomes*—Affected by use of one or more prevention as intervention modes (primary, secondary, and/or tertiary) to confirm client prescriptive change. Short-term goal outcome influences intermediate and long-term goal setting and possibility of reformulation of short-term goals.
Assessment Basis	Extent to which client is able to meet basic needs, perform daily activities, cope with health and illness, and function in a social role.	Extent to which there is actual or potential penetration of normal line of defense of the client by stressors which may be intra, inter, or extrapersonal in nature.
Data	Personal System *Perception:* Patient's perception of the event, sensory system integrity, chrono-	Client/Client System Data *Stressors:* Identification of actual and/or potential

(*Continued on page 62*)

Orem	Rogers	Roy
situation which involves 3 steps: (1) determination of why a patient needs nursing care, (2) design of a nursing system specific to the patient's needs, (3) initiation, conduction, and control of assisting actions addressed to meeting the therapeutic self-care demand or to regulate the exercise in development of self-care agency.	modalities directed toward actualizing maximum well-being for the individual, family, and society.	nurse provides which includes diagnosing patient adaptation problems and planning, carrying out and evaluating care.
Determination of why a person requires nursing in relation to therapeutic self-care demand: capabilities for engaging in self-care agency, potential for further development of self-care agency and quantity of self-care deficit in relation to therapeutic self-care demand.	Evaluation of the nature of human and environment field patterns as manifest in correlates of field patterning. The integrality of human and environmental fields is a basic premise. Evaluation is relative and probabilistic, continuously innovative, and charac-terized by nonrepeating rhythmicities.	Extent to which the patient has achieved an adaptive state within four adaptive modes and cognator/regulator effectiveness in bringing about that adaptation.
Therapeutic Self-Care Demand *Universal Self-Care Requisites:* Adequacy of air intake,	Correlates of Patterning Include: Higher frequency field patterns, growing diver-sity, etc., manifest in	First Level Adaptive Modes: Identification of patient behaviors in each adap-tive mode and recogni-

(*Continued on page 63*)

TABLE 6. (Continued)

	King	Neuman
Data (cont.)	logic age, developmental level, sex, educational level, nurse's perception of patient's perceptions *Stress:* Patient's stress and nurse's stress, potential anxiety, positive force in life, energy use, interference with perceptual system, drug and diet history *Self:* Client's perception of self, current health status, body image *Growth and Development Status:* Client's background, ability to carry out developmental tasks, ability to carry out activities of daily living *Body Image:* Client's perception, influence of body image on lifestyle, family members' perception of body image *Space:* Perception of personal space, cultural interpretation of space *Time:* Perception of time, altered perception of time Interpersonal Systems *Communication:* Patterns, communication between client, family, and caregiver *Interaction:* Purposeful, information component of interactions *Transaction:* Value component of interactions, perceptions of client and nurse *Role:* Perception of role of nurse, client, other professionals	stressors, intra, inter and extrapersonal in nature *Client/Client System:* Basic structure factors, energy resources, flexible line of defense, normal line of defense, lines of resistance, potential for reconstitution *Client/Client System Stability:* Past, present, and future life process factors, coping patterns, expectations *Client/Environment Interactions:* Intrapersonal, interpersonal and extrapersonal interactions under the influence of the four variables of man: physiologic, psychologic, sociocultural, developmental *Resources:* Internal, external *Perceptions:* Caregiver, Client

(Continued on page 64)

Orem	Rogers	Roy
adequacy of water intake, adequacy of food intake, elimination and excretion processes, balance–rest and activity, balance–solitude and social interaction, existence and potential hazards to human life functioning and well-being, evidence of need for action to protect normal functioning *Developmental Self-Care Requisites:* Living conditions: supportive, nonsupportive of life processes; conditions that promote, interfere with developmental processes; deleterious effects of conditions that affect human life and development *Health Deviation Self-Care Requisites:* Evidence of need to seek appropriate medical assistance, effects and results of pathologic conditions and status that set up requirements for care, effects and results of medically prescribed diagnostic, therapeutic and rehabilitation measures, evidence of discomforting or deleterious effects of medical measures, evidence of ability to accept self in a particular state of health or with specific forms of treatment, evidence of maintaining a lifestyle with pathologic status which promotes continued personal development *Self-Care Agency and Potential for its Development:*	such attributes as: sleeping, waking, beyond waking; slower to faster rhythms; experience of time passing; and many others *Principles of Homeodynamics* *Principle of Resonancy:* The continuous change from lower to higher frequency wave patterns in human and environmental fields *Principle of Helicy:* The continuous innovative, probabilistic, increasing diversity of human and environmental field patterns characterized by nonrepeating rhythmicities *Principle of Integrality:* The continuous mutual human field and environmental field processes	tion of person's position on health–illness continuum *Basic Physiology Needs:* Nutrition, elimination, fluid and electrolyte, oxygen, circulation, regulation, exercise and rest *Self-Concept:* Physical self, personal self, interpersonal self *Role Function:* Role conflict, role failure, role mastery *Interdependence:* Need for affiliation, need for achievement, independency/dependency *Second Level:* Identification of focal, contextual, and residual stimuli relative to ineffective response behavior of client *Focal Stimuli:* Degree of change, stimulus is cause *Contextual Stimuli:* All other stimuli which contribute to behavior *Residual Stimuli:* Stimuli having an undetermined effect on behavior

(Continued on page 65)

TABLE 6. (*Continued*)

	King	Neuman
Data (*cont.*)	*Stress:* Environmental, present disturbance, past experience, coping mechanism *Social System— Environment:* One of client/caregiver, concepts of organization, power, authority and decision making, understanding of background of nurse/client, demographic variables	
Nursing Diagnosis	Deviations from health resulting from disturbances in the client's personal, interpersonal, and social systems	Consists of variances from wellness as determined by analysis of a comprehensive client/client system data base and theoretical considerations. Hypothetical interventions are postulated to reach the desired client stability or wellness level
Planning	Setting of mutual goals between client and caregiver to move the individual toward health in the social system and joint planning on how the goals can be reached together. Interaction is critical; goals are influenced by client's and nurses' perceptions, backgrounds, values and health status. Priority setting is carried out mutually whenever possible.	Negotiation with the client for desired prescriptive change to correct variances from wellness, based on classified needs and resources identified in the nursing diagnosis. Appropriate nursing (action) intervention strategies are postulated for retention, attainment, and/or maintenance of client/client system stability or desired outcome goals.

(*Continued on page 66*)

Orem	Rogers	Roy
Repertoire of self-care practices, usual components of patient's self-care system, abilities and limitations for deliberate actions, knowledge, skills, and motivation to meet *each* self-care requisite; what patient is able to do and does do meeting prescribed therapeutic self-care demand; what patient should do, should not do, is willing to do, in meeting prescribed therapeutic self-care demand; potential for future exercise of self-care agency and continued development		
Existence or potential self-care deficits by associated factors or combinations of factors	Based on principles of homeodynamics, manifests variations in rhythms, patterns, diversity and other mutual human and environmental field processes	A statement of the client's adaptive behavior with the most relevant influencing factors as determined from the assessed data base
Based on why person needs nursing and the nurse's judgment about the kind of nursing required. Contains details regarding time, place, and roles of nurse and patient for performance of nurse–patient activities. Designation of a system of nursing assistance based on patient defined self-care deficit: wholly compensatory; partially compensatory; supportive-educative. Goal of action—compensate for patient self-care limitations to insure that self-care is	Developed on the basis of nursing evaluation with nursing interventions determined accordingly with the goal of attainment of optimum health for the individual and group. Intervention is predicated upon irreducible wholeness of the human being and derives its safety and effectiveness from a unified concept of human functioning. Goal setting encompasses both preservation and enhancement of a meaningful life and meaningful transitions	Setting goals determined by relative importance of the problem with intent of changing ineffective adaptive response to adaptive behavior or of reinforcing adaptive behavior. Intervention actions are selected on the basis of influencing stimuli that can be managed. To effect change and stabilize adaptation, possible approaches are listed with the highest probability of achieving the goal selected.

(Continued on page 67)

TABLE 6. (*Continued*)

	King	Neuman

Planning (*cont.*)

Implementation

A Transaction
Personal:
Help patient maintain self-esteem and interact in ways that give patient choices to exert some control over environment; control environment and protect against too much intrusion on patient's personal space; schedule activities to meet the needs of the individual; control environment to limit unneccessary disruption in Circadian rhythms
Interaction:
Goal-oriented interaction, move toward reciprocally contingent interaction, decrease stressors on patient and family, provide information, assist patient to verbalize concerns and expectations, minimize stress when carrying out procedures.

One or more of three prevention as intervention modes are used to confirm prescriptive change for the client as follows:
Primary Prevention:
Action required to retain client/client system stability, i.e., maintain the integrity of the flexible line of defense by strengthening resistance to stressors
Secondary Prevention:
Action required to attain client/client system stability, i.e., mobilize client's internal and external resources to reduce reactions to stressors
Tertiary Prevention:
Action required to maintain client/client system stability, i.e., mobilize and utilize client internal and external resources to maintain the highest possible level of wellness following secondary prevention as intervention.

Evaluation

Identified goals and attainment of goals provides a measure of effectiveness of care. Client's perception in evaluating effects. Nurse's perception of changes. Goal-oriented nursing record is an information system that if implemented provides a permanent record for research studies and documents care to measure effectiveness.

Client outcome following nursing intervention reflects the degree of confirmation of prescriptive change. For example, nursing goals, designed in the planning phase, are measurable in terms of increased resistance to stressors, decreased degree of reaction and maintenance of a desired level of wellness following intervention because of a

(*Continued on page 68*)

given and is therapeutic and to enable patient to develop adaptive behavior.

Modes of helping are: acting for, teaching, guiding and directing, supporting (physical and psychologic), providing developmental environment, initiation, conduction, and control of assisting actions to achieve nursing results that are related to identified therapeutic self-care requirements and to self-care limitations and ability.

According to nursing system: compensate for patient's self-care limitations, overcome when possible self-care limitations of patient and family so future short-term and long-term therapeutic self-care requisites can be met effectively, foster and protect patient self-care abilities and prevent development of new self-care limitations.

from life through death. Individual participates in the goal setting.

Implementation based on principles of homeodynamics and other theories. It includes individualization of services coupled with creativity in integrating nursing knowledge for continuously novel evaluative and interventive modalities. Tools of practice require intellectual skill for their safe and competent identification and use. Tools include technical and manual skills, therapeutic touch, and multiple other means.

Intervention attempts to manage the environment by removing, increasing, decreasing, and/or altering stimuli related to ineffective response. When possible, focal stimulus is channeled first. Nurse is the external regulatory force to modify stimuli affecting adaptation on the part of the patient.

Can patient realize self-management and provide continuing therapeutic self-care? Is there a decrease self-care deficit and increase self-care agency when possible? What evidence of personal development and human well-being? Use evidence in evaluating results achieved against results specified in the nursing system design.

Appraisal is continuous and dynamic. Assessment of the nature and direction of change in the human and environmental field patterning as manifest in correlates of field patterning is a necessary adjunct to determining interventive effectiveness. Client participation is essential.

Effectiveness of nursing intervention in client goal achievement: behavior—adaptive, movement toward peak health, individual needs of biologic, social, and psychologic integrity are met. Basis of judging effectiveness by result that nursing approach had regarding the client's adaptive behavior. If behavior still ineffective adaptation, reassess

(Continued on page 69)

TABLE 6. *(Continued)*

	King	Neuman
Evaluation *(cont.)*		reaction. Evaluation of nursing outcome following intervention (action) confirms the degree of goal attainment. Reformulation or further goal planning may be desirable for subsequent nursing intervention. Client outcome thus validates the nursing process and the model from which it was derived.

nursing diagnoses derived from comprehensive and accurate data, has no meaning for a particular client.

Bruner's notion of teaching the *structure* of a subject is particularly relevant to the teaching of nursing process, for it provides the student very quickly with a sense of the essence of nursing practice. Bruner (1963) states: "Grasping the structure of a subject is understanding it in a way that permits many other things to be related to it meaningfully. To learn structure, in short, is to learn how things are related" (p. 7). The ability to transfer knowledge of the subject to a more complex phenomenon is a function of the individual's ability to know the structure of the subject. Bruner suggests the notion of a spiral curriculum, whereby the structure of the subject once learned, is related to increasing complex phenomena.

Nursing process needs to be introduced to students early in the educational program in terms of its structure as a holistic, interrelated activity which addresses simple to complex health problems. The repertoire of knowledge and skills inherent in each step increases in complexity as the student carries out the process with increasing numbers or complexity of variables. The skill of the process remains constant; it is the different parameters with which the process is used that are the changeable element. The tendency to emphasize the complexity of the substance and of the skills of each step as discrete items separate from the total process destroys the integrity of the process and precludes the ability of the student to see the unitary nature of the process. The tendency to view nursing process primarily in terms of complex variables negates the essence of the process and interferes with the student's ability to see its interrelationships.

The following vignette describes the experience of a student in her beginning clinical practical experience:

Orem	Rogers	Roy
		influencing stimuli to see if nursing approach should be modified by managing another stimuli.

(The theories presented in this table appear with the approval of Imogene King, Betty Neuman, Dorothea Orem, Martha Rogers and Sister Callista Roy.)

I noticed that my patient was sad, for she was very quiet and did not want to see anyone. When I questioned her about her sad expression, she told me that she was embarrassed at the way she looked. Usually she went to the hairdresser weekly, but she had been in the hospital over a week and she knew she looked terrible. I asked her if she would like to learn to set her hair while in the hospital so that she could do it at night and her hair would look nice in the daytime. She expressed interest, so I bought some curlers and showed her how to use them. The next day when I went into her room, I saw her smiling and she commented on how proud she was of her new accomplishment.

Did the student experience the nursing process?

1. Assessment
   Data gathering:
      Client quiet; did not want to see anyone; stated distress over appearance of hair.
      Hospitalization interfered with pattern for hair care.
   Interpretation:
      Failure to maintain usual hair care resulted in lessening of self-image.
   Nursing diagnosis:
      Withdrawal from interaction with others because of poor self-image due to inability to provide for usual hair care.
2. Planning
   Goal:
      Meet client's need for hair care.
   Interventions:
      Mutually agreed to by nurse and client.
      Teach client to set her own hair.

3. Implementation
   Curlers purchased.
   Client taught to set her own hair.
4. Evaluation
   Client's self-image regained.
   Greeted student with a smile.
   Expressed pride in new skill.

This simple example is developed to emphasize the point that the teaching of nursing process in its entirety is not dependent upon a vast array of knowledge and skills. There are many opportunities to assist the beginning student to care for a client in terms of the nursing process so that the interrelationships among the steps can be perceived before more complex judgments and decisions are involved. That is, the structure of the process and its relationship to the practice of nursing must be taught early in the first clinical experience. As the parameters with which the process is used increase, so do the cognitive, psychomotor, and affective skills to carry out the process. Regardless of the character of the parameters, the integrity of the nursing process as a holistic activity is maintained in the teaching.

Skills in Nursing Process. As noted in the discussion thus far, nursing process entails multiple and diverse skills in the three domains of learning, namely cognitive, psychomotor, and affective. The charge to teachers of clinical nursing is that each of the relevant skills are mastered so that they can be synthesized into this critical process for delivery of nursing care. Subsequent chapters address the teaching of these skills within the clinical field, which are relevant not only to nursing process, but to the other dimensions of roles that nurses assume within the practitioner role.

Cognitive Skills in Nursing Process. Because nursing process is itself a cognitive activity which addresses not only what nurses do, but how they arrive at what they do, special consideration is given here to the issues in teaching cognitive skills that are directly related to nursing process, particularly in the crucial step of making a nursing diagnosis. As the process of categorizing nursing diagnosis proceeds in professional arenas, the process by which nurses make nursing diagnoses for clients has become of concern to nursing educators, practitioners, and researchers.

Skill in diagnosing requires more than data collection and a decision for action. It requires the ability to attach meaning to the data, not each datum as an entity in itself, but rather, meaning to the conglomerate of data obtained so that some sense of the client's health status is determined. Diagnosing is an abstract concept which entails cognitive information processing skills, which involve clustering of cues and making inferences so that a valid meaning is established. Concept formation in nursing diagnosis is a complex process, for it is a disjunctive concept attainment task. This task, as described by Bruner, Goodnow, and Austin (1956) entails analysis of cues, not all of which are related. That is, a diagnosis that is made does not preclude the notion that other diagnoses also must be made. In working with client data in nursing, more than one diagnosis is the usual rather than the unusual. This activity contrasts with the conjunctive concept attainment task where all data are related to each other and one diagnosis is possible.

It is the process between data collection and action that the instructor must stress, for studies at this time suggest that nurses are not engaging in a theoretical process of diagnosing. Aspinall (1976) found nurses lacking the ability to make nursing diagnoses that extended beyond physiologic problems. She noted that nurses are generally action oriented and proceed directly from what is seen to do to an action without engaging in the deliberative processes which may evidence different meanings to what is observed.

DeBack (1982) studied senior nursing students' ability to make nursing diagnoses from a case history. Three criteria were used in evaluating the diagnosis skill:

1. Client rather than disease centered.
2. Stated in terms of client concerns and level of competence in dysfunction.
3. Statement of client concerns, competence in dysfunction that can be altered or maintained through nursing action. (pp. 29–30)

Results of the 200 analyses suggest there is much work to be done in teaching diagnostic skill. While 56 percent of respondents could meet the first criterion, only 34 percent could meet the second criterion. It is this criterion that is especially critical, for it directs the intensity and strategy selection for nursing care. It also requires skills of concept formation, inferential reasoning, and knowledge recall. The third criterion was obtained by less than half (49 percent) of the respondents. While one may accept the notion that some of the difficulty is a function of the state of the art in nursing diagnosis, data from the study suggest more emphasis on management of client data is in order. This notion is further supported by Matthews and Gaul (1979) in their study, which demonstrated that nurses' ability to deal with abstract concepts as measured by the Concept Mastery Test was considerably below the national average.

Cognitive skill development is essential for nursing diagnosis and, thus, must be of considerable concern to the instructor because of the role nursing diagnosis assumes in directing client care. The nursing instructor needs to reckon with what the student does with the data as well as what data were collected. Acknowledgement of the impact of one's own biases, preconceived ideas, and knowledge limitations is essential in helping students examine data. Simon (1947) speaks of "bounded rationality" as limiting the ability to make accurate decisions. This concept refers to the limitation of completely objective rationality. Of particular note is the danger of limitation on data collection and cue interpretation when students have preconceived notions of what ought to be the cues that accompany certain dysfunctional states.

In addition to concern about the data themselves and the way they are interpreted is the process by which they are clustered and inferences made. It is the information processing skills that are often lacking in the educational process. Many nursing care plans which are developed as learning experiences, in contrast to those used in practice, do not provide for demonstrating cue clustering and inferential reasoning. Data are presented as discrete items, each described and interpreted from some scientific perspective. A quantum leap is then required to state a nursing diagnosis (although even this step is often omitted) and to design plans of action, often related to each datum collected. The critical step which demonstrates the information-processing behavior before nursing diagnosis or action is seldom seen in such a plan. Nursing plans of this type foster the notion of nurses as "doers" who respond to what they see without the deliberative processes that provide a reasonable validation of clients' needs on the basis of accurate and relevant data.

Cognitive skills are the baseline for competency in using the nursing process. Of particular concern in this chapter are the information processing skills that are essential if a valid nursing diagnosis is to be made. The process of teaching these cognitive skills within the clinical field is described in Chapter 6.

SUMMARY

Nursing process is a methodology of practice. It is the mechanism through which a theory or concept of nursing is operationalized into the delivery of nursing care. Because it is a practice modality, its mastery is attainable in the clinical setting where the learner is a participant in the care of real clients with real or potential health problems. The client may be an individual, a family, a group, or a community.

Nursing process is primarily a cognitive activity encompassing cognitive, psychomotor, and affective skills. Each of its four steps (assessment, planning, implementation, and evaluation) has its own constellation of skills that must be learned and synthesized into the total process.

The teaching of the nursing process requires the need to protect the integrity of the total process so that its steps are not viewed as separate phenomena, but rather as interrelated activities producing a whole. Introduction to nursing process early in the education program emphasizes its structure; its relationship to other dimensions of nursing. The principle of teaching from simple to complex is relevant as the student learns to use the process with increasingly complex variables necessitating increasingly complex skills.

The movement of the profession toward establishing a nursing diagnosis classification system places a particular challenge to instructors in the clinical field to facilitate the learner's development of cognitive skills essential for handling client data so that valid nursing diagnoses can be made and the planning and delivery of care is congruent with the diagnoses. Nursing process addresses not only doing for or with the client, but also the means by which the nurse arrives at the decisions to take a particular course of action.

REFERENCES

Abdellah, F. G., Beland, I., Martin, A., & Matheny, R. (1960). *Patient centered approaches to nursing.* New York: MacMillan.

Aspinall, M. J. (1976). Nursing diagnosis—the weak link. *Nursing Outlook, 7,* 433–37.

Bower, F. (1982). *The process of planning nursing care* (3rd ed.). St. Louis: C. V. Mosby.

Bruner, J. S. (1963). *The process of education.* New York: Vintage Books.

Bruner, J. S., Goodnow, J., & Austin, G. (1956). *Study of thinking.* New York: Wiley.

Campbell, C. (1978). *Nursing diagnosis and intervention in practice.* New York: Wiley.

Carnevali, D. (1983). *Nursing care planning: Diagnosis and management* (3rd ed.). Philadelphia: Lippincott.

Carpenito, L. (1983). *Nursing diagnosis: Application to clinical practice.* Philadelphia: Lippincott.

Chinn, P. L., & Jacobs, M. (1983). *Theory and nursing.* St. Louis: C. V. Mosby.

DeBack, V. (1982). The relationship between senior nursing students' ability to formulate nursing diagnosis and the curriculum model. In B. J. Brown, & P. L. Chinn (Eds.), *Nursing education: Practical methods and models* (pp. 21–36). Rockville, Md.: Aspen Systems.

Donabedian, A. (1969). Medical care appraisal—quality and utilization. In *Guide to medical care administration,* vol 2. (pp. 2–96). New York: American Public Health Assoc.

Fawcett, J. (1984). *Analysis and evaluation of conceptual models of nursing.* Philadelphia: F. A. Davis.

Gordon, M. (1982). *Nursing diagnosis: Process and application.* New York: McGraw-Hill.

Griffith, J., & Christensen, P. (1982). *Nursing process.* St. Louis: C. V. Mosby.

Guzzetta, C., & Forsyth, G. (1979). Nursing diagnostic pilot study: Psychophysiologic stress. *Advances in Nursing Science, 2*(1), 27–44.

Hall, L. E. (1955). Quality of nursing care. *Public Health News,* New Jersey State Department of Health.

Henderson, V. (1966). *The nature of nursing.* New York: MacMillan.

Johnson, D. E. (1959). A philosophy of nursing. *Nursing Outlook, 7,* 198–200.

Jones, P. (1979). A terminology for nursing diagnoses. *Advances in Nursing Science, 2*(1), 73–80.

Kim, M. J., McFarland, G. K., & McLane, A. M. (1984). *Classification of nursing diagnosis: Proceedings of the fifth national conference.* St. Louis: C. V. Mosby.

King, I. (1981). *A theory for nursing* (2nd ed.). New York: Wiley.

Kritek, P. B. (1979). Commentary: The development of nursing diagnosis and theory. *Advances in Nursing Science, 2*(1), 73–80.

Marriner, A. (1983). *The nursing process* (3rd ed.). St. Louis: C. V. Mosby.

Matthews, C. A., & Gaul, A. L. (1979). Nursing diagnosis from the perspective of concept attainment and critical thinking. *Advances in Nursing Science, 2*(1), 17–26.

Mayers, M. (1983). *A systematic approach to the nursing care plan* (3rd ed.). Norwalk, Conn: Appleton-Century-Crofts.

McCain, R. F. (1965). Nursing by assessment—not by intuition. *American Journal of Nursing, 65*(4), 82–84.

Neuman, B. (1982). *The Neuman systems model.* Norwalk, Conn: Appleton-Century-Crofts.

Nursing, a social policy statement. (1980). Kansas City, Mo: American Nurses Association.

Nursing Theories Conference Group. (1980). *Nursing theories: The base for nursing practice.* Englewood Cliffs, N.J.: Prentice-Hall.

Orem, D. (1980). *Nursing concepts of practice* (2nd ed.). New York: McGraw-Hill.

Orlando, I. J. (1961). *The dynamic nurse patient relationship.* New York: Putnam.

Peplau, H. (1952). *Interpersonal relationships in nursing.* New York: Putnam.

Phaneuf, M. (1976). *The nursing audit: Self regulation in nursing practice* (2nd ed.). New York: Appleton-Century-Crofts.

Reilly, D. E. (1975). Why a conceptual framework? *Nursing Outlook, 23,* 566–69.

Reilly, D. E. (1980). *Behavioral objectives: Evaluation in nursing.* New York: Appleton-Century-Crofts.

Rogers, M. (1970). *An introduction to the theoretical basis of nursing.* Philadelphia: F. A. Davis.

Roy, C. (1976). *Introduction to nursing: An adaptation model.* Englewood Cliffs, N.J.: Prentice-Hall.

Simon, H. A. (1947). *Administrative behavior.* New York: MacMillan.

Standards: Nursing practice. (1973). Kansas City, Mo.: American Nurses Association.

Wiedenbach, E. (1964). *Clinical nursing, a helping art.* New York: Springer.

Yura, H., & Walsh, M. (1983). *The nursing process* (4th ed.). Norwalk, Conn: Appleton-Century-Crofts.

REFERENCE NOTES

1. From *Nursing diagnosis: Process and application.* (1982). By M. Gordon. New York: McGraw-Hill. Reprinted with permission.

BIBLIOGRAPHY

Aspinall, M. J., & Tanner, C. A. (1981). *Decision making for patient care.* New York: Appleton-Century-Crofts.

Broderick, M. E., & Ammentorp, W. (1979). Information structures: An analysis of nursing performance. *Nursing Research, 28,* 106–10.

Brown, M. M. (1974). The epidemiological approach to study of clinical nursing diagnosis. *Nursing Forum, 13,* 347–59.

Chinn, P. L. (Ed.). (1979). Nursing diagnosis. *Advances in Nursing Science, 2*(1).

Chinn, P. L. (Ed.). (1980). Nursing theories and models. *Advances in Nursing Science, 3*(1).

Donaldson, S. K., & Crowley, D. (1978). The discipline of nursing. *Nursing Outlook, 26,* 113–20.

Fawcett, J. F. (1980). A framework for analysis and evaluation of conceptual models of nursing. *Nurse Educator, 5,* 10–14.

Field, L. (1979). The implementation of nursing diagnosis in clinical practice. *Nursing Clinics of North America, 14*(3), 497–505.

Flaskerud, J. H. (1983). Utilizing a nursing conceptual model in basic level curriculum development. *Journal of Nursing Education, 22,* 224–27.

Goodwin, J. O. (1980). A cross-cultural approach to integrating nursing theory and practice. *Nurse Educator, 5,* 15–20.

Gordon, M., & Sweeney, M. A. (1979). Methodological problems and issues in identifying and standardizing nursing diagnosis. *Advances in Nursing Science, 2*(1), 1–5.

Hall, L. E. (1966). Another view of nursing care and quality. In K. S. Parker (Ed.), *Continuity of patient care: The role of the nurse* (pp. 47–66). Washington, D.C.: Catholic University Press.

Henderson, B. (1978). Nursing diagnosis: Theory and practice. *Advances in Nursing Science, 1*(1), 75–83.

Johnson, D. E. (1980). The behavioral system model for nursing. In J. P. Riehl & S. C. Roy (Eds.), *Conceptual models for nursing practice* (2nd ed.) (pp. 207–216). New York: Appleton-Century-Crofts.

Laros, J. (1977). Deriving outcome criteria for a conceptual model. *Nursing Outlook, 25,* 333–36.

Levine, M. E. (1973). *Introduction to clinical nursing* (2nd ed.). Philadelphia: F. A. Davis.

Kim, M. J., MacFarland, G. K., & McLane, A. M. (1984). *Pocket guide to nursing diagnosis.* St. Louis: C. V. Mosby.

Kissinger, J. F., & Munjas, B. A. (1981). Nursing process: Student attributes and teaching methodologies. *Nursing Research, 30,* 242–46.

McMurry, P. H. (1982). Toward a unique knowledge base in nursing. *Image, 14,* 12–15.

Mollick, M. J. (1983). Nursing diagnosis and the novice student. *Nursing and Health Care, 4,* 455–59.

Newman, M. A. (1979). *Theory development in nursing.* Philadelphia: F. A. Davis.

Price, M. R. (1980). Nursing diagnosis—making a concept come alive. *American Journal of Nursing, 80,* 668–71.

Riehl, J. P., & Roy, C. (1980). *Conceptual models for nursing practice.* New York: Appleton-Century-Crofts.

Schaefer, J. (1974). The interrelationship of decision making and nursing process. *American Journal of Nursing, 74,* 1852–56.

Shamensky, S. L., & Yanni, C. R. (1983). In opposition to nursing diagnosis, a minority opinion. *Image, 15*(2), 47–50.

Spector, R. (1979). *Cultural diversity in health and illness.* New York: Appleton-Century-Crofts.

Stantis, M. A., & Ryan, J. (1982). Noncompliance, An acceptable diagnosis? *American Journal of Nursing, 82,* 941–42.

Stevens, B. J. (1984). *Nursing theory: Analysis, application, evaluation* (2nd ed.). Boston: Little, Brown.

Tucker, S. M., Breedy, M. A., Canobbio, M. M., et al. (1984). *Patient care standards* (3rd ed.). St. Louis: C. V. Mosby.

Walker, L. O., & Nicholson, R. (1980). Criteria for evaluating nursing process models. *Nurse Educator, 5*(5), 8–9.

Watson, J. (1981). Nursing's scientific quest. *Nursing Outlook, 29,* 413–20.

4

Clinical Milieu:
A Learning Environment

Teaching is an interactive process that requires involvement of teacher and learner in a supportive and facilitative milieu. Milieu refers to the psychosocial climate within which teaching and learning take place. This milieu is a major contributing factor to the learning responses of students and ability of the teacher to carry out educational responsibilities. The milieu may support these individuals, impede them, or limit options for learning. A supportive milieu, essential for learning, is characterized by valuing learning; exhibiting a caring relationship for all concerned; providing for student freedom within structure for exploring, questioning, and trying out different approaches; accepting differences in others; and fostering the development of each individual.

In a profession like nursing, the milieu needs to provide for the development of new patterns of thinking, feeling, and doing that serve not only the individual but also the greater society. New knowledge is meant to be used by the nurse for the benefit of others. It is in the practice setting where the student develops knowledge and learns how to use it in service for others. In order for the reality of practice to be experienced by students, learning must take place in clinical settings which have goals other than educational. Service goals and learning goals may or may not be in competition, but their relationship greatly influences the character of the milieu in which the student and faculty function.

CLINICAL FIELDS FOR NURSING EDUCATION

In the clinical field, the student learns to apply theories of action to real clinical problems, learns how to learn, develops skill in handling ambiguity, and becomes socialized into the profession. These purposes of clinical practice can be achieved in any setting where the student is involved in the practice of nursing.

Types of Clinical Settings

Traditionally, clinical practice in nursing programs has taken place in hospitals and public health departments (Graham & Gleit, 1981). The present scope of nursing practice and that projected for the future have resulted in a wide range of practice fields appropriate for use in an educational program. These include homes, schools, industries, rehabilitation centers, ambulatory care centers, hospices, nursing homes, senior citizens programs, day care centers, practitioners' offices, and other agencies and community programs with a primary or secondary health care focus. The directions of developing patterns of health care delivery suggest that the hospital setting will become a center for highly acute care with most care provided in the home, ambulatory settings, and other community agencies. Any setting in which the student is involved with health care, in concert with the stated objectives of the experience, is appropriate for use in a nursing education program.

Purposes of Clinical Fields

Clinical fields have their own purposes, which may be delivery of health care for selected populations, education for practitioners and students in different disciplines, and in many settings conduction of research. Each setting has its own priorities among these various purposes which, in turn, dictate the options available for learning. In some settings, such as schools, health care delivery is secondary to a product goal; i.e., education. Health care is viewed as having a supporting role toward the ultimate goal of the organization.

Nature of Clinical Field

The multipurpose goals of clinical settings have much to do with the kinds of services provided in the agency and types of personnel functioning there. Although the ultimate goal of health care agencies is the welfare of the client served, there is much potential for dissonance and discord as each group of individuals seeks its own territory and method of operation. This is particularly true in health care settings where there are two types of authority: (1) administrative authority and (2) professional authority. Administrative authority includes responsibility for the organization and functioning of the institution in terms of institutional goals, such as delivery of a service, efficiency, and cost effectiveness. Professionals may have other goals, such as developing their own knowledge, skills, and professional practice and contributing to the body of knowledge of their disciplines.

The authority of professionals is necessary for effective practice. Etzioni (1964) states, "Only if immune from ordinary social pressures and free to innovate, to experiment, to take risks without the usual social repercussions of failure, can a professional carry out his work effectively" (p. 76). Professionals act independently in the use of professional knowledge; their decisions are their own, not dictated by institutional authority. "The ultimate justification for a professional act is that it is, to the best of the professional's knowledge, the right act. He might consult his colleagues before he acts, but the decision is his" (p. 77). An organization, health care or otherwise, needs to make accommodations between competing goals of the institution and professionals who function within it. The milieu is influenced by this accommodation of goals.

Individuals meeting service goals of an institution represent various levels of practice and accountability, generally with reasonably defined functions and expectations. The relationships among individuals within any group, for example nurse aides and registered nurses, and between groups, such as physicians and nurses, may interfere with effective functioning within the organization, particularly when responsibilities are perceived differently by the parties involved. Such conflicts often arise because of problems in communication and changing demands on a professional group by expanding knowledge and technology and political, social, and economic decisions.

Every clinical field has its own cultural values, norms, and expected behaviors. This cultural dimension serves to control the behavior of various individuals in the setting and provides sanctions for those who deviate. The cultural norms are directed primarily toward those who are providers of service. New entrants, such as students and clients, need to learn the expected behaviors and accommodate accordingly if they are to be accepted in the organization.

The clinical field in which learner and teacher are to enter is multigoal-directed and multidisciplinary. It has potential for competition and conflicting forces influencing its activity at any one moment.

Rationale for Use of Clinical Field in Nursing Education

Clinical practice provides experiences with real clients and real problems which enable learners to use knowledge in practice, develop skill in problem solving and decision making, learn how to learn, and develop a commitment to be responsible for one's own actions. Only in the field are there experiences for applying theories of action to real problems. According to Argyris and Schön (1976), a theory of action has not been learned unless it can be put into practice. Concrete situations to which these theories correspond are available in the field.

The field, however, is more than a place to apply theory to practice. It provides opportunity for developing problem-solving and decision-making skills and for collaborating with other disciplines in finding solutions to clinical problems. Experiences in the field facilitate development of skill in divergent thinking and ability to deal with the ambiguities inherent in clinical practice. Unpredictability in the field, multiple distractions and variable time demands, sometimes interfering with learning, help prepare the student for reality.

In the field, learners observe variations in the responses of clients and encounter situations that challenge them to develop their knowledge and skills further. The practice field is a place to learn how to learn because it fosters independence with learning and self-reliance and provides opportunity for questioning and seeking new knowledge. In the field students are challenged to explore alternate modalities of care. Schein (1972) argues that professions need innovators to improve practice. In the clinical setting, the student has an opportunity to examine and try out these new approaches with clients and staff.

Field experiences also provide the means through which the student becomes socialized into the profession and its values and learns to accept the notion of professional responsibility. Accompanying this socialization is the experiencing of role discontinuity and ambiguity. Role discontinuity results from the transition from the role of student in the classroom and laboratory setting to the field. This transition creates the need for learners to develop new ways of defining their roles in the practice setting and selecting their behaviors (Hursh & Borzak, 1979). In the field, the student also experiences role ambiguity, unclear role definition, which necessitates acquiring behaviors associated with the role of professional practitioner. Hursh and Borzak believe that role discontinuity and ambiguity create "in students a pronounced 'readiness for learning,' an openness to new perspectives and new information, and the need to experiment with new behaviors in order to function adequately in the situation" (p. 74).

Field practice provides opportunity for the student to develop a commitment to be responsible for one's own actions. In any clinical setting, the learner must be willing to accept responsibility for his or her own actions and for fulfilling commitments relative to practice. Even with beginning practice, it is important for the student to be accountable for identifying where further learning and guidance are needed and for carrying out the clinical activities for which responsibility was given and accepted. Argyris and Schön (1976) believe that developing a commitment to be responsible for one's own actions "is best achieved through field experience because of its real problems, real clients, high-risk situations, deadlines, and demands for performance and accountability" (p. 192).

DEVELOPMENT OF MILIEU FOR LEARNING

A field rich in learning experiences but lacking a supportive milieu discourages learners in seeking experiences and results in the loss of many opportunities for growth. Likewise, a field with potentially limited experiences but rich in a supportive milieu may provide opportunity for students to examine new health care needs and ways of addressing them. Regardless of the setting for clinical practice, the milieu is a factor in determining student achievement and satisfaction with the learning experience. The teacher and agency personnel influence the nature of the milieu and degree to which it supports learning.

Faculty Responsibilities

Development of a climate for learning requires a teacher who is knowledgeable, clinically competent, skillful as a teacher, and committed to clinical teaching. It is important for faculty to examine their own beliefs and values about teaching and learning, their role in promoting learning, and the role of the student, for these influence how the instructional process is carried out and also the quality of the milieu for learning. The teacher's attitudes toward students and staff affect interactions and the type of relationships established in the setting.

In a supportive learning milieu, the teacher encourages independence with learning and self-reliance rather than fostering dependence and reliance on the teacher for sanctions, information needed for practice, solutions to problems, and evaluation of learning. With this independence the student learns how to learn.

In the field, students need freedom to explore, question, and dissent because without this critical thinking is inhibited. The field is a place in which the student can experiment in applying concepts and theories to practice, solving problems, and evolving new modes of care. To foster such experimentation, the learner needs freedom to try out different approaches with clients and staff. Taking calculated risks means that the decision to try a different approach was carefully made after considering the consequences. Teachers may not be sure enough of themselves to encourage such experimentation and thus may stifle the innovative potential of students. Teachers as advocates of students often must intervene with staff to facilitate student opportunities for trying out the "new."

Fear of making an error limits student development and willingness to experiment with care. Teachers, fearful themselves of student mistakes, often place unrealistic demands on learners for perfect practice. Mistakes are an inherent part of the learning process and in most clinical situations there is room for error. It is the faculty's responsibility to intervene in the decision-making process and in delivery of care to minimize the chance of the student making an error that would result in harm to the client. Argyris and Schön (1976) suggest that failure is a predictable consequence of early practice of untested behaviors to be learned. The clinical milieu needs to be one in which teacher and student together examine failures and learn from them. Unless failures and mistakes are valued, there will be no learning from the experience. For the student to admit error, seek guidance from faculty, and value the feedback given, the relationship between teacher and student must be characterized by trust and mutual respect.

In a supportive learning milieu, the teacher accepts differences among students in their approaches to solving clinical problems and in the ways they analyze situations. Research suggests, for instance, that field-independent and -dependent learners vary in these approaches and style of interacting. Field-independent learners are high in analytical skills and favor tasks that require analysis rather than those that emphasize the interpersonal dimension. Field-dependent learners, in contrast, demonstrate less analytical skills and prefer situations involving interactions with others. Both types of competencies are needed in clinical practice.

In a milieu which fosters independent learning, experimentation, and risk-taking behavior, students are still held accountable for their actions and for fulfilling commitments relative to practice. Learners in any clinical setting must assume responsibility for providing quality care, whatever the extent is of that care, and for carrying through with activities for which they accepted responsibility. Students must also be accountable for identifying their abilities and limitations in practice. It is important to emphasize that a supportive learning milieu does not permit students to be free of responsibility.

Relationships with Agency Personnel

Development of a supportive milieu depends on the relationships established between the teacher and agency personnel and between students and staff. These relationships influence the practice experience in terms of learning and the satisfaction of students, faculty, and staff with the experience. Development of collaborative relationships between faculty and agency personnel is essential for a supportive learning milieu.

> Collaboration means true partnership, in which the power on both sides is valued by both, with recognition and acceptance of separate and combined spheres of activity and responsibility, mutual guarding of the legitimate interests of each party, and a commonality of goals that is recognized by both parties. This is a relationship based upon recognition that each is richer and more truly real because of the

strength and uniqueness of the other. (American Nurses Association, 1980, p. 7)

Knowledge of the objectives of clinical practice enables staff to assist faculty in identifying experiences available in the setting which might be appropriate. The teacher, in turn, needs to be sensitive to requests of staff in relation to client care and other kinds of learning experiences. In many practice settings, staff has contact with students from various types of programs, including nursing and other health professions, who are at different levels of development, who have varying objectives to be achieved, and who engage in a wide range of learning experiences. It is no surprise that, at times, service personnel become weary regarding student experiences. Faculty should be sensitive to the purposes and priorities of the clinical setting and cognizant of the adaptations by staff necessary for implementing student experiences there. Agency personnel, in turn, need to recognize that because of varying clinical objectives and levels of students, the responsibilities of students and types of experiences in which they engage will differ.

There are a variety of efforts to blend education and practice in order to strengthen the ties between schools of nursing and clinical settings. The unification models at Rush University, University of Rochester, and Case Western Reserve University provide mechanisms for combining teaching, practice, and research. Although differences exist among these models, faculty has responsibility, in varying degrees, for teaching of students, client care, and research. Joint appointments with commitments to both education and service provide another means of enhancing the relationship between the two settings. Other strategies have been identified for strengthening this relationship (Blazeck, Selekman, Timpe, & Wolf, 1982).

Regardless of the organizational relationship of faculty with the practice setting, the teacher is responsible for assisting students in working with staff. This requires clarifying the role and expectations of staff in relation to student learning and supervision in the field and establishing lines of communication among faculty, students, and agency personnel. The role of staff varies according to the objectives and type of experience. Preceptors, for instance, assume a different role with students than do staff nurses in a setting where the teacher provides on-site supervision.

Development of working relationships with agency personnel begins with the initial contacts made with the clinical setting and planning with agency staff for the practice experience. Initial meetings with agency representatives serve to clarify the nature of the practice experience, overall objectives to be achieved, and faculty role and responsibilities and provide opportunity for agency personnel to present requirements of the clinical setting and the agency's

TABLE 7. CONTRACT WITH CLINICAL AGENCY[a]
Agreement

XYZ
University of Washington
School of Nursing

We, the undersigned, representatives of the University of Washington SCHOOL OF NURSING and XYZ, enter into the following cooperative agreement to provide educational experiences for students of the SCHOOL OF NURSING.

IT IS HEREBY AGREED:

1. The SCHOOL OF NURSING, through a designated faculty member for each student or group of students, will be responsible for instruction and administration of the students' educational program.

2. Within the scope of health care services provided by XYZ, the students will be given a desirable clinical learning experience. During this experience, the students shall in no sense be considered employees except if they are employed during time designated as not part of their educational program and will not be relied upon for patient care services to maintain the quality of patient care.

3. XYZ will retain full responsibility for the care of patients and will provide administrative and professional supervision of the students insofar as their presence affects provision of health care services and/or the direct or indirect care of patients. For placements under supervision of a preceptor, the preceptor will be responsible for administrative and professional supervision of the students while providing care for patients/clients.

4. The students and faculty of the SCHOOL OF NURSING will comply with the policies and procedures established by XYZ.

5. XYZ will make available to the students basic supplies and equipment necessary for the care of patients/clients and will make available, within the limitations of facilities, office and conferencing facilities for the students and, if applicable, faculty of the SCHOOL OF NURSING.

6. XYZ and the SCHOOL OF NURSING will plan jointly the evaluation of the students' learning experience.

7. The SCHOOL OF NURSING will require, at the beginning of each student's program, evidence of a recent physical exam and current immunizations against diphtheria, tetanus, poliomyelitis, and rubella (or have a positive rubella titer) for students who will be engaged in the delivery of nursing care. Also required will be a yearly PPD with follow-up X ray and medication for any positive results.

8. The University of Washington will hold harmless XYZ from any loss, claim, or damage arising out of acts or omissions of students or faculty associated with the educational programs of the University of Washington SCHOOL OF NURSING except for any such loss, claim, or damage arising out of acts or omissions taken or made at the direction of XYZ pursuant to paragraph three above.

9. There will be no discrimination against any participant in the program covered by this agreement, or against any applicant for participation, because of race, religion, color, sex, handicap, age, or national origin, or status of disabled veteran or Vietnam era veteran, nor shall there be any such discrimination in the employment practices and personnel policies of either party.

10. This agreement is to provide an educational experience for (student) for (000) Quarter 198(X) and may be extended by letter to include additional student placements for subsequent quarters.

or

10. This agreement will continue from quarter to quarter and will be reviewed at the request of either party. Prior to each quarter student placements are to be made, the SCHOOL OF NURSING will provide a list of students and the name of the responsible faculty member to XYZ for concurrence. This agreement may be canceled by written notice one full academic quarter prior to termination.

or

10. This agreement will continue from year to year and will be reviewed at the request of either party. The SCHOOL OF NURSING and XYZ will jointly plan in advance student placement, taking into account the needs of the SCHOOL OF

TABLE 7. (*Continued*)

NURSING for clinical placements, maximum number of students for whom XYZ can provide educational experiences, and the needs of other disciplines or schools desiring clinical placements. This agreement may be canceled by written notice one year prior to termination.

XYZ	By	**University of Washington School of Nursing**	By
(Name of Administrator)	Date	(Name of Administrator)	Date

[a]This contract is from the School of Nursing at the University of Washington, Seattle, and has been reprinted here in its entirety with the permission of Dr. Rheba de Tornyay, Dean.

expectations of faculty and students. These meetings provide the basis for establishing a contract or formal agreement between the clinical setting and nursing program, usually negotiated by administrative personnel of both settings. Often, the nature of the practice experience influences whether a contract is necessary or if a letter of agreement is sufficient. A contract, usually stated in general terms, may be followed by a letter of agreement where the arrangements for the experience are detailed (Jones, 1983). A sample contract is shown in Table 7.

Subsequent planning conferences, involving the teacher and staff with whom the students will interact, are necessary to complete the arrangements and deal with the specifics of the experience. Orientation of staff to the objectives, student role and responsibilities, level of the learner, times in clinical setting and in contact with clients, faculty role, expectations of staff, and other details is accomplished in these planning meetings. The roles and responsibilities of the involved parties and specifics of the experience need to be mutually agreed upon and not dictated by either faculty or staff.

SELECTION OF CLINICAL SETTINGS

The clinical setting selected for field practice is important in achieving the objectives and purposes of clinical practice in a nursing education program. In some communities, selection of clinical sites is a difficult process because of competition among nursing programs for use of clinical settings, particularly hospitals and community health agencies. Access to patients has even become a problem in some ambulatory settings where nursing students compete for placement with medical, social work, and other students in the health professions (Jones, 1983).

Many of the settings traditionally used by nursing programs may not be appropriate for the diversity of objectives to be achieved in clinical practice, such as health promotion, care of families, and management of chronic health problems. Use of multiple sites for field practice is often needed to meet these program objectives and provide opportunity for the student to care for clients with varying health concerns and participate with other disciplines in the provision of that care. Unfortunately, diversity places demands on faculty for expertise in practicing in different kinds of settings, for development of collaborative relationships with staff from multiple agencies, for obtaining information about the settings (their expectations and requirements, the availability of learning experiences and preceptors, and other specifics important in planning the experience), and for completion of arrangements with each agency. Use of multiple settings for field practice may also result in increased cost for the nursing program in terms of number of faculty, faculty time in planning for the clinical experiences, and travel time for faculty and students. It is important for faculty to weigh the benefits of using a large number of clinical settings with the associated demands on faculty and resources.

Criteria for Selection

The setting selected for field practice should facilitate student achievement of the objectives and purposes of clinical practice in a nursing program. Hawkins (1981) suggests that this selection process often focuses "on time and place rather than on objectives for the experience" (pp. 13–14). The teacher's habits and beliefs, convenience, and established contractual arrangements may influence the evaluation and selection of clinical sites (Bevil & Gross, 1981).

Several major criteria need to be considered in selecting settings for field practice. Critical in any setting is maintaining faculty responsibility for the practice experience. Hawkins (1981) reported this was one criterion faculty was not willing to compromise when choosing clinical agencies. The criteria are organized in four areas: (1) overall: setting and faculty, (2) clients, (3) staff, and (4) resources for students and faculty.

Overall: Setting and Faculty

1. Setting is licensed or accredited, as applicable
2. Faculty is responsible for field practice experience
3. Administrative personnel and staff are flexible as to learn-

ing experiences, student time in agency, faculty role, on-site time of faculty, and other aspects of learning experience
4. Philosophy of clinical setting and nursing department is consistent with values and beliefs of faculty
5. Faculty is available to teach in setting
6. Faculty recognizes rights and responsibilities of setting
7. Evaluation of prior experience of faculty and students in setting reflects standards of nursing program
8. Costs associated with use of clinical setting are acceptable to nursing program

Clients
1. Client population is appropriate for objectives to be attained
2. Client population is sufficient in number for number of students to be placed in setting
3. Clients are present in setting an adequate amount of time for achievement of objectives
4. A range of learning experiences is available in setting
5. Nursing care practices are current
6. Nursing care reflects standards of practice and faculty values and beliefs
7. Resources (e.g., social service) for care of clients are available in setting and accessible to students
8. Client records are accessible to students and reflect current practices

Staff
1. Nursing staff is available to serve as preceptors, mentors, and in other roles, depending on the objectives
2. Staff collaborates with faculty and students in selection of learning experiences
3. Staff participates in orientation by faculty to experience and expectations and in evaluation of experience
4. Faculty and/or students are oriented by staff to clinical setting

Resources for Students and Faculty
1. Resources for student learning (e.g., staff development, library, reference materials, multimedia laboratory) are available in setting
2. Experts (e.g., clinical specialist, nurse practitioner, patient educator, nurse researcher) in setting are accessible to students for consultation
3. Space is provided for faculty and students to store personal belongings and have conferences
4. Setting includes dining facilities if none are available nearby.

88

TABLE 8. INSTRUMENT FOR ASSESSMENT OF CLINICAL SETTING

General Information:
Name of clinical setting _____

Location _____

Purpose _____

Contact persons (Name, title, and telephone number) _____

_____

_____

_____

Type of setting _____

    Client population (Describe) _____

    _____

    _____

    _____

Agency staff (Describe qualifications of staff with whom students would be working, include potential preceptors in setting)

_____

_____

_____

_____

Other disciplines practicing in setting _____

Restrictions of setting (e.g., number of students, student time in setting, on-site time of faculty)

_____

_____

Requirements for students and faculty (e.g., health screening, dress, name tags, list of students to be forwarded to setting)

_____

_____

_____

_____

_____

Resources for students and faculty (e.g., for learning, dining, parking)

_____

_____

_____

TABLE 8. (*Continued*)

Contractual agreement: (1) Yes   (2) No   (3) Pending

Information given to clinical setting (e.g., school of nursing bulletin, course materials, clinical evaluation instrument)

_____

_____

_____

_____

_____

	Yes	No	N/A[a]
Overall: Setting and Faculty:			
1. Is the clinical setting licensed or accredited, if relevant for this type of setting?	___	___	___
2. Will faculty be responsible for the field practice experience?	___	___	___
3. Are administrative personnel and staff flexible as to learning experiences, student time in agency, faculty role, on-site time of faculty, and other aspects of the learning experience?	___	___	___
4. Is the philosophy of the clinical setting and nursing department consistent with the values and beliefs of faculty?	___	___	___
5. Is faculty available to teach in the clinical setting?	___	___	___
6. Does faculty recognize the rights and responsibilities of the setting?	___	___	___
7. Do the evaluations of prior experience of faculty and students in the setting reflect standards of the nursing program?	___	___	___
8. Are the costs associated with use of the clinical setting acceptable to the nursing program?	___	___	___
Clients:			
1. Is the client population appropriate for the objectives to be attained?	___	___	___
2. Is the client population sufficient in number for the number of students to be placed in the setting?	___	___	___
3. Are clients present in the setting an adequate amount of time for student achievement of the objectives?	___	___	___

(*Continued*)

90

TABLE 8. (*Continued*)

	Yes	No	N/A[a]
4. Is there a range of learning experiences available in the setting?	___	___	___
5. Are nursing care practices current?	___	___	___
6. Does the nursing care reflect standards of practice and faculty values and beliefs?	___	___	___
7. a. Are resources (e.g., social service) for the care of clients available in the setting?	___	___	___
b. Are these resources accessible to students?	___	___	___
8. a. Do client records reflect current practices?	___	___	___
b. Are client records accessible to students?	___	___	___

Staff:

1. Is nursing staff available to serve as preceptors, mentors, and in other roles, depending on the objectives?	___	___	___
2. Is the staff willing to collaborate with faculty and students in the selection of learning experiences?	___	___	___
3. Will the staff participate in orientation by faculty to the experience and expectations and in the evaluation of the experience?	___	___	___
4. Will the staff orient faculty and/or students to the clinical setting?	___	___	___

Resources for Students and Faculty:

1. Are there resources for student learning (e.g., staff development, library, reference materials, multimedia laboratory) in the clinical setting?	___	___	___
2. Are experts (e.g., clinical specialist, nurse practitioner, patient educator, nurse researcher) in the clinical setting accessible to students for consultation?	___	___	___
3. Is there a place for faculty and students to store personal belongings and have conferences?	___	___	___
4. Are there dining facilities if none are available nearby?	___	___	___

Other:

1.	___	___	___

(*Continued*)

TABLE 8. (*Continued*)

	Yes	No	N/A[a]
2.	___	___	___
3.	___	___	___
4.	___	___	___
5.	___	___	___

[a]Not applicable

Some criteria are of greater importance than others in relation to the objectives, and faculty needs to make this determination prior to reviewing potential settings. It may be necessary to add to the criteria presented here more specific ones depending on the philosophy of the nursing program, objectives to be attained in practice, and specific type of setting being considered. An instrument that incorporates the selection criteria and collects general information about the clinical setting as a whole, shown in Table 8, facilitates selection by providing a systematic way of reviewing potential sites and recording the data obtained.

Evaluation of Clinical Setting

The decision to continue with use of a setting for field practice needs to be based on an evaluation of the setting and extent to which learners achieved the objectives for clinical practice there. Criteria for the selection of clinical settings may be used for their evaluation. The identification of factors which promoted or impeded student learning provides a basis for modifying the practice experience if the decision is made to use the setting again.

Evaluation incorporates agency personnel, particularly staff most directly involved with the experience, and students. Inclusion of staff provides a means of identifying issues to be resolved and gives staff an opportunity to evaluate the experience and its role in it. Evaluation by learners of the clinical setting and of the experiences in which they engaged provides another source of data important in making the decision to continue or not with use of the setting. Sharing learner evaluations with members of the staff reinforces the importance of their role in the experience and assists them in modifying subsequent experiences. Evaluation by staff and students is particularly significant for those clinical settings in which there is minimal on-site faculty supervision, such as ones involving graduate students and preceptors.

When the setting no longer provides experiences for learners to attain the goals of clinical practice and when the objectives change

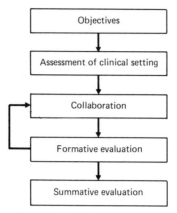

Figure 1. Selection and evaluation of clinical setting.

and different characteristics of the practice setting become important, faculty needs to examine alternate sites for field practice. The decision to change clinical settings might also be based on continuing problems in the agency unable to be resolved by faculty, students, and staff.

The process of selecting a clinical agency and evaluating the experience there may be viewed as a sequence of events, depicted in Figure 1, beginning with the objectives of the experience. An assessment of the setting determines its appropriateness for promoting attainment of these objectives and whether or not it meets other criteria for selecting clinical sites. Through collaborative efforts of faculty and staff, a milieu for learning is established, and service and educational goals are both achieved. Formative evaluation carried out by faculty, students, and staff takes place throughout the field practice experience and provides continuous feedback to them. Formative evaluation is diagnostic in nature, informing faculty, students, and staff of problems with the practice experience needing resolution and confirming positive aspects. Summative evaluation, conducted periodically, serves to ascertain whether or not the clinical setting has provided the necessary experiences for achievement of the objectives and the impact on the agency of student experience there.

QUALITIES OF TEACHER IN CLINICAL FIELD

Much has been written about attributes that constitute effective and ineffective teaching. Certainly students are able to differentiate teachers who facilitated or interfered with their learning and the related characteristics of those teachers. Teacher behavior can contribute to or discourage student learning and, therefore, is an important variable in establishing a learning milieu in the clinical setting.

Characteristics of Teacher

Characteristics of an effective clinical teacher may be grouped into four areas: (1) knowledge and clinical competence, (2) teaching skill, (3) relationships with students, and (4) personal characteristics. Knowledge of the subject matter pertains to the teacher's breadth and depth of understanding as it relates not only to the topic at hand but also to the larger sphere where that knowledge interfaces with other knowledges. Ability to analyze theories and synthesize from multiple sources, emphasis on conceptual understanding, willingness to discuss points of view other than one's own, and currency in the field are characteristics of a teacher who possesses this knowledge (Hildebrand, Wilson, & Dienst, 1971). Effective clinical teaching requires competence in the teacher role and as a clinician. Maintenance of clinical competence is essential in assisting students in the development of knowledge and skill and providing expert supervision in the field.

Teaching skill involves the ability to diagnose learning needs, plan instruction in terms of learner characteristics and goals to be achieved, supervise students, and evaluate learning. An effective teacher presents information in an organized manner, gives clear explanations and directions to students, answers questions clearly, and demonstrates procedures and other care practices effectively. Jacobson (1966) emphasized that a teacher in nursing must be well-informed and also must be able to communicate that knowledge to students.

The ability of the teacher to interact with students and staff is another important teacher behavior. Hildebrand, Wilson, and Dienst (1971) indicate that this ability involves relating to the group of students as a whole and developing mutual respect and rapport between the teacher and individual learner.

Other characteristics of effective teaching relate to personal attributes of the teacher, which in many ways are associated with the dynamism of the faculty and enthusiasm for teaching in the field. This flair and enthusiasm come with enjoyment in working with students and confidence in one's own teaching ability and clinical skills. Eble (1972) believes one of the benefits of self-confidence is that it enables the teacher to display genuine enthusiasm for teaching, a major factor in motivating students and maintaining their interest in learning. In a study of teacher behaviors which either facilitate or interfere with student learning in the clinical setting in nursing education, O'Shea and Parsons (1979) found friendly, understanding, supportive, and enthusiastic behavior of the teacher promoted learning.

Teaching requires a great deal of caring for others and giving of the self as well as energy, time, skill, and knowledge (Eble, 1972). The teacher of nursing must have knowledge of and be competent in many areas. Honesty, ability to admit errors and limitations, and lack of pretense of omnipotent knowledge are as important as possessing the necessary knowledge and skills for teaching.

Pugh (1980) surveyed nursing faculty and students to identify their beliefs about the importance of different clinical teaching behaviors. Students reported that they expected faculty to demonstrate behaviors associated with teaching activities and ones related to the role of the nurse. Behaviors pertaining to the role of the nurse included assisting students to synthesize patient data, interact with clients and others, develop as professional practitioners, and function in the clinical situation. From this study, Pugh identified three patterns of teacher behavior in the clinical setting: (1) nurse: faculty who enact primarily behaviors related to the role of the nurse; (2) teacher: those who demonstrate behaviors associated with teaching activities; and (3) nurse–teacher: faculty who integrate behaviors of both roles.

Effective clinical teaching places many demands on faculty— demands for knowledge and clinical expertise, skill in interacting with students and others in the setting, and personal characteristics which promote learning. Knowledge of the subject matter and clinical competence are critical, but knowing *how* to teach is as important. A teacher with knowledge and expertise in clinical practice is not a teacher if unable to communicate that knowledge to students and facilitate their learning in the practice setting.

Teacher–Student Relationship

A humanistic climate that supports the process of learning is dependent on a caring relationship between teacher and student. The success of any clinical learning experience rests heavily on this relationship as learners pursue educational goals leading toward their development as professional practitioners.

Just as the nurse–patient relationship is a helping one, so is the teacher–student relationship. Carl Rogers (1983) identified certain qualities of this relationship that facilitate learning. These qualities, similar to those necessary for any therapeutic encounter, include realness or genuineness, trust and respect for the learner, and empathetic understanding.

The teacher who exhibits realness or genuineness in a relationship is honest and open with students and willing to express his or her own feelings. Genuineness implies an ability to admit mistakes and acknowledge limitations.

Other qualities of this relationship include trust (important in promoting risk-taking behaviors in the field), and respect; i.e., accepting learners as they are. Trust communicates confidence in student ability to achieve in clinical practice; and, in a trusting relationship with faculty, learners are more inclined to discover and seek out new experiences. Judgment of performance occurs, but feedback from faculty is viewed as a means of helping students learn and further develop their skills, not as a punitive process addressing negative aspects of performance as an end in itself.

Empathetic understanding is also a significant attribute of a strong teacher–student relationship. Empathy means the teacher can view a situation from the learner's perspective (King & Gerwig, 1981). The development of a helping relationship requires teacher responsiveness to the feelings of students and an ability to communicate that understanding to them. Carl Rogers (1983) writes, "When the teacher has the ability to understand the student's reactions from the inside, has a sensitive awareness of the way the process of education and learning seems *to the student*, then again the likelihood of significant learning is increased" (p. 125).

Studies by Aspy and Roebuck (1974) have demonstrated that the interpersonal skills of the teacher influence student learning. These researchers found that empathy, congruence (genuineness), and positive regard (respect), which Rogers identified as critical dimensions of any interpersonal relationship, were significantly related to cognitive learning. High levels of empathy, congruence, and positive regard provided by the teacher tend to enhance learning, and conversely, low levels of these conditions may impede it. Although these studies were conducted with elementary school students and teachers in a classroom setting, they have implications for nursing faculty in that Aspy and Roebuck have been able to demonstrate a relationship between teachers' interpersonal skills and student learning.

Using Aspy's scales for evaluating the interpersonal skills of the teacher, Karns and Schwab (1982) examined nursing students' perceptions of teaching behaviors that promote a positive relationship between the teacher and student. Although the sample was small, most of the behaviors identified by students were ones relating to the conditions of empathy, congruence, and positive regard.

Field practice is inherently stressful for students. The environment cannot be fully controlled, and the student is faced with unexpected occurrences and uncertainties. Often, the clinical setting, client population, teacher, and even peers are unfamiliar to the learner. Field practice places the student in a vulnerable position in that learning occurs as a public event, in front of others—the teacher, clients, peers, agency staff, and sometimes even individuals from other disciplines. Perception of faculty as a threat forces students into "playing games" in an effort to survive in the system. Survival, rather than learning, becomes the emphasis. A trusting relationship between teacher and student is a prerequisite to reducing some of this stress and to the students' use of faculty as a resource for learning.

Teaching in the field requires a supportive learning milieu, planning with agency personnel for the practice experience, development of caring relationships with learners, and use of effective teaching behaviors. The teacher has responsibility for selecting learning experiences for students that reflect the objectives and take into consideration the goals and priorities of the clinical setting.

SELECTION OF LEARNING EXPERIENCES

Selection of learning experiences in the field requires collaboration of faculty, students, and agency staff but remains the responsibility of faculty. Retention of this responsibility by the teacher is important to fulfill the educational purposes of field practice. With some experiences, students are responsible for choosing the learning activities in which they will engage, and planning for these experiences then occurs between students and staff.

Criteria for the selection of learning experiences in the field include:

1. Appropriateness for the objectives of the experience
2. Availability of faculty
3. Appropriateness for learner's level of knowledge and skill, learning needs, and individual characteristics of learner
4. Provision for progressive development and continued growth of the learner
5. Compatibility with the philosophy and conceptual framework of the nursing program
6. Provision for variety

Learning experiences in the field are selected for the purpose of achieving the objectives for clinical practice. These experiences might involve interviewing a client or family, health teaching, providing care, conducting a conference, completing written assignments, and participating in other types of activities. The learning experiences vary according to the objectives regardless of whether these objectives are established by faculty or reflect personal learning goals of students.

Availability of faculty, or preceptors in the setting, with expertise in the area of practice and in sufficient number for student supervision represents another criterion in selecting experiences. The student–faculty ratio is dependent upon the objectives and level of the learner. Preceptorships, for example, allow for larger student–faculty ratios than do others requiring direct faculty supervision.

Beginning students and those entering a new clinical area need closer supervision by the teacher than do learners who have experience in the practice specialty.

Selection of experiences in field practice depends on the learner's present level of knowledge and skills and individual learning needs. Not all students will have similar learning needs, and, therefore, it is unreasonable to expect them to complete the same learning activities.

Individual differences of students also must be considered in the selection of clinical experiences. One important difference relates to the student's aptitude or time required for mastery of a particular learning task. The time available for learning should reflect that required by the learner. Research has clearly demonstrated that students learn at different rates. Not only are there rate variations among students, but the rate at which a person learns is not constant over different learning tasks. According to Carroll (1971), the "rate of learning may be quite specific to a given task, dependent as it is on specific attributes and prior learnings" (p. 37). The amount of time needed to learn is a function of the prerequisite knowledge and skills possessed by the student. If the learning experience assumes certain prerequisites that the student lacks, additional time is necessary in order to acquire these entry behaviors. This means that the learning experience initially should assist the student in acquiring entry behaviors in which he or she is deficient and then should provide for individual differences in rates of learning. It is recognized that with perseverance and time allowed for learning, students with varying aptitudes can achieve the objectives; but in most nursing programs, some time frames within which clinical objectives must be met to progress in the program need to be established.

Collaboration with learners as to the selection of experiences provides for individual styles of learning, interests, and preferences. It is important for students to participate actively in choosing experiences meaningful to them.

Learning experiences in the field provide for progressive development of knowledge, skills, and values and for continued growth of the learner. A sequence of experiences that has both continuity and connection is important in providing for this progressive development (Guinée, 1978). Experiences build on preceding ones and modify those that follow. The nature of and way in which the experiences are organized are important in promoting continued growth of the learner.

The philosophy of the nursing program, with respect to statements about learning and teaching, influences the selection of clinical experiences. A philosophic statement that the learner is self-directed and actively involved in the learning process may be reflected in field practice in provisions for the student to participate in selecting experiences and to direct his or her own learning in accord with the stated goals of the experience. In the field, students learn the practice of nursing as described in the conceptual framework of the nursing program. The experiences selected should be congruent with this description of the nature of nursing practice. For instance, if the nursing program is based on a stress–adaptation framework, experiences in the field should assist learners in using this framework with clients.

Learning experiences in the clinical field should provide for variety. Gow (1976) suggests to maintain student interest and promote independent inquiry, variety should be introduced into the instruction. The very nature of nursing itself, with its multiple activities and skills required, demands variation in clinical experiences.

INSTRUCTIONAL PROCESS

The instructional process may be viewed in terms of five interrelated components: clinical objectives, assessment of learner, instruction, formative evaluation, and summative evaluation. These follow a sequence of events as depicted in Figure 2.

Clinical Objectives
The first component relates to the clinical objectives established for the practice experience. These objectives provide the basis for teaching in the clinical setting because they specify the outcomes to be attained there. The clinical objectives are part of the overall course objectives and represent those behaviors to be attained in practice. While the clinical objectives are developed by the teacher, students

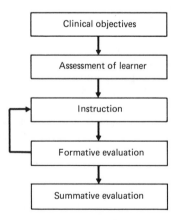

Figure 2. Instructional process in the clinical field.

set individual goals for learning in field practice, which are also representative, then, of this first component.

Assessment of Learner

Instruction begins at the level of the learner, so the second component necessarily deals with assessment in terms of (1) entry behaviors, the prerequisite knowledge and skills for learning a particular task, and (2) relevant characteristics of the learner. These prerequisites constitute the necessary link between the students and attaining the objectives because without them students are unable to adequately learn the task under consideration (Bloom, 1976). Given this view, the learner must possess or acquire the necessary entry behaviors to achieve the clinical objectives established for the practice experience.

Assessment determines if learners possess the necessary prerequisites for accomplishing the objectives. This is an important step in the instructional process for if students lack the entry behaviors for a given learning situation, even high-quality instruction will not overcome the effect of this lack unless that teaching is directed toward remedying these deficiencies (Bloom, 1976). Assessment reveals to the teacher whether or not the instruction needs to assist the learner in acquiring the prerequisite behaviors. Assessment might also reveal that some students have already achieved certain objectives and are able to move on to other learning tasks. Huckabay (1980) emphasizes that "assessment of entering behavior determines where the instruction must begin" (p. 18).

Assessment also includes determining the affective characteristics of the learner, "a complex compound of interests, attitudes, and self-views" (Bloom, 1976, p. 75), which vary greatly among students. Learning is facilitated when students are interested in the practice experience and have a desire to learn. Bloom believes that individuals tend to like activities which they perceive they have done or can do successfully. This perception is determined by previous experiences with similar learning tasks. If students perceive they have completed prior related tasks successfully, they are likely to approach the next similar learning situation with a positive affect. This raises the question as to the influence of student perception of the relationship with the teacher and success with learning in the field on subsequent related clinical experiences. Students who believe they have performed unsuccessfully in the past with interviewing, for instance, may approach subsequent learning experiences involving interactions with clients with some degree of negative affect.

Another related matter is whether students view the clinical experience as relevant to their individual goals. The learner who perceives some relationship between the present learning situation and experiences and future goals is more likely to have a positive affect (Bloom, 1976). Student establishment of own goals for learning provides a strategy for maintaining interest and motivation to learn.

Assessment also reveals differences in rates of learning, cognitive styles, and cultural patterns among students, relevant to planning the instruction. These differences influence teaching methods, types of learning experiences, time allowed for learning, and teacher behavior.

Learner assessment may be carried out by: (1) questioning, (2) observation of performance, (3) written tests, and (4) student self-evaluation.

Instruction

Instruction, the third component, pertains to the actual teaching process. This phase involves the selection of teaching methods and learning experiences for facilitating attainment of the objectives or initially assisting the student in acquiring any lacking prerequisite behaviors, development of the learning milieu, and interaction with students and staff in the process of carrying out the instruction. Research continually reminds faculty of the wide range of differences among students and need for these to be taken into account in the instruction.

Regardless of the specific experiences in which students engage, the instruction should provide for clear directions and explanations to learners, active involvement of the student in the experience, practice of behaviors to be learned, and reinforcement for learning (Bloom, 1976). The teacher adapts the extent of the directions, amount of participation and practice, and use of reinforcement to the individual's needs.

Formative Evaluation

The remaining two components of the instructional process refer to evaluation of the learner. Formative evaluation provides feedback to students as to their progress in achieving the objectives and is continuous throughout the practice experience. Evaluation which is formative in nature serves a diagnostic purpose because it informs students as to areas where further learning is necessary. This information is then used to plan additional instruction. For this reason, formative evaluation is depicted in Figure 2 with a connecting line to the instructional component. Formative evaluation alone only improves learning to a small degree, and therefore needs to be accompanied by supplemental instruction whereby students can correct their learning difficulties. Airasian (1971) suggests "the aim (of formative evaluation) is to foster learning mastery by providing data which can direct subsequent or corrective teaching and learning" (p. 79). Since formative evaluation is an integral part of the instruction, the resulting data are not subjected to the grading process.

Summative Evaluation

Summative evaluation, in contrast, is conducted at the conclusion of certain clinical experiences or the course to determine if the objectives have been achieved. This type of evaluation provides data for arriving at grades in clinical practice. Airasian (1971) writes: "Summative evaluation is concerned with how students have changed. The implication is that the changing process is for the most part completed and that little correction of identified deficiencies is possible" (p. 78).

The instructional process is depicted here in terms of five components beginning with the identification of clinical objectives and proceeding through assessment of the learner, planning and carrying out the instruction, and evaluating student learning in relation to the objectives. For the instruction to be effective, individual differences of learners must be taken into account in each phase of the process.

SUMMARY

Through experiences in the clinical field, the learner acquires the knowledge, skills, and values necessary for professional practice and becomes socialized into the profession. In clinical practice, students apply theories of action to real problems, develop skill in problem solving and decision making, learn how to learn, and develop a commitment to be responsible for their own actions. Learning is enhanced in a milieu which supports student independence and freedom to learn and provides opportunity for experimentation. The relationships established among faculty, students, and staff are important in creating a supportive milieu.

The purposes of clinical practice in a nursing program may be achieved in any setting in which the student is involved in the practice of nursing. There are many clinical settings appropriate for use in a nursing education program—hospitals, homes, community health agencies, schools, industry, ambulatory care centers, hospices, nursing homes, senior citizens programs, day care centers, and other agencies and community programs with a health focus. Since experiences in the field are critical in developing a practitioner capable of formulating a theory of practice, selection of clinical settings is a major faculty responsibility. Other responsibilities of the teacher in the setting involve development of collaborative relationships with agency personnel and planning with them for the practice experience, periodic evaluation of the setting, and selection of learning experiences for students. Criteria for selecting these experiences include: (1) appropriateness for the objectives of the experience, (2) availability of faculty, (3) appropriateness for learners, (4) provision for progressive development and continued growth of the learner, (5) compatibility with the philosophy and conceptual framework of the nursing program, and (6) provision for variety.

In the clinical field, the teacher, through interaction with the learner, facilitates student attainment of the objectives, providing the supportive milieu required for learning to take place. Effective clinical teaching requires knowledge and clinical competence, skill in teaching and in developing relationships with students and others in the setting, and personal characteristics which promote learning. Knowledge of nursing and clinical competence are important, but the teacher must also be able to teach. The process of instruction may be viewed in terms of five components: development of clinical objectives, assessment of the learner, instruction, incorporation of formative evaluation as an integral part of the instruction, and provision for summative evaluation.

The practice field is rich in learning experiences for students; granted a supportive milieu, learners will be encouraged to engage in them. The teacher carries the major, but not the sole, responsibility for developing and maintaining such a milieu.

REFERENCES

Airasian, P. W. (1971). The role of evaluation in mastery learning. In J. H. Block (Ed.), *Mastery learning: Theory and practice* New York: Holt, Rinehart & Winston.

American Nurses' Association. (1980). *Nursing: A social policy statement.* Kansas City, Mo.

Argyris, C., & Schön, D. A. (1976). *Theory in practice: Increasing professional effectiveness.* San Francisco: Jossey-Bass.

Aspy, D. N., & Roebuck, F. N. (1974). From humane ideas to human technology and back again many times. *Education, 95,* 163–71.

Bevil, C. W., & Gross, L. (1981). Assessing the adequacy of clinical learning settings. *Nursing Outlook, 29,* 658–61.

Blazeck, A. M., Selekman, J., Timpe, M., & Wolf, Z. R. (1982). Unification: Nursing education and nursing practice. *Nursing & Health Care, 3,* 18–24.

Bloom, B. S. (1976). *Human characteristics and school learning.* New York: McGraw-Hill.

Carroll, J. B. (1971). Problems of measurement related to the concept of learning for mastery. In J. H. Block (Ed.), *Mastery learning: Theory and practice.* New York: Holt, Rinehart & Winston.

Eble, K. E. (1972). *Professors as teachers.* San Francisco: Jossey-Bass.

Etzioni, A. (1964). *Modern organizations.* Englewood Cliffs, N.J.: Prentice-Hall.

Gow, D. T. (Ed.). (1976). *Design and development of curricular materials.*

Pittsburgh: University Center for International Studies, University of Pittsburgh.

Graham, B. A., & Gleit, C. J. (1981). Clinical sites used in baccalaureate programs. *Nursing Outlook, 29,* 291–94.

Guinée, K. K. (1978). *Teaching and learning in nursing.* New York: Macmillan.

Hawkins, J. W. (1981). *Clinical experiences in collegiate nursing education: Selection of clinical agencies.* New York: Springer.

Hildebrand, M., Wilson, R. C., & Dienst, E. R. (1971). *Evaluating university teaching.* Berkeley, Calif.: Center for Research and Development in Higher Education, University of California.

Huckabay, L. M. (1980). *Conditions of learning and instruction in nursing.* St. Louis: C. V. Mosby.

Hursh, B. A., & Borzak, L. (1979). Toward cognitive development through field studies. *Journal of Higher Education, 50,* 63–78.

Jacobson, M. D. (1966). Effective and ineffective behaviors of teachers of nursing as determined by their students. *Nursing Research, 15,* 218–24.

Jones, C. (1983). Negotiating student placements in ambulatory settings. *Journal of Nursing Education, 22,* 255–58.

Karns, P. J., & Schwab, T. A. (1982). Therapeutic communication and clinical instruction. *Nursing Outlook, 30,* 39–43.

King, V. G., & Gerwig, N. A. (1981). *Humanizing nursing education: A confluent approach through group process.* Wakefield, Mass.: Nursing Resources.

O'Shea, H. S., & Parsons, M. K. (1979). Clinical instruction: Effective/and ineffective teacher behaviors. *Nursing Outlook, 27,* 411–15.

Pugh, E. J. (1980). Factors influencing congruence between beliefs, intentions, and behavior in the clinical teaching of nursing (Doctoral dissertation, Northwestern University, 1980). *Dissertation Abstracts International, 41*(6), 2521A–22A.

Rogers, C. R. (1983). *Freedom to learn for the 80's.* Columbus, Ohio: Chas. E. Merrill.

Schein, E. H. (1972). *Professional education: Some new directions.* New York: McGraw-Hill.

BIBLIOGRAPHY

Aspy, D. N. (1972). *Toward a technology for humanizing education.* Champaign, Ill.: Research Press.

Baker, C. M. (1981). Moving toward interdependence: Strategies for collaboration. *Journal of Nursing Administration, XI*(4), 34–39.

Block, J. H. (Ed.), (1971). *Mastery learning: Theory and practice.* New York: Holt, Rinehart & Winston.

Brown, S. A. (1981). Faculty and student perceptions of effective clinical teachers. *Journal of Nursing Education, 20*(9), 4–15.

Carpenito, L. J., & Duespohl, T. A. (1981). *A guide for effective clinical instruction.* Rockville, Md.: Aspen Systems.

Centra, J. A. (Ed.). (1977). *Renewing and evaluating teaching.* San Francisco: Jossey-Bass.

Craig, J. L., & Page, G. (1981). The questioning skills of nursing instructors. *Journal of Nursing Education, 20*(5), 18–23.

Daggett, C. J., Cassie, J. M., & Collins, G. F. (1979). Research on clinical teaching. *Review of Educational Research, 49,* 151–69.

Eschbach, D. (1983). Role exchange: An exciting experiment. *Nursing Outlook, 31,* 164–67.

Fitzpatrick, L. M., & Heller, B. R. (1980). Teaching the teachers to teach. *Nursing Outlook, 28,* 372–73.

Griffith, J. W., & Bakanauskas, A. J. (1983). Student–instructor relationships in nursing education. *Journal of Nursing Education, 22,* 104–7.

Haukenes, E., & Mundt, M. H. (1983). The selection of clinical learning experiences in the nursing curriculum. *Journal of Nursing Education, 22,* 372–75.

Irby, D., & Rakestraw, P. (1981). Evaluating clinical teaching in medicine. *Journal of Medical Education, 56,* 181–86.

Johnson, J. (1980). The education/service split: Who loses? *Nursing Outlook, 28,* 412–15.

Kadushin, A. (July, 1968). Games people play in supervision. *Social Work,* pp. 23–32.

Lawrence, R. M., & Lawrence, S. A. (1980). Student experience in voluntary health care agencies. *Nursing Outlook, 28,* 315–17.

McKeachie, W. J. (1979). Student ratings of faculty: A reprise. *Academe, 65,* 384–97.

O'Shea, H. S. (1982). Role orientation and role strain of clinical nurse faculty in baccalaureate programs. *Nursing Research, 31,* 306–10.

Pugh, E. J. (1983). Research on clinical teaching. In W. L. Holzemer (Ed.), *Review of research in nursing education.* Thorofare, N.J.: Slack.

Seigel, H. (1984). Up the down staircase in nursing education: An analysis of the nurse educator as a professional. *Journal of Nursing Education, 23,* 114–17.

Sorensen, G., Gassman, A., & Walters, M. (1984). An experiment in a working relationship between nursing education and nursing service. *Journal of Nursing Education, 23,* 81–83.

Strauss, S. S., & Hutton, E. B. (1983). A framework for conceptualizing stress in clinical learning. *Journal of Nursing Education, 22,* 367–71.

Styles, M. M. (1984). Reflections on collaboration and unification. *Image,* XVI, 21–23.

5

Teaching Methods

The multipurpose nature of the clinical field, types of learning outcomes, diversity of nursing competencies, and differences among learners and teachers require various methods for teaching in the practice setting. Teaching method refers to a way of organizing and presenting the instruction reflective of a theoretical perspective of teaching and learning and directed toward achieving specific learning outcomes. No one method is sufficient for teaching nursing in the clinical field. The teacher, therefore, chooses from a repertoire of methods depending on the objectives, individual characteristics of the learner, and his or her own teaching abilities and conceptual framework of the teaching–learning process. Methods particularly relevant to teaching in the clinical field are the focus of this chapter.

The chapter is organized according to eight classifications of teaching methods. Each category is presented as follows: First, a discussion of the theoretical base for the classification; second, a description of the teaching methods included in it; and third, an identification of guidelines for use of the methods.

CRITERIA FOR SELECTION OF TEACHING METHODS

Planning for the clinical practice experience includes the decision as to methods to use for promoting achievement of the objectives. Such a decision reflects consideration of the nature of the objectives, entry behaviors and characteristics of the learner, qualities and skills of the teacher as well as availability in relation to the teacher–student ratio, characteristics of the clinical field, and particular attributes and limitations of the teaching method itself. Criteria for the selection of teaching methods for field practice include:

1. Appropriateness for the objectives of the practice experience in relation to the particular attributes of the method.
2. Appropriateness for learners in terms of abilities, experience, and other characteristics.

3. Compatibility with the teacher's skill and conceptual framework of the teaching–learning process.
4. Suitability in terms of availability of resources and constraints of the clinical setting.
5. Congruence with the philosophy of the nursing program in relation to faculty beliefs about teaching and learning.
6. Provision for variety, in accord with the various competencies to be achieved.

The particular attributes of each method make some strategies more appropriate than others for fostering certain types of learning. The question for faculty is which methods are the best ones for achieving the clinical objectives? For many objectives, several methods might be used, thereby allowing for individual differences among learners and teacher preference. For example, assisting students to apply concepts of teaching and learning to patient education may be accomplished through experiential methods such as a simulation or a patient assignment in which the student carries out instruction with a client, through use of media, or by observation of patient teaching combined with discussion. Other objectives, however, such as those relating to psychomotor skill development, are more limited as to the methods that are appropriate in terms of the performance aspect.

Knowledge of the learner provides another source of data for making the decision as to teaching strategies. Methods should be appropriate for the learners who will participate in them in terms of abilities, experience, cognitive styles and other relevant characteristics. Role play may not be suitable if students lack the necessary concepts for analyzing the outcomes of the role play situation and are unfamiliar with the other participants. Use of experiential methods, such as patient assignment, for instance, depends on the learner's present level of knowledge and skill and on the kinds of related experiences the student has had in field practice. Teaching methods also need to reflect individual differences among learners. Field-dependent learners, for instance, prefer methods that involve interactions with others more so than do learners who are field-independent.

Choice of methods is ordinarily made by the teacher but might also be made cooperatively by teacher and learner or even, in some situations, by the learner. Student input into selection of methods provides a means and evidence of attending to the interests of the learner and preferences for a teaching method if more than one is appropriate for the objectives.

Methods should capitalize on faculty strengths and should be compatible with teaching abilities. This is not to say that faculty should avoid trying out new strategies, but with some methods, the teacher may need further development of his or her own skills before using a method in the clinical setting. The selection of methods also reflects the faculty's own style of teaching, preference for particular strategies, and one's own beliefs about clinical teaching and ways of promoting learning in the practice setting. One component of the faculty's conceptual framework of teaching and learning is the relationship between various teaching methods and the learning process.

Teaching methods for clinical practice must reflect the resources available and be within the constraints of the setting and clinical teaching situation. Knowledge of the requirements of the methods for effective implementation, therefore, is important in the selection of strategies. Considerations in relation to this criterion include: (1) the time required for use of the teaching method and faculty time in preparing for it; (2) requirements of the method, such as space within the clinical setting and related equipment and supplies; (3) costs entailed with purchase, continued use, and administration; and (4) number of participants that permit effective implementation. Faculty might also consider the context of the teaching situation in terms of the time when the method will be used. Late afternoon of a day in which students engaged in field practice may not be an appropriate time for a teacher-centered method; one where learners participate actively in the instruction may be better suited.

The philosophy of the nursing program influences the selection of clinical teaching methods. Strategies should be congruent with the beliefs expressed in the philosophy regarding teaching and learning.

Variety in teaching methods, as long as it is in accord with the competencies to be achieved, may be advantageous in maintaining student interest. Selection of methods for the sake of variety alone, however, is rarely appropriate (Cooper, 1978).

CLINICAL TEACHING METHODS

Clinical teaching methods available to faculty are classified in relation to the primary purposes served by each strategy in the field. These categories are:

1. Experiential
2. Problem solving
3. Conference
4. Observation
5. Media
6. Self-directed
7. Preceptorship
8. Systems for concentrated practice

Some teaching methods can serve several purposes and are not confined by the basic categorization. For example, patient assignment, while classified as an experiential method because it provides for actual participation in the events to be learned, also promotes problem-solving learning with real clients and problems.

Experiential

Experiential teaching methods provide for direct experiencing of events, either through clinical practice involving interaction with real clients and others in the field or through contrived experiences of reality such as with simulations and role play. Learning results from actual participation in the events to be learned.

Experiential methods are based on a phenomenologic concept of learning. They provide for interaction of learners with the environment from which the learners derive personal meaning reflective of uniqueness of the individual and their own cognitive ability. Learners differ in their perception of events in the environment and the meanings given to phenomena, and thus, the learning outcomes evolving from the experience vary with the learner. Experiential methods recognize the importance of perception, insight, and cognitive structure formation in learning. They involve the whole learner, in cognitive, psychomotor and affective aspects of the learning event. Because of this involvement, there is an important affective dimension to the learning, regardless of whether the experience is directed toward cognitive or psychomotor outcomes. Experiential methods provide for actual participation of the learner in the events to be learned and recognize the ability of the individual to derive personal meaning from the experience.

Experiential clinical teaching methods include:

1. Clinical assignment
2. Written assignments, which often accompany experiences in the practice setting
3. Simulation and game

Clinical Assignment. Clinical assignment involves patient care; other kinds of experiences with clients; and practice experiences with peers, nursing staff, and members of other disciplines. Clinical assignment is essential in assisting students to use concepts and theories in practice, learn how to learn, develop skill in handling ambiguity, and become socialized into the profession. Experiences in care of clients and with others in the clinical setting facilitate the development of problem-solving and decision-making skills; provide opportunity for moral and ethical decision making relative to client, setting, and self; and enable learners to develop and refine psychomotor skills. Nursing is people oriented, and experiences in practice enable students to learn to work with others.

The nature of the clinical assignment is dependent upon the objectives, individual learning needs, and knowledge base of the learner. In some instances, the assignment may be care of a client or group of clients. In other instances, students may be assigned specific types of learning experiences with clients or others in the setting. This is particularly true in early stages of clinical experience. For example, when the goal is the development of communication skills, the clinical assignment emphasizes interacting with clients rather than their care per se. Faculty needs to decide whether an assignment involving complete care of the client is the most appropriate strategy for the given practice experience.

Guidelines for Use

1. Clinical assignments should provide for progressive development of the learner.
2. A clinical assignment should be based on specific clinical objectives and should reflect the learner's needs and abilities in terms of knowledge and skill.
3. The rationale underlying a patient assignment or other experience in the clinical setting should be clear to the learner so as to emphasize the relationship between the particular experience and intended learning outcomes.
4. When learners choose their own experiences, which provides a means of attending to personal learning goals and individual preferences, it is important for faculty to assure that these experiences promote attainment of the objectives.
5. Clinical assignments for the group of learners for whom faculty is responsible must take into account the time needed for supervision.
6. Clinical assignments are best developed when faculty and agency personnel concur on goals, types of experiences, specific responsibilities of students, and the length of time learners are in the clinical setting.
7. Student preparation for a clinical assignment may involve library research, laboratory practice, and visitation in the clinical setting.
8. At the conclusion of clinical assignments, conferences are necessary to assist learners in examining the experiences and setting directions for future learning.

Written Assignments. Written assignments may be used effectively to promote problem-solving learning in relation to clients and other problems encountered in the practice setting. They help learners to identify and reflect upon their values and beliefs, improve understanding of a particular aspect of clinical practice, and develop written communication skills. Written assignments may be preliminary to clinical practice, concurrent with practice, or subsequent to it. Types of written assignments relevant to clinical practice include nursing care plans, case studies, teaching plans, process recordings, experiential diaries, learning logs, reports, and other forms of written work.

Nursing Care Plans. Nursing care plans enable the learner to analyze the client's health care problems and develop a plan which incorporates goal setting and a selection of care activities as well as provides direction for evaluation. The format of the care plan may be that of a specific clinical agency in which the student is involved in practice or one developed by faculty for use as a learning strategy, a learning care plan, in a particular course or throughout the program. The intent of the learning care plan, which tends to be more detailed and comprehensive than the practice plan, is to assist in the development of the knowledge base for practice. The number of learning care plans is dependent upon the student's learning needs, for the ultimate goal of teaching here should be to move the student to the practice model as soon as possible.

Case Study. Case study represents a holistic picture of a client's health care problems and requires more in-depth analysis of these problems than a care plan. At best, it requires from the learner an explanation of relevant theories and principles. When used as a clinical teaching strategy, the case study is based on a client for whom the student is responsible for care or is derived from a clinical situation in which the student has been previously involved. The case study might be presented in conference for peer review.

Analysis of a case provides opportunity for the students to: (1) examine the interrelationships of multiple phenomena in the clinical situation, (2) enlarge own knowledge base, (3) acquire skill in problem solving, (4) examine creative approaches to the solutions of problems and present a supporting rationale for them, and (5) organize ideas logically in written form. When using case studies, it is important that students possess sufficient depth of understanding and the theoretical background necessary for analyzing the clinical situation under review.

Teaching Plan. A written teaching plan enables learners to apply concepts of learning and teaching in providing for client educational needs. The teaching plan is part of the total plan of care which addresses teaching as an intervention strategy. There are many formats with which teaching plans may be developed; in general, there are five major parts: objectives, content, teaching methods, learning activities, and evaluation.

Process Recording. For objectives relating to the development of skill in interacting with others, the process recording provides a means for learners to record and then analyze their communications. A process recording consists of a written record of the communication that occurred between the learner and client, peer or another member of the health care team (Reilly, 1980) and an analysis of that interaction. With this method, the learner is able to examine the client's and his or her own verbal and nonverbal behaviors, thereby increasing understanding of the client and improving learner's interaction skills.

The focus of the process recording depends on the purposes to be accomplished. If the objectives relate to nonverbal communication, for instance, then the written report and subsequent analysis of the interaction may emphasize nonverbal behaviors of the participants. Because this assignment is time consuming for students and for faculty who review it and provide feedback, the number of recordings should be determined by the needs of the student. Continuance of the assignment beyond its value for learning results in boredom for students which, in turn, may precipitate careless or less-than-honest completion of the process recording. Learners must also have time immediately following the interaction for writing the report. One format for a process recording is presented in Table 9.

Experiential Diary and Learning Log. Similar to a process recording, experiential diaries and learning logs also provide a means of recording experiences related to field practice. Diary writing is a dialogue with the self, representing a record of the student's feelings, reactions, attitudes, perceptions and activities regarding experiences in the field. Diary writing prepares learners for working with clients and families and enables them to reflect on their experiences and derive personal meaning from them. Spontaneous responses result when there are no instructions as to the format of the presentation. The message, "write as though you were writing your own diary," suffices.

Reilly (1958) demonstrated the use of diaries in determining the nature of learning experiences in the clinical field. Students wrote a diary after their first experience in the clinical setting, one month later, and at the time they entered a new setting. A content analysis of the diaries provided faculty with cues for planning subsequent learning experiences.

Learning log, a form of diary, is a sequential record of learning experiences usually documented in relation to specific clinical objectives. Students may be directed by faculty as to notations to be made in the log, depending on the objectives associated with the experience, or may be encouraged to formulate their own notations relevant to the objectives.

Other Assignments. Other written assignments appropriate for clinical practice include reports, such as those of field trips; papers;

TABLE 9. GUIDELINES FOR NURSE–PATIENT PROCESS RECORDING[a]

Milieu	Patient	Nurse
Describe environment in which patient and nurse are interacting. Include physical and social aspects and feeling tone of environment. Indicate changes in the milieu that occur throughout the interaction.	Describe patient's appearance.	Describe nurse's nonverbal communication.
	Describe patient's nonverbal communication. Record patient's verbal communication, using direct quotes whenever possible.	Record nurse's verbal communication, using direct quotes whenever possible.
Identify effects of milieu on the interaction.		
Identify modifications in milieu planned by nurse.		

[a]Adapted from Wayne State University College of Nursing.

and written work students complete about observations made in the field and of practice experiences in which they have engaged.

Guidelines for Use
1. Objectives for the assignment should be clearly identified.
2. Written assignments should assist learners in applying theory to practice and should reflect the conceptual framework of the nursing program.
3. Written assignments should reflect the learner's background and ability.
4. Instructions for completing the assignment should be clear and understood by the learner.
5. Consideration should be given as to the number required of each type of written assignment, particularly in relation to the objectives to be achieved and individual learner needs.

Feelings	Analysis
Describe nurse's *feelings,* e.g., anger, fear, relief, comfort, pleasure. Identify changes in feelings as interaction progresses.	1. Analyze nonverbal and verbal meanings of patient's communication. 2. Analyze nurse's responses to client's behavior, both verbal and nonverbal. 3. Identify specific communication skills used by nurse (e.g., open-ended questions, reflection, etc.). 4. Identify use or nonuse of empathetic responses by nurse. 5. Identify blocks nurse may have used and why such blocks may have occurred. 6. Describe effects of nurse's feelings, needs, attitudes, values and beliefs on nurse's behavior and on the interaction. 7. Identify physical, environmental, and cultural variables that may have affected the interaction. 8. Describe effect of client's behavior on nurse and on the interaction. 9. Describe implications for nursing actions.

6. The expectations of faculty as to the comprehensiveness of the written work and depth of analysis should be communicated clearly to the learner.
7. An important component of any written assignment is faculty feedback, which needs to be given as close as possible to the time the assignment is completed.
8. Faculty should be supportive of new and creative approaches taken by students with their written work.

Simulation and Game. Another category of experiential teaching methods includes simulations and games. While not replacing direct involvement with clients, simulations and games prepare learners for clinical practice by providing opportunity to develop and test cognitive skills in a relatively risk-free environment where the consequences of any mistakes are less costly than they would be with real clients, to apply theories of action before required to use those theories in practice, to learn complex skills in a more controlled setting than the field, to practice psychomotor skills, and to gain a perspective of what a clinical situation might be like for others. Experiencing an event in a simulated situation or through a game before encountering it in the field promotes learning in that the student is more confident as to possible ways of handling the situation and is more sensitive to the client's perspective.

With simulations and games, students learn a combination of: (1) facts and concepts taught by the simulation or game, (2) processes simulated by the experience, and (3) effects of alternate decision-making strategies (Hyman, 1974). Hyman also suggests that simulations and games encourage critical thinking by having the learner analyze possible moves and probable consequences of them. While there is less agreement and evidence as to specific benefits of simulations and games in terms of cognitive learning, there is wide support for these methods in relation to increasing motivation and interest (Greenblat, 1977); promoting affective learning, for example, changing attitudes and increasing empathy; and improving one's self-awareness.

Simulation. A simulation creates an experience that represents reality; in essence, it mimics a real-life situation. There are, in general, four types of simulations: (1) active case study (Clark, 1978), (2) models, (3) simulated patients, and (4) role play.

In the active case study method, information relative to a clinical situation is presented to the learner and usually requires that some decision be made. Information is gradually added to the case, often reflecting the consequences of the learner's decision, thereby simulating the progression of events in the real clinical situation. In this way, students learn how to solve clinical problems in a contrived setting and receive immediate feedback on the consequences of their decisions. The simulation may also provide opportunity for practice of psychomotor skills relevant to the clinical situation and client problems being simulated. deTornyay and Thompson (1982) have referred to this type of simulation, in written form, as the Patient Management Problem.

With the active case study method, the simulation may be presented in paper and pencil format, through audiovisual media (frequently involving videotaping), and by computer. In a computer simulation of a clinical problem, the student responds to data presented by the computer, makes a decision, and receives feedback on the consequences of that decision. With some computer programs, the patient's status is altered by the decisions made which vividly communicates to the learner the outcomes of the decision-making process. Hales (1984) describes the concept of computer-assisted interactive video instruction which combines the computer simulation with videotape in such a way that video segments are shown, depending on the learner's response to the material presented in the computer simulation. The student is thus able to view the client's progress in this simulated situation and respond to visual and aural scenarios, creating an experience that more closely mimics a real-life dilemma than would use of either a computer simulation or videotape alone.

A second type of simulation common in nursing education involves the use of models of the human body for teaching clinical skills, such as in the form of manikins, like "Mrs. Chase," for practicing basic nursing procedures. Many other models are available for teaching specific skills—breast examination, intramuscular and intravenous injections, and urinary catheterization, to name a few. Models enable students to practice skills in a safe environment and increase their confidence in performing them before having to use and often adapt those skills with clients.

Another type of simulation involves the use of peers and other persons who act in the role of client and behave as a patient would in that situation. Simulated patients may be used for the practice of psychomotor skills, taking a health history, physical assessment, and other experiences where a live patient is needed to represent effectively the real-life situation. The simulation may be videotaped so that participants are able to analyze their own behaviors or to permit evaluation by others.

In role play, another type of simulation, the learner portrays a specific individual and is generally given much freedom to act out that role spontaneously. Role play is particularly appropriate for objectives related to developing interpersonal relationships with clients, peers, and other health care providers. In general, two students act out the roles and the rest of the students in the clinical group observe, analyze, and provide feedback to the role players. Role play may be combined with videotaping to allow for learner analysis at the completion of the activity. Guidelines for using role play are presented in summary form in Table 10.

Game. In comparison to a simulation, a game is a contest among participants that has rules, goals, activities to perform, constraints on the activities, and pay-offs (Clark, 1978). Games, therefore, involve competition among players or with oneself if played individually. Games for clinical teaching include crossword puzzles to teach medical terminology, question and answer games on clinical problems and care of clients (Crancer & Maury-Hess, 1980), and board games on clinical topics and nursing management.

Simulation Games. A simulation game mimics aspects of the real world but is patterned in a game format (Cooper, 1979). Combining

TABLE 10. GUIDELINES FOR ROLE PLAY

1. Planning
   a. Describe the clinical situation and identify the roles to be played (may be identified by teacher or student).
   b. Discuss the situation with students to assure understanding of the roles portrayed and context, without overbriefing them.
   c. Ask for volunteers to act out the roles.
   d. Describe the role of the rest of the students and observations to be made.
2. Role Play
   a. Keep the time for the role play to approximately 10 to 15 minutes, which should allow for sufficient portrayal of the roles.
   b. Halt the role play when time expires, the objectives have been achieved, or problems arise.
3. Discussion (Debriefing)
   a. Have students discuss their observations and analysis of the role play, beginning with the players.
   b. Ask the players to share insights and feelings they had in portraying the roles.
   c. Assist students in relating the outcomes of the role play to the objectives and to clinical practice.
   d. Limit discussion to the role play experience, not the acting ability or individual characteristics of the players.
   e. Provide for evaluation of the role play experience.

properties of simulations and games allows learners to experience aspects of the real world and at the same time "have goals, sets of activities to perform, constraints on what they can and cannot do, and positive and negative pay-offs, as consequences of their actions" (Greenblat, 1977, p. 6). Some illustrations of simulation games include: *Starpower* (Simile II) in which participants learn about power and the distribution of wealth through the trading of chips, simulating a society of have and have nots; *Terminex,* designed to help learners deal with the dying patient and work with staff (Smoyak, 1977); *Pediatrix,* simulating the experience of children in the hospital (Barham et al., 1977); *Into Aging* (Slack), for demonstrating how an older person is influenced by health professionals and other persons with negative attitudes and information about aging; *Blood Money* (Gamed/Simulations Inc.) which teaches about some of the problems faced by hemophiliacs within the health care system; and *Assylumation* on the legal rights of mental patients (Caracappa, Nagy-McMenamin, & Yuschak, 1977).

Simulations and games provide for experiential learning with an experience that represents a real-life situation in various ways. They have potential for raising motivation and interest in an area of clinical nursing, sensitizing students to what a situation might be like for others, assisting learners in developing decision-making skills, and enabling them to practice in a relatively safe environment.

Discussion, referred to as debriefing, following a simulation and game is important for students to (1) identify the concepts learned, (2) relate their learning to the objectives, (3) discuss application to clinical practice, and (4) evaluate the experience. The format of and questions for the debriefing session should be identified by the teacher prior to the activity. With some types of simulations and games, debriefing is in written form for completion independently by the learner or is part of the computer program.

Guidelines for Use

1. The simulation/game should promote attainment of the objectives.
2. Consideration should be given to the requirements of the simulation/game, for example, number of participants, time for preparing for and engaging in the simulation/game, equipment, props, cost, and space and to the constraints of the teaching situation.
3. The teacher should be familiar with the simulation/game— how it is played, equipment and any materials needed, directions to be given to students, and the teacher's own role.
4. Pretesting the simulation/game with a group of students familiarizes faculty with it, which facilitates implementation and provides a means of evaluating its usefulness.
5. Students should have the necessary theoretical background and skill level for participating in the simulation/game and learning from it.
6. Learners must understand the purpose of engaging in the simulation/game and how it relates to the objectives.
7. Directions given to the students for participating in the simulation/game should be clear and if complex, should be in written form for each learner.
8. The teacher is responsible for halting the simulation/game when time expires, play ceases, problems arise with implementation, or students are no longer benefitting from the experience.
9. Debriefing should follow the simulation/game.

Some considerations by faculty in planning for use of a simulation/game are included in Table 11.

Problem Solving

Problem-solving methods assist learners in analyzing a clinical situation with the intent of defining problems to be solved, deciding on actions to be taken, applying knowledge to a clinical problem, and clarifying one's own beliefs and values. They encourage divergent thinking, the derivation of more than one solution to a problem, which is essential for effective problem solving in practice, and

TABLE 11. PLANNING CONSIDERATIONS FOR USE OF SIMULATION/GAME

Objectives:
Does the simulation/game relate to the objectives to be attained by learners?
What other goals might be met through the simulation/game?
Cost:
Is the cost of the simulation/game, for purchase (if commercially available), development (if to be developed by faculty), and continued use within the budgetary constraints of the nursing program?
Participants:
What is the minimum and maximum number of learners to participate in the simulation/game?
Is this number within the constraints of the teaching situation in which the simulation/game will be used?
What roles might other students assume if unable to engage in the simulation/game?
Do the intended learners have the necessary theoretical background and skill level for engaging in and learning from the simulation/game?
What preparation will be needed on the part of students to participate in the simulation/game?
Time:
What are time requirements for use of the simulation/game: preparation time for faculty? time for the simulation/game? time for debriefing after it is completed?
Are these within the constraints of the teaching situation?
Setting:
How much space is required for the simulation/game?
Is the required space available in the setting in which students will be?
Materials:
What equipment, supplies, props, and other materials are required by the simulation/game?
Are these available in the setting, or may they be easily transported there?
Debriefing:
Does the simulation/game have guidelines for debriefing?
What are important questions to be explored in the debriefing session?

transfer of learning, stressing the connection between previous experiences and learning with new problems.

Problem-solving methods derive much of their theoretical base from cognitive-field theory. They also draw upon information processing theory and decision theory.

Problem-solving teaching methods appropriate for clinical practice include:

1. Problem-solving situation
2. Decision-making situation
3. Incident process

Problem-solving Situation. A problem-solving situation represents a written description of a clinical event for the purposes of defining problems to be solved as indicated in the situation, identifying relevant data significant to understanding the nature of the problem, proposing hypotheses, identifying appropriate nursing actions to be taken in the situation and underlying theoretical bases for such actions, and applying theory to practice. This method serves as one means of assisting students in applying the conceptual model of nursing upon which the curriculum is based to issues and problems in clinical practice.

Problem-solving situations may be client, staff, or setting oriented or may represent issues affecting nursing practice and care delivery. They may be completed individually by students or in small groups and in combination with media. Questions directed toward the problem situation may be in a written form or raised by the teacher or students in discussion of the situation. The following example illustrates a problem-solving situation.

Problem-solving Situation

Objectives

Identifies universal, developmental, and health deviation self-care requisites.

Relates concepts of self-care theory to client situation.

Identifies nursing measures for meeting client's self-care needs.

Situation

Mr. A. is a 60-year-old patient who recently had a laryngectomy. His incision is healing and only requires a dressing change once daily. He has been unable to sleep for the last two evenings because of pain in his neck radiating to his shoulder. Mr. A. admits to being a problem drinker and to having a long history of smoking. Over the past two years, he has lost a significant amount of weight. He lives alone and is presently unemployed.

Mr. A. rings the call bell for the nurse and writes on his memo pad, "I can't stand it anymore—the pain is too much for me."

1. What are Mr. A.'s universal, developmental, and health deviation self-care requisites?
2. On the basis of this information, what are the probable self-care demands?
3. What questions would you ask Mr. A. and what observations would you make to determine Mr. A.'s potential capability for self-care?
4. What actions should the nurse take in regard to Mr. A.'s statement?

Decision-making Situation. A decision-making situation is a form of problem solving in which a decision is required. Learners examine the data presented, identify alternatives for action and consequences of each, establish priorities, and then make a decision. Reilly (1980) describes another type of decision-making situation in which the decision is stated and learners indicate agreement or disagreement with it and provide a supporting rationale for the position chosen.

Decision-making situations may involve decisions relative to clients, staff, and communication with other disciplines. Like problem solving, the questions for discussion may be in written form or may be raised by the teacher during conference. Students may complete the decision-making situation individually or in small groups, but it is important that they have an opportunity for discussion to capture the thought process used in responding to the situation.

The following example illustrates a decision-making situation.

Decision-making Situation

Objectives

Uses the decision-making process in identifying nursing actions.

Situation

In reviewing a patient's chart, Ms. C., a registered nurse, finds that the order for Digoxin is considerably larger than the usual dose. She confirms this in a reference book and explains the situation to the head nurse. After reviewing the order on the patient's chart, the head nurse tells Ms. C., "Give the medication. I'm sure Dr. Smith had a reason for ordering this dose."

1. What is your assessment of the situation?
2. Identify three possible courses of action that might be taken.
3. Describe the possible consequences of each source of action.
4. Which course of action would you choose?
5. Why did you select the course of action you did?

Incident Process. The incident process, also designed to assist students in developing skill in reflective thinking, is built around a single incident or clinical event. Through group discussion, learners seek information about the incident, identify the problem, describe their approach and supporting rationale, and then generalize from the incident to other clinical experiences. The incident process, originated by Pigors and Pigors, encourages students to gather necessary data for making a decision, develop skill in asking appropriate questions, learn from their peers, and apply their learning to other clinical situations (Cooper, 1981).

Generally, the incident is described briefly in written form, although it might be presented verbally by the teacher or by a student. The incident should be generated from a practice experience in which the learner or faculty has recently been involved, although it is possible to propose a hypothetical situation providing it reflects a likely clinical event. Incidents may be client, staff, or setting oriented or may involve student responses to the learning situation. The person directing the discussion, the teacher or one of the students, should have knowledge of the incident.

Cooper describes five phases of the incident process:

1. Studying the incident and formulating questions to gather more information about it.
2. Asking questions in an effort to acquire sufficient information to identify the problem. In this phase, the discussion leader provides only facts relative to the incident under study.

3. Identifying the problem.
4. Exploring possible alternative actions and making a decision individually as to which alternative to select, including a rationale for the choice. After learners defend their individual choices to the group, the group, in turn, comes to agreement as to the most appropriate action to be taken, followed by a report by the discussion leader as to what actually occurred.
5. Generalizing from the incident to other clinical experiences, considering ways in which the concepts learned are applicable to other situations, and reflecting on the case as a whole.

There are many incidents associated with field practice that could be used. A few illustrations are included.

Incidents

Mr. B., 75 years old, was diagnosed recently with inoperable metastatic lung cancer. In a home visit, the nurse notices that Mr. B. has continued smoking.

John, a 17-year-old diabetic, comes to the clinic with a blood sugar of 360. He tells the nurse, "I was partying and maybe had too much to drink. My doctor said I could eat whatever I wanted since I'm still growing."

Guidelines for Use

Because of similarities in use of problem-solving situations, decision-making situations, and the incident process, one set of guidelines is included.

1. The clinical situation should be within the level of understanding and experience of the students.
2. The description of the clinical situation should be sufficient to assure understanding of the problem and questions posed.
3. The situation described for problem solving or decision making should be of reasonable length and complexity to achieve the purposes for which it is designed without making it necessary for students to devote extensive time to reading and rereading the description.
4. Extraneous information should be excluded from the incident, and the description should focus primarily on factors that have a direct influence on the event itself.
5. The teacher, or student if functioning as discussion leader, should keep the discussion centered on the clinical situation without giving learners the answers or making the decisions for them.

Conference

The clinical conference is a form of group discussion about some aspect of clinical practice. Conferences promote problem-solving learning in that the group undertakes critical analysis of a problem and explores alternate and creative approaches. With this method, students are able to talk through the problem-solving process and receive immediate feedback from peers and the teacher. Schweer and Gebbie (1976) write, "The nursing care conference viewed as a creative act provides a learning environment that fosters opportunities for students to *think through* challenging and worthwhile problems, allowing for their completion and evaluation while simultaneously learning new subject matter" (p. 119). In a conference, the group of learners gains exposure to varied clinical situations, many of which students may not encounter themselves. Conferences also provide opportunity for peer review, discussion of concerns and issues relative to clinical practice, and problem solving by different disciplines.

In addition to these outcomes, group discussions are effective in producing noncognitive changes in the learner (McKeachie, 1962). In a conference, students have a chance to interact with one another and with the teacher, using each other as resources for learning. Discussion enhances the ability to formulate ideas and express them clearly; gives learners an opportunity to be recognized for their contributions; increases confidence in interacting in a group format; and provides a place for them to explore feelings, attitudes, and values affecting practice. Students can develop, in a discussion format, skills in group membership and leadership (McKeachie, 1962).

The relationships between the teacher and learner and within the group are significant in promoting discussion, for learners need to be comfortable with peers and other participants and particularly with the teacher to express their views and feelings and take risks in responding to questions. The teacher's behavior often influences whether or not students will participate in a conference and their willingness to be honest and open. The faculty's general stance can invite or discourage student participation.

There are four types of conferences relevant for teaching in the clinical field:

1. Preconference and postconference
2. Peer review
3. Issue
4. Multidisciplinary

Preconferences and postconferences relate directly to the field practice experience. Preconferences prepare students for their experiences in the practice setting; assist them in identifying client problems, planning care, and evaluating outcomes; and provide a means for students to discuss with faculty (and with peers if in a group format) questions about their clients. These conferences enable the teacher to identify concerns and feelings of students regarding the practice experience. Preconferences may be one-to-one or in a group depending on learner needs, teacher preference, and context within which the clinical experience takes place.

Postconferences take place following clinical practice, such as the end of an experience in which students have been in the field, or after a specific learning experience completed by an individual or group of learners; for instance, an observational experience. These postclinical discussions provide an opportunity for group problem solving, in relation to problems in which students are involved in practice, and for sharing of clinical experiences among the group.

Clinical conferences may also be used for reviewing and critiquing each other's work. Peer review enables learners to gain experience and skill in the process of evaluating another's practice, similar to what takes place in the work setting. In a conference intended for peer review, the criteria for critique of another's work should be explicit and understood by learners. In addition, students must be comfortable with one another and value feedback from peers for such a review to be effective. Experience in peer review within the educational process prepares learners for carrying this out in their own practice.

Conferences also provide an opportunity for discussion of issues affecting nursing practice not necessarily generated from the clinical experience but relevant to it as in a postconference. In a conference learners can explore a range of economic, political, and social issues and their implications for nursing practice and care delivery in general and in the particular clinical setting in which they are having experience.

Multidisciplinary conferences emphasize the process of collaborative decision making in which plans for client care are developed, evaluated, and revised; and implementation of the plan by different disciplines is examined. As early as 1958, Reilly described the value for student learning of multidisciplinary conferences in her study of clinical conferences attended by nursing and medical students. Students reported that these conferences "contributed to improved patient care by furthering mutual understanding" among disciplines (Reilly, 1958, p. 24).

Multidisciplinary conferences also enable learners and practitioners to explore different perspectives of issues affecting care and the delivery of that care, such as, the impact of prospective payment according to diagnosis-related groups on client care and the practice of different health care professionals. Schein (1972) emphasizes the need for greater collaboration among professionals for solving problems. "Many of the more pressing problems that face society today are so complex that no *single* profession can ever hope to deal with them effectively" (p. 34).

Guidelines for Use

1. At the outset, the objectives for the conference should be clarified.
2. The discussion should reflect principles of group process and dynamics.
3. The teacher has an important role in keeping the discussion focused, without dominating it, and providing necessary feedback to learners.
4. The teacher should emphasize periodically the major points made.
5. The atmosphere of the discussion should encourage participation, learner willingness to take risks in responding, and acceptance of different approaches and opinions.
6. Group size should generally be limited to approximately ten to twelve participants to allow for adequate exchange of ideas among them.
7. The physical arrangement should provide for face-to-face discussion.
8. At the conclusion of the conference, a summary should be given by teacher or student of the learning outcomes and applicability to other clinical situations.

Observation

Observation of an actual experience in the field or of a demonstration provides for learning through modeling. According to social learning theory (Bandura, 1977), modeling promotes learning by informing the learner of what the behavior to be developed is like. From observation of others, the learner forms an image of how new behaviors are performed which serves as a guide for future learning.

Observational teaching methods include:

1. Observation in the field
2. Field trip
3. Nursing rounds
4. Demonstration

Observation in the Field. Observation in the clinical setting (1) prepares learners for future experiences with clients, giving them a perspective of what the care or specific intervention is like; (2) enables them to view others in practice, which serves as a guide for development of their own behaviors; (3) makes it possible for students to observe a clinical situation with which they may not have an opportunity to be involved themselves; and (4) provides a means for improving their own observation skills. Participatory observation, in which learners participate in activities as they are observing, minimizes the effects of their presence by making them less noticeable and setting clients and others at ease. A balance needs to be established between such participation and attending to the observations so the participation does not interfere with making skillful observations.

Observation may be done individually or in small groups, depending on the situation being observed. With group observation, it is particularly important that careful consideration be given to the effect on those observed.

Field Trip. The field trip provides an opportunity for observations outside of the clinical setting in which students are presently involved in practice. Students gain experiences that are generally not available in their own setting to augment current knowledge and acquire a broader perspective of the health care issue under discussion.

A field trip may be taken to any site pertinent to the clinical objectives. Arrangements must be made by faculty with the clinical agency to clarify the purpose of the field trip, kinds of observational experiences desired, level and number of students, length of time in the agency, and other specifics of the experience. Evaluation by faculty, students, and clinical agency personnel of the observational experience is critical in planning for subsequent field trips to the particular setting.

Guidelines for Use

The following guidelines pertain to use of observation in the field and field trip:

1. Students need to understand the purpose and objectives of the experience so they may be attentive to and may selectively focus their observations on relevant activities.
2. For some experiences, a written guide is valuable to assist learners in focusing their observations.
3. Faculty should plan carefully with clinical agency personnel for the observational experience and with practitioners who will be involved in it.
4. When the observation is of clients or families, permission should be obtained from them and/or the practitioner responsible for care.
5. Written or verbal reports of the experience and observations made assist learners in evaluating their observational skills.
6. Discussion of the observations provides an opportunity for sharing among learners, having questions answered regarding the observational experience, relating the experience to future practice and behaviors to be performed, evaluating the experience, and proposing recommendations regarding future observations of a similar nature.

Nursing Rounds. Nursing rounds involve the observation and often interview of a client or several clients in the setting, generally followed by group discussion. Through an actual visit to the client, students are able to observe the client's condition, review the care provided, and collect information from the patient. Rounds also provide an opportunity for demonstrating a particular nursing intervention or the result of an intervention and for learners to observe interaction of the teacher, peer, or nursing staff (if participating in the rounds) with the client. Observing the client in the client's own environment contributes to discussion about that individual's care.

Rounds may be conducted by the teacher, by students (of their own clients), or by nursing staff. After arrangements have been completed for the nursing rounds, Cooper (1982b) recommends that the rounds begin with an introduction of the patient to the students, emphasizing the client's contribution to their learning, followed by discussion with the client, observations, and any demonstrations. Discussion of the observations made should take place following the nursing rounds and out of the client's presence. In the discussion, students are able to reflect on their observations; review the patient's problems and care, considering additional data obtained in the rounds; propose alternate interventions if appropriate; apply knowledge to the particular client situation; and relate their observations to other patients and to future learning.

Major difficulties in use of nursing rounds concern respecting the client's privacy during the observation and interview and assuring that the client desires to participate. Permission from the client must always be obtained in advance, and clients must understand their right to refuse participation. Clients should also be encouraged to indicate when they no longer desire to continue with the nursing rounds.

Guidelines for Use
1. The purpose of the nursing rounds and observations to be made should be clearly identified for learners.
2. Students should be prepared for participating in the nursing rounds, which might include review of the client's health history, outside readings, and other relevant learning activities.
3. The client selected for nursing rounds should reflect the objectives to be achieved.
4. The teacher or learner should obtain permission from the client in advance of the nursing rounds and prepare the client, which includes: (a) purpose of the rounds; (b) kinds of questions to be asked, observations to be made, and activities to be performed; (c) roles of the teacher, nursing staff, student, and client; (d) time for initiating the rounds; and (e) total amount of time involved.

5. Opportunities should be provided for the client to ask questions and participate in the rounds if desired.
6. The individual conducting the rounds should be continually aware of the client's response and should be prepared to stop the experience when necessary.
7. Consideration should be given to the number of learners who may be accommodated on the nursing rounds in relation to client status, room, and ability of learners to see and hear.
8. Discussion to reflect on the observations made and learning outcomes should be held away from the client following the nursing rounds.

Demonstration. Demonstration involves a presentation of how to perform a procedure or task, how to use equipment, or how to interact with clients or others (Cooper, 1982a). It provides for learning through visual and auditory modes and thus enables students to observe a procedure and its component steps while having those steps and underlying principles explained. A demonstration may be performed in the learning laboratory or clinical field. In the laboratory, the teacher has greater control over the demonstration, there are fewer distractions than in the field, and students are able to practice the procedure more easily than usually possible in the clinical setting. Some demonstrations are best taught with patients, real or simulated. For those carried out with real clients, it is important that they be selected and prepared for the experience similarly as in the instance of nursing rounds. Regardless of the setting, the presentation may be in small groups or with an individual learner. The demonstrator may be the teacher, a staff nurse, or others with expertise in the procedure; or the demonstration may be presented in media, such as, a videotape recording, film, or filmstrip.

As with other observational teaching methods, students need information as to the purpose of the demonstration and important points on which to focus attention. Verbal directions of the teacher during the presentation serve as a means of emphasizing these relevant aspects. Explanations of the underlying principles, while important to the demonstration, need to take place before the demonstration begins and following it, not during the actual presentation, where the focus should be on the procedure itself.

For some procedures, particularly if they are complex or require advanced skill, the demonstration in its entirety or selected segments may need to be repeated. Practice is essential to allow learners to try out the procedure observed, receive feedback and additional instruction from the teacher, and develop confidence in performance. Because learning occurs at different rates, the amount of practice needed will differ among students. Practice may be completed independently once the procedure has been performed satis-

TABLE 12. GUIDELINES FOR PRESENTING A DEMONSTRATION

Preparation:
1. Identify relevant readings and other activities to prepare learners for demonstration.
2. For complex procedures, develop written guidelines for focusing observations during demonstration.
3. Practice demonstration beforehand so skilled in performing procedure and manipulating any related equipment.
4. Time demonstration beforehand including time for:
    Preparation
    Introduction to demonstration
    Actual demonstration
    Discussion following demonstration
    Practice by learners
    Clean up

Before Demonstration:
1. Prepare materials and equipment before learners arrive and test equipment to assure working order.
2. Arrange materials and equipment so they can be visualized by all learners.
3. Introduce purpose of demonstration and provide overview of procedure to be demonstrated.
4. Review materials and equipment used in procedure.
5. Discuss underlying principles prior to beginning demonstration.
6. Identify important features to be observed in demonstration.
7. Check that all learners can see demonstration and hear related explanation.

Demonstration:
1. Demonstrate steps of procedure in same sequence as would be followed in practice.
2. Describe procedure as demonstrating it with emphasis on procedure itself and important points in performing it.
3. Avoid details that are not essential to proper performance.
4. Emphasize how procedure is performed rather than how not to perform it.
5. Monitor pace of demonstration.

After Demonstration:
1. Repeat demonstration or segments of it if students need further observation of procedure.
2. Discuss procedure immediately following demonstration and review again important points in performing it.
3. Provide opportunity for supervised practice considering individual differences of learners as to amount of practice, feedback, and reinforcement needed.
4. Take into consideration left-handed learners if relevant to performance of procedure.
5. Evaluate demonstration and identify areas for modification with subsequent ones.

factorily. Additional guidelines for carrying out a demonstration are presented in Table 12.

Guidelines for Use
1. Learners should have an understanding of the procedure demonstrated and underlying principles.
2. The teacher needs to be skillful in performing the procedure.
3. All learners must be able to see the demonstration and hear the related explanation.

4. Discussion of the procedure and underlying principles should take place before and after the actual demonstration.

5. During the demonstration, the teacher's explanation should focus on the procedure itself and should draw attention to important aspects.

6. Learners should have an opportunity to practice the procedure immediately following the demonstration and receive feedback from the teacher or from another person with expertise in the procedure as they are learning how to perform it.

7. If the demonstration is shown in media, arrangements should be made for supervised practice by learners following viewing.

8. As learners are practicing, the teacher should provide feedback and reinforcement without additional questions or discussion to allow them to focus on the steps of the procedure.

9. The amount of practice and feedback needed will differ among learners.

Media

Media provide for multisensory learning. Depending on the form, they communicate a message to the learner through varied sensory modes: visual, such as with slides and filmstrips; auditory, as with audiotapes; tactile with use of models and other objects to be manipulated; and often through a combination of these. In general, the more senses involved the easier it is for learners to conceptualize the message communicated. Auditory learning requires students to visualize internally what is heard. Combining auditory and visual modes enables learners to hear and see the message simultaneously, which permits visualization of the concept or activity to be learned and provides an accompanying description of it. Media create a vicarious experience for learners. They give learners an idea of what a situation is like, which is important in preparing them for clinical practice and for their own experiencing of that situation.

Media have an advantage of being able to show remote and inaccessible processes and events, close-up pictures, and procedures in which learners may not have an opportunity to observe or participate in themselves. They are appropriate for teaching problem solving and decision making. With psychomotor skills, media provide a means of demonstrating the skill and emphasizing the critical elements in performing it. Media also promote affective learning by introducing learners to clinical situations that can be examined for value connotations. Situations depicted through media lend themselves to critical analysis by learners, individually or in small groups, from an affective perspective.

There is a wide range of print and nonprint media available for clinical teaching, as indicated in Table 13. It is important for learn-

TABLE 13. TYPES OF MEDIA

Print	Nonprint
Handout	Audiotape/record
Pamphlet	Computer
Programmed instruction (printed)	Film
Textbook	Filmloop
Workbook/study guide	Filmstrip
	Model
	Multimedia program
	Overhead transparency
	Photograph
	Real object
	Slide
	Television
	Videotape

ers to develop skill in evaluating the quality of care as seen in the media, judging the appropriateness of specific interventions and procedures for one's own setting and practice, and adapting, if necessary, what they have learned in the media for use with clients and others in the clinical setting.

Guidelines for Use

1. Selection of appropriate media must be based on the objectives to be achieved in practice and individual learner needs.
2. The media should reflect the level of the learner in terms of knowledge, skill, and clinical practice experience.
3. The quality of the media and applicability to clinical practice must be evaluated by the teacher prior to use.
4. The media may be completed in the learning laboratory or clinical setting individually by learners or in small groups.
5. Students need assistance in applying and often adapting what they learn through media to their own practice.
6. The purpose for use of the media and how the media relate to the clinical experience and to their own learning needs should be clear to learners.
7. Group discussion following completion of media provides a way of judging appropriateness for the setting, applying concepts learned to clinical practice, exploring the affective dimension, and evaluating the quality of the media.
8. Media should be integrated within the total learning experience to complement other teaching methods used in the field and to avoid excessive repetition with these strategies.
9. With use of media, particularly when completed independently, the teacher should identify with students where further learning and additional experiences are necessary.

Self-directed

Self-directed teaching methods are based on a phenomenologic concept of learning that recognizes learning as an individual process requiring active involvement of the learner. This view acknowledges the uniqueness of the individual and his or her ability to make choices and decisions about learning. There is sufficient evidence to support the wide range of individual differences among learners. Students enter the learning situation with different levels of knowledge and skill, past experiences, cultural backgrounds, cognitive styles, teaching preferences, and rates of learning. Self-directed teaching methods attempt to reflect individual differences and needs among learners. With these methods, the responsibility for learning rests with the learner.

There are multiple strategies for self-directed learning. The degree of learner choice and control over the learning experience differs with the method. Learning contract and independent study, for example, are designed and controlled by the learner while other strategies, such as modules, multimedia programs, and computer-assisted instruction, are developed by the teacher or are available commercially. Even though the teacher may be responsible for the design or selection of the instructional materials, the learner can still choose alternate or additional learning activities, select the setting (home, work, library, or elsewhere) in which the learning will take place, and control the amount of time in learning and pace (Bell & Bell, 1983).

Four self-directed teaching methods are described:

1. Learning contract
2. Independent study
3. Self-paced module
4. Computer-assisted instruction

Learning Contract. A learning contract represents a written agreement between the teacher and learner specifying their responsibilities in terms of outcomes to be achieved. The learner then fulfills the contract independently. Contracts enable learners to pursue individual objectives related to clinical practice, which are compatible with overall program and course goals, according to their preferred styles of learning and with learning activities and resources identified by them. They also provide for choice in evaluation methods and process. In discussing the use of contracts, Carl Rogers (1983) writes: "Contracts provide a sort of transitional experience between complete freedom to learn whatever is of interest and learning that is relatively free, but that is within the limits of some institutional demand and course requirement" (p. 149).

The contract, developed by the learner in collaboration with faculty or a preceptor, generally includes the following components:

1. Goals and objectives to be achieved in field practice upon completion of the contract.
2. Types of learning activities to be carried out within a designated time frame.
3. Expectations of the faculty/preceptor and student.
4. Evaluation methods and materials and other evidence to be submitted.
5. Credit allocation and grading, if applicable.
6. Date for completion of the contract.

A format for a learning contract is illustrated in Table 14.

Guidelines for Use

1. The objectives to be achieved through the learning contract should be congruent with the clinical objectives.
2. Learners need to be oriented to the use of the contract method in field practice, elements to be included, and the relationship to clinical evaluation and to the grade.
3. The teacher should assist the learner in developing the contract and assessing whether the objectives and learning activities are realistic, considering the level of the learner, time for learning, and other constraints.
4. The contract should be negotiated by the teacher and learner and should be mutually acceptable.
5. Periodic conferences should be held between teacher and learner to provide for formative evaluation.
6. The contract may be modified under special circumstances if the alterations are agreed upon by those who signed it.

Independent Study. In independent study the learner is given freedom to manage his or her own learning without the formalized procedure of negotiating a learning contract. The objectives to be achieved through independent study may be determined by the learner in collaboration with the teacher or by the teacher with the student then independently pursuing relevant experiences. Independent study is valuable in meeting individual learning needs of students relative to field practice, assisting them in preparation for a clinical experience, and enabling them to investigate a particular clinical problem in depth.

Guidelines for Use

1. An orientation to independent study and how to proceed with it is important in preparing learners for use of this method in field practice.

2. Some learners may need guidance from the teacher as to the process of independent study and identification and use of resources for learning.
3. Learners should be held accountable for meeting the objectives identified for learning through independent study.
4. Periodic conferences between faculty and learner are needed to provide for formative evaluation.

Self-paced Module. Self-paced modules represent another means of individualizing instruction and providing for self-directed learning. A module is a self-contained unit of instruction which is completed independently by the learner. Students progress through the module at their own rates of learning, taking as much time as necessary to achieve mastery. Depending on their learning needs, students may omit learning activities, repeat them, or participate in additional ones. The learning activities often represent various strategies, such as media and readings. Through pretests that enable them to identify objectives already attained, learners are able to determine the most appropriate point in the module at which to begin the instruction.

For field practice, a module may be used for acquisition of knowledge and development of skills as a prerequisite to practice, preparation for specific clinical experiences, review of content or skills, and for learning beyond any particular clinical requirement. Modules are appropriate for use in orientation of nurses to a clinical setting and for updating their knowledge and skills in practice.

A self-paced module generally contains the following components:

1. Purpose of module.
2. Pretest for determining objectives already met.
3. Objectives,including any prerequisites.
4. Learning activities, allowing for choice and assisting in application of content to clinical practice, and resources for learning.
5. Posttest or other evaluation strategy for determining if students attained the objectives.

It also is important that a strategy, such as use of questions, be incorporated in the module to allow for periodic assessment of progress toward meeting the objectives and provide feedback to learners as they are completing the instruction.

Guidelines for Use
1. Modules used for field practice should reflect the clinical objectives and individual learner needs.
2. Faculty should evaluate the quality of the module and relevance to clinical practice prior to use with learners.

TABLE 14. LEARNING CONTRACT

Name _____   Course _____
Dates:
   Started _____   Clinical Agency _____

   Completed _____   Faculty _____

Credits _____   Preceptor _____

Grade _____

Nature of field practice experience: _____

_____

_____

_____

_____

Section I: Goals and Objectives

A. *Goals:* Write a statement of your goals for this field practice experience. Identify how these goals relate to your professional goals. _____

_____

_____

_____

_____

B. *Objectives:* Write the objectives for this experience that you expect to achieve. ____

_____

_____

_____

_____

Section II: Learning Activities

A. *Learning Activities:* Identify learning activities which you will carry out to achieve these objectives. Code each activity in relation to the objectives stated above. ____

_____

_____

_____

_____

B. *Schedule of Activities:* Project a calendar of activities. (Consult with faculty/preceptor where relevant). _____

_____

_____

_____

_____

TABLE 14. (*Continued*)

Section III: Student–Faculty/Preceptor Expectations

A. *Student:* Describe your expectations of the faculty/preceptor in this field experience. _____

_____

_____

_____

_____

B. *Faculty/preceptor:* Describe your expectations of the student in this field experience. _____

_____

_____

_____

_____

Section IV: Evaluation

A. *Evaluation Methods:* Identify evaluation methods and materials to be submitted. ___

_____

_____

_____

_____

B. *Evaluation Report:* Prepare a written evaluation report of the field practice experience in terms of stated goals and objectives. _____

_____

_____

_____

_____

Section V: Agreement

This agreement is considered fulfilled when all elements of the contract are met. If circumstances arise which inhibit fulfilling this agreement within the designated time, an incomplete grade will be received and terms for the extension of the contract will be negotiated. If changes in the agreement are indicated, negotiation for these changes will occur with the student, faculty, and preceptor.

Student Signature _____ Date _____

Faculty Signature _____ Date _____

Preceptor Signature _____ Date _____

3. With modular learning, faculty, preceptor, student assistant, or peer with expertise in the area should be available to assist with learning and practice of behaviors, answer questions, and recommend additional learning experiences if necessary.
4. It is important to assist students in applying to clinical practice what they have learned in modular format and practiced independently.
5. The teacher is responsible for assessing if further learning and practice are needed.

Computer-assisted Instruction. Computer-assisted instruction (CAI) provides for active involvement of the learner in responding to questions asked by the computer and making decisions regarding clinical situations presented. CAI also allows for differing rates of learning. CAI may be used to assist learners in acquiring knowledge needed for care of clients, analyzing data, deciding on clinical problems, selecting intervention strategies, and evaluating care.

There are several types of CAI: drill and practice, tutorial, and simulation.

In *drill and practice* questions are presented to learners seeking a response from them. The computer program then provides immediate feedback in terms of the response. Factual information, such as definitions of terms, laboratory values, and calculating dosages of medications, is particularly appropriate for drill and practice.

Tutorial provides for more feedback than with drill and practice. The computer presents information to the learner, then asks questions about the material, branching forward if the student responds correctly or backward if remediation is necessary (Hassett, 1984).

A *computer simulation* presents a real-life situation enabling the learner to make a series of clinical decisions similar to ones necessary in actual practice. The learner's decisions influence the information presented subsequently. Simulations are particularly appropriate for assisting students in analyzing client data or that related to a situation involving staff, identifying nursing diagnoses or staff-oriented problems from the data presented, proposing interventions, and evaluating the effectiveness of the approaches.

Guidelines for Use
1. There must be sufficient hardware available to support CAI.
2. Selection of the computer program should be based on the objectives and individual learner needs.
3. The program should be appropriate for the learner in terms of knowledge, skill, and clinical practice experience.
4. The quality of the computer program should be evaluated by faculty prior to use.

5. Discussion following completion of CAI provides a way of reviewing the information presented, clarifying students' questions, and assisting them in relating the information to clinical practice.
6. The teacher should identify with students where further learning and additional experiences are necessary.
7. The time and cost required for use of CAI should be justified in terms of learning and student and faculty satisfaction with the method.

Preceptorship

Clinical preceptors are staff nurses and other nursing practitioners in a clinical setting who serve as role model and teacher for students, new graduates, and other nurses through a one-to-one relationship. Preceptorships are based on the concept of modeling. Learners acquire or modify behaviors by observing vicariously a model who has the behaviors needed by the learner, and having an opportunity to practice those behaviors. Through modeling one acquires both the skills and professional style (for instance manner and attitudes) of the person observed, often with style emerging out of the acquisition of skills (Adelson, 1962). In this way, the student progresses from the development of necessary skills for practice to professional style.

In the role of teacher, the preceptor provides instruction for learners based on identified objectives and individual learner needs, provides feedback, assists learners in integrating education and work values, and is involved in their evaluation. The learner, in turn, has an opportunity to work and identify with a competent role model involved in decisions of clinical and unit management and ideally one who derives satisfaction from the work setting (Friesen & Conahan, 1980).

Many of the experiences involving preceptors, whether for students or new graduates, are designed to facilitate the transition from the student role to that of staff nurse. By working on a one-to-one basis with a practitioner functioning in the role, students and new graduates are able to model behaviors of the practitioner and become socialized into the professional role. Preceptors provide an opportunity for the development of a mentor relationship with the learner, important in facilitating role transition. Limón, Bargagliotti, and Spencer (1981) report that this close relationship which develops between the preceptor and learner promotes role acquisition and represents a positive experience for both the preceptor and learner.

There are various ways in which preceptors may be incorporated within nursing education programs depending on the goals to be achieved. Clinical courses, particularly those offered in the student's final semester or during the summer preceding the last year of study, may be designed to include the use of preceptors who act as role model and teacher for the student to whom assigned. Waters, Limón, and Spencer (1983) describe a four-week preceptorship program for associate degree in nursing students where the student is paired with a clinical preceptor to ease the transition from school to work and to develop skills in nursing management and caring for groups of patients. During the preceptorship, students are in the clinical setting the equivalent of full-time employment.

Experiences involving preceptors may also focus on the development of knowledge and clinical skills in a particular area of nursing practice. Often, students select their own area of practice and clinical setting, depending upon their objectives. The kinds of experiences in which students engage and the amount of time spent in the agency vary with the nursing program and objectives to be achieved.

When preceptors are used for clinical teaching, faculty functions in a different role than with other clinical courses. In general, the teacher is responsible for: (1) planning the experience with agency personnel and with the preceptor; (2) orienting students to the course, use of preceptors for clinical instruction, and faculty role; (3) assisting preceptors with educational problems that arise; (4) monitoring the experience and student achievement of the objectives; and (5) participating in evaluation. Although preceptors provide the clinical instruction, faculty has overall responsibility for the experience and an important role in monitoring it so student and program objectives are attained.

In clinical agencies, preceptors as part of an orientation program or a nurse internship facilitate role transition of the new graduate and entry into the work setting. Preceptors have also been used to assist experienced nurses in changing roles in the setting or moving into a new area of clinical practice.

Guidelines for Use
1. The objectives for the experience should be clearly identified.
2. The roles and responsibilities of the preceptor, learner, and faculty should be specified, particularly in relation to the selection of learning experiences, instruction in the setting, and evaluation of learning.
3. Lines of communication should be established among preceptor, learner, faculty, and other involved personnel in the clinical agency.
4. Preceptors, learners, and other personnel should be oriented to and prepared for the experience.
5. Recruitment of preceptors is a responsibility of clinical agency personnel, but the selection of preceptors, based on specific criteria, is a joint responsibility of faculty and agency staff.

6. For a preceptor program to be effective, preceptors need appropriate work schedules for carrying out their additional responsibilities, administrative support, and recognition for their efforts.
7. For programs involving students, contractual arrangements and the extent of preceptor liability should be clarified.

Systems for Concentrated Practice

Concentrated clinical practice is aimed at facilitating the transition from the student role to staff nurse role and increasing the learner's clinical and leadership skills and confidence in his or her own ability in practice. Concentrated practice is developed within some kind of system or pattern that includes experience with the practitioner role. Such practice, by enabling learners to function in the role for which they are preparing, provides a means of bridging the gap between school and work. This intensive clinical experience provides for experiential learning and the development of problem-solving and decision-making skills and reflects concepts of modeling, particularly with those strategies in which the student or new graduate is involved in a mentor relationship with a practitioner.

Three systems offering concentrated clinical practice include:

1. Externship
2. Work study
3. Internship

Externship. An externship provides opportunity for students to gain experience in a practice setting and receive both academic credit from the college/university and a salary from the agency, frequently at the rate of ancillary personnel, for the experience. Often offered in the summer preceding the final year of study, externships vary as to the number of credit hours, extent of time in the clinical setting, kinds of experiences in which students engage, and supervision of the learner. Students are frequently supervised by preceptors, with periodic contact with faculty who retains responsibility for planning, monitoring, and evaluating the experience.

Work Study. A work study program provides flexibility for the student to leave the educational setting for a period of time to engage in concentrated clinical practice, although usually in an ancillary position, and obtain experience with other systems of care. In this type of experience, employment is arranged by the nursing program or student and is limited to a specified length of time, for instance, a semester, generally coinciding with the student's academic schedule (Waters, Limón & Spencer, 1983). Faculty has a role in counseling students in the selection of clinical settings and type of experience so that the work study is an integral part of the total nursing program.

Internship. An internship refers to a work period immediately following formal education (Schein, 1972). With this model, the practice experience takes place after completion of an educational program rather than during it, as with externship and work study, and thus is arranged by the clinical setting in which the new graduate is employed. An internship represents a supervised orientation program aimed at facilitating the transition from student to staff nurse (Roell, 1981). Internships generally range in length from two to six months (Lewison & Gibbons, 1980).

Guidelines for Use

One set of guidelines is included for use of externship, work study, and internship.

1. Objectives for the experience should be clearly stated.
2. Learners must have the necessary knowledge base and skills for participating in concentrated clinical practice.
3. The kinds of experiences in which the learner is to engage and the person responsible for supervision should be clearly identified.
4. The nature and degree of supervision should be adapted according to the needs of individual learners.
5. Roles and responsibilities of the student or new graduate and others involved in the experience should be clarified.
6. Clear lines of communication among participants are essential for effective implementation.
7. Sharing of experiences among students and new graduates during their involvement in concentrated clinical practice is important in promoting learning; providing support among learners; and enabling them to share frustrations, concerns, and achievements.

SUMMARY

Planning for the field practice experience includes the decision as to teaching methods for promoting achievement of the objectives. No one teaching method is inclusive because of the multipurpose nature of the field, multiple activities inherent in nursing, variation in purpose and objectives for a specific clinical experience, and differences among learners and teachers. Teaching methods are classified as experiential, problem solving, conference, observation, media, self-directed, preceptorship, and systems for concentrated practice.

Experiential methods provide for direct experiencing of events either through clinical practice involving interaction with real clients and others in the field or through contrived experiences of reality, such as with simulations and role play. These methods include clinical assignment, various written assignments, and simulation/game.

Problem-solving methods assist learners in analyzing a clinical situation to identify problems to be solved and relevant actions to be taken and in applying knowledge to a clinical problem. There are three types of problem-solving methods appropriate for teaching in the field: problem-solving situation, decision-making situation, and incident process.

Clinical conferences are group discussions about some aspect of clinical practice. Pre- and post-conference, peer review, issue, and multidisciplinary are types of conferences relevant for clinical teaching.

Observational teaching methods include observation in the field, field trip, nursing rounds, and demonstration. A wide range of print and nonprint media is also appropriate for teaching in the field.

Self-directed methods recognize learning as an individual process requiring active involvement of the learner. Strategies classified as self-directed include learning contract, independent study, self-paced module, and computer-assisted instruction.

Preceptorships and systems for concentrated practice, externship, work study and internship, facilitate transition from the student role to staff nurse role. These methods also promote the development of the learner's clinical skills and confidence in his or her own ability in practice.

Criteria assist faculty in relating teaching methods to the demands of the learning situation. The teacher's task is to choose from these classifications methods that fit with the objectives, learners, teacher, and clinical setting in which the practice takes place.

REFERENCES

Adelson, J. (1962). The teacher as model. In N. Sanford (Ed.). *The American college: A psychological and social interpretation of the higher learning.* New York: Wiley.

Bandura, A. (1977). *Social learning theory.* Englewood Cliffs, N. J.: Prentice-Hall.

Barham, B., Gaffney, D. A., Larsen, C., et al. (1977). *Pediatrix.* Mimeographed.

Bell, D. F., & Bell, D. L. (1983). Harmonizing self-directed and teacher-directed approaches to learning. *Nurse Educator, VIII*(1), 24–30.

Blood money. (1975) New York: Gamed/Simulations.

Caracappa, M., Nagy-McMenamin, D., & Yuschak, M. G. (1977). *Assylumation.* Mimeographed.

Clark, C. C. (1978). *Classroom skills for nurse educators.* New York: Springer.

Cooper, S. S. (1978). Methods of teaching—revisited. *The Journal of Continuing Education in Nursing, 9*(4), 24–26.

Cooper, S. S. (1979). Methods of teaching—revisited: Games and simulation. *The Journal of Continuing Education in Nursing, 10*(5), 14, 47–48.
Cooper, S. S. (1981). Methods of teaching—revisited: The incident process. *The Journal of Continuing Education in Nursing, 12*(6), 22–24.
Cooper, S. S. (1982a). Methods of teaching—revisited: The demonstration. *The Journal of Continuing Education in Nursing, 13*(3), 44–45.
Cooper, S. S. (1982b). Methods of teaching—revisited: Nursing rounds and bedside clinics. *The Journal of Continuing Education in Nursing, 13*(5), 19–21.
Crancer, J., & Maury-Hess, S. (1980). Games: An alternative to pedagogical instruction. *Journal of Nursing Education, 19*(3), 45–52.
deTornyay, R., & Thompson, M. A. (1982). *Strategies for teaching nursing* (2nd ed.). New York: Wiley.
Friesen, L., & Conahan, B. J. (1980). A clinical preceptor program: Strategy for new graduate orientation. *Journal of Nursing Administration, X*(4), 18–23.
Greenblat, C. S. (1977). Gaming-simulation and health education: An overview. *Health Education Monographs, 5*(1), 5–10.
Hales, G. D. (1984). *Interactive video in nursing: Review of concepts and projects.* Paper presented at the annual meeting of The Society for Research in Nursing Education, San Francisco, Calif.
Hassett, M. R. (1984). Computers and nursing education in the 1980s. *Nursing Outlook, 32,* 34–36.
Hyman, R. T. (1974). *Ways of teaching* (2nd ed.). Philadelphia: Lippincott.
Into aging. (1978). Thorofare, N. J.: Charles B. Slack, (developed by T. L. Hoffman & S. Dempsey).
Lewison, D., & Gibbons, L. K. (1980). Nursing internships: A comprehensive review of the literature. *The Journal of Continuing Education in Nursing, 11*(2), 32–37.
Limón, S., Bargagliotti, L. A., & Spencer, J. B. (1981). Who precepts the preceptor? *Nursing and Health Care, II,* 433–36.
McKeachie, W. J. (1962). Procedures and techniques of teaching: A survey of experimental studies. In N. Sanford (Ed.), *The American college: A psychological and social interpretation of the higher learning.* New York: Wiley.
Reilly, D. E. (1958). *Nursing student responses to the clinical field.* New York: Columbia University, Department of Nursing.
Reilly, D. E. (1980). *Behavioral objectives—evaluation in nursing* (2nd ed.). New York: Appleton-Century-Crofts.
Roell, S. M. (1981). Nurse-intern programs: How they're working. *Nurse Educator VI*(6), 29–31.
Rogers, C. R. (1983). *Freedom to learn for the 80's.* Columbus, Ohio: Chas. E. Merrill.
Schein, E. H. (1972). *Professional education.* New York: McGraw-Hill.
Schweer, J. E., & Gebbie, K. M. (1976). *Creative teaching in clinical nursing* (3rd ed.). St. Louis: C. V. Mosby.
Smoyak, S. A. (1977). Use of gaming simulation by health care professionals. *Health Education Monographs, 5*(1), 11–17.
Starpower. (1969). Del Mar, Calif.: Simile II.

Waters, V., Limón, S., & Spencer, J. B. (1983). *Ohlone transition: Student to staff nurse.* Battle Creek, Mich.: W. K. Kellogg Foundation.

BIBLIOGRAPHY

Ball, M. J., & Hannah, K. J. (1984). *Using computers in nursing.* Reston, Va.: Reston.

Billings, D. M. (1984). Evaluating computer assisted instruction. *Nursing Outlook, 32,* 50–53.

Burke, R. L. (1982). *CAI sourcebook.* Englewood Cliffs, N.J.: Prentice-Hall.

Christian, P. L., & Smith, L. S. (1981). Using video tapes to teach interviewing skills. *Nurse Educator, VI*(4), 12–14.

Clark, C. C. (1976). Simulation gaming: A new teaching strategy in nursing education. *Nurse Educator, I*(4), 4–9.

Cooper, S. S. (1982). Methods of teaching—revisited: Experiential diaries and learning logs. *The Journal of Continuing Education in Nursing, 13*(6), 32–34.

Corbett, N. A., & Beveridge, P. (1982). Simulation as a tool for learning. *Topics in Clinical Nursing, 4*(3), 58–67.

Craig, J. L., & Page, G. (1981). The questioning skills of nursing instructors. *Journal of Nursing Education, 20*(5), 18–23.

Dear, M. R., & Bartol, G. (1984). Independent study as a learning experience in baccalaureate nursing programs: Perceptions and practices. *Journal of Nursing Education, 23,* 240–44.

DiRienzo, J. N. (1983). Before client care—An interactive conference. *Journal of Nursing Education, 22,* 84–86.

Eble, K. E. (1976). *The craft of teaching.* San Francisco: Jossey-Bass.

Farrell, J. J. (1981). Media in the nursing curriculum. *Nurse Educator, VI*(4), 15–19.

French, P. (1980). Academic gaming in nursing education. *Journal of Advanced Nursing, 5,* 601–12.

Huckabay, L. M. D. (1981). The effects of modularized instruction and traditional teaching techniques on cognitive learning and affective behaviors of student nurses. *Advances in Nursing Science, 3*(3), 67–82.

Kirchhoff, K., & Holzemer, W. L. (1979). Student learning and a computer-assisted instructional program. *Journal of Nursing Education, 18*(3), 22–30.

Limón, S., Bargagliotti, L. A., & Spencer, J. B. (1982). Providing preceptors for nursing students: What questions should you ask? *The Journal of Nursing Administration, XII*(6), 16–19.

Limón, S., Spencer, J. B., & Waters, V. (1981). A clinical preceptorship to prepare reality-based ADN graduates. *Nursing & Health Care,* 267–69.

Martens, K. H. (1981). Self-directed learning: An option for nursing education. *Nursing Outlook, 29,* 472–77.

Mirin, S. (1981). The computer's place in nursing education. *Nursing & Health Care, II,* 500–6.

Mitchell, C. A., & Krainovich, B. (1982). Conducting pre- and postconferences. *American Journal of Nursing, 82,* 823–25.

Oermann, M. (1984). An instrument for analyzing curriculum materials in nursing. *Journal of Nursing Education, 23,* 404–6.

Oermann, M. H. (1984). Analyzing and selecting audiovisual materials. *Nurse Educator, 9*(4), 24–27.

Olson, R. K., Gresley, R. S., & Heater, B. S. (1984). The effects of an undergraduate clinical internship on the self-concept and professional role mastery of baccalaureate nursing students. *Journal of Nursing Education, 23,* 105–8.

Pigors, P., & Pigors, F. (1966). The incident process—A method of inquiry. *Nursing Outlook, 14*(10), 48–50.

Plasterer, H. H., & Mills, N. (1983). Teach management theory—Through fun and games. *Journal of Nursing Education, 22,* 80–83.

Redman, B. K. (1983). *The process of patient teaching in nursing* (5th ed.). St. Louis: C. V. Mosby.

Sasmor, J. L. (1984). Contracting for clinical. *Journal of Nursing Education, 23,* 171–73.

Schleutermann, J. A., Holzemer, W. L., & Farrand, L. L. (1983). An evaluation of paper-and-pencil and computer-assisted simulations. *Journal of Nursing Education, 22,* 315–23.

Sleet, D. A., & Hileman, L. (1981). *Guide to health instruction: Simulations, games, and related activities.* Irvine, Calif.: Human Behavior Research Group.

Sleet, D. A., & Stadsklev, R. (1977). Annotated bibliography of simulations and games in health education. *Health Education Monographs, 5*(1), 74–90.

Stuart-Siddall, S., & Haberlin, J. M. (Eds.), (1983). *Preceptorships in nursing education.* Rockville, Md: Aspen Systems.

Swedsen, L. A. (1981). Self instruction: Benefits and problems. *Nurse Educator, VI*(6), 6–9.

Wolf, Z. R., & O'Driscoll, R. (1979). How useful is the preclinical conference? *Nursing Outlook, 27,* 455–57.

6

Cognitive Learning in the Clinical Field

Individuals function as total integrated beings in all human experiences. The learning process engages the learner in a holistic fashion along cognitive, psychomotor, and affective dimensions. In education, there is reference to these three areas; i.e., cognitive, psychomotor, and affective, as domains of learning. Although most learning involves a composite of behavioral responses from all three domains, educators have found it helpful to consider the domains separately for instructional purposes. Because of the special characteristics of performance for each domain, this chapter and chapters 7 and 8 address separately the specific theoretical constructs and teaching processes of each area. Although each domain of learning is emphasized as a separate entity, the teacher must constantly bear in mind that the domains are interrelated, and indeed, this interrelationship may be essential for expert performance of any one skill.

Knowledge has always been recognized as essential to nursing, but how has the term knowledge been generally used? Does it mean "know about something?" or does it refer to an inherent action, "knowing how?" Today's nursing practice must encompass both "knowing about" and "knowing how," for nursing is a discipline that practices in concert with other health professionals, all influenced by the impact of exploding knowledge and technology. The expanding boundaries of knowledge create the need for disciplines like nursing to reexamine its roles and responsibilities and the nature of preparation of its practitioners.

Historically, nurses were receivers of information from others. This information then served as a basis for nursing knowledge. The discrepancy between nursing and medical knowledge occurred as a result of medical education moving into the university, where it began to develop its scientific base, while nursing maintained the practice mode of apprenticeship learning. Nursing then "adopted" the physician's knowledge and incorporated it into nursing knowledge. The usual learning experiences entailed lectures by the physician on a given pathologic phenomenon followed by a class on nursing of that phenomenon. Nursing knowledge was predominantly prescriptive for the medical state of the patient. The authoritarian structure of the hospital setting, modeled from the religious and military influences of nursing's beginnings, left little margin for creative thinkers among nurses in terms of designing nursing care or patterns by which the care was delivered.

Indeed, nursing still does borrow theories, but a new direction is underway as nursing research is generating nursing knowledge. In pursuit of this knowledge, "knowing how" has become a significant factor. This "knowing how" entails the cognitive processes of concept attainment, problem solving, decision making, critical thinking, and clinical judgment, which addresses skills in using and validating both nursing and borrowed knowledge. Emphasis is now on cognitive skill development, which considers knowledge as a dynamic factor to be developed and constantly tested. Solutions to problems in patient care and the delivery of this care are more complex and require different cognitive skills than in the past. In this chapter, each of these cognitive processes is explored and its relationship to teaching in the cognitive domain in nursing is demonstrated.

CONCEPT LEARNING

Although the acquisition of facts and specific information relevant to nursing practice represents an important outcome of a nursing education program, it certainly is not the primary goal of teaching. The fragile nature of facts in an information society requires that students learn concepts and theories of knowledge domains pertinent to nursing. The use of this knowledge depends upon the development of intellectual skills for analyzing and evaluating situations encountered in the practice field. Concepts provide a means for individuals to group together facts and organize their perceptions and experiences. Through the learning of concepts, students are able to categorize new information. Since theories consist of concepts, concept attainment is a prerequisite to the acquisition of theories for use in practice.

There are many concepts to be learned for the practice of nursing. Some concepts relate to the client, such as health, aging, and pain; others pertain to nursing actions, for instance, nursing process and more specifically, positioning and touch. Still others reflect the physical, social, and symbolic environment, such as territory, social support, and power (Kim, 1983).

Learning would be a difficult process if information was acquired through memorization alone. Students, especially in the health fields, are continually faced with a mass of details to be learned, and the management of this can only be accomplished through the learning of concepts. Concept learning refers to the classifying of somewhat different events or objects into a single category (Ellis, 1972). The process of conceptualization, placing events or objects into categories, serves to reduce the complexity of the environment and enables learners to identify different events and objects in it. Concepts also reduce the need for constant learning and give direction as to actions to be taken (Bruner, Goodnow, & Austin, 1956). For example, once students have learned the concept of pain, they do not have to relearn this concept with each client and instead only need to assess whether or not the essential defining properties are present. If the patient exhibits these defining properties, then "it" is pain. To know that the patient is in pain also provides direction as to appropriate nursing actions to be taken. Concepts enable learners to relate different classes of events and objects to one another to form systems. Bruner and colleagues (1956) write:

> For we operate . . . with category *systems*—classes of events that are related to each other in various kinds of superordinate systems. We map and give meaning to our world by relating classes of events rather than by relating individual events. (p. 13)

Definition of Concept

Concept refers to a general *idea* reflecting a group of events or objects that share common characteristics. It represents a generalization about particulars (Norris, 1982). Martorella (1972), drawing upon research by Bruner and colleagues (1956) and Viaud (1960), defines concept as a "continuum of inferences by which a set of observed characteristics of an object or event suggests a class identity" (p. 5). Inferences are made from observations by the learner which in turn suggest additional inferences about other unobserved characteristcs.

Characteristics of Concepts

Concepts may be considered as categories of events or objects which have certain attributes, a rule which defines the category, and exemplars or positive instances of the concept. Attributes are "those characteristics which are the identifying features of a concept, and which enable one to distinguish between exemplars and nonexemplars" (Martorella, 1972, p. 7). An attribute, then, is a characteristic of the event or object relevant for grouping it into a category. The concept of patient refers to someone receiving health care. Whether or not such a person is male or female or is young or old are attributes irrelevant to the concept of patient. In learning a concept, one identifies the relevant attributes and learns to ignore irrelevant ones.

The greater the number of irrelevant attributes, the more difficult it is to learn the concept since it becomes harder to identify the relevant ones (Ellis, 1972). "The addition of even a single irrelevant attribute adds considerably to the difficulty of the learning task" (Glaser, 1969, p. 723).

Attributes combined in certain ways represent a rule. The rule states the essential attributes for defining the concept; it is how the attributes are combined. In the preceding example, patient refers to a person receiving health care. The rule here is that the person must be receiving health care.

Exemplars are positive instances or examples of the concept, while nonexemplars are negative instances. Exemplars carry important information to assist the learner in identifying what the concept is. Research indicates that individuals learn more efficiently from positive instances of the concept than from negative ones (Glaser, 1969). Learning the concept of empathy proceeds more efficiently if examples of empathy are given emphasis rather than instances of a lack of empathy. Yet, it is also important, particularly with concepts that are difficult to acquire, that learners attend to the negative instances as well as the positive in order to use all of the information available to identify the concept. Concepts are learned more efficiently when the positive and negative examples are distinct from one another (Travers, 1972). For instance, the concept of pain is difficult to learn because instances of pain vary and sometimes there is not a clear distinction between pain and a lack of it.

Types of Concepts

Bruner and colleagues (1956) identified three types of concepts or categories: conjunctive, disjunctive, and relational. These three classes of concepts are basically different types of rules for grouping attributes. A conjunctive concept, which is relatively easy to learn, is the joint presence of several attributes or characteristics. Consider the concept of nursing team. Essential attributes of this concept are that it consists of a group of at least two persons who represent nursing personnel. If either of these characteristics is not present, then "it" is not a nursing team.

In contrast, disjunctive concepts are categories where the events or objects share alternate attributes; one or another of the attributes defines the concept. A professional organization with a membership requirement such as "any nurse residing in a certain region or employed in a particular type of clinical agency" exemplifies a disjunctive category. The difficulty with disjunctive concepts is that the attributes are not necessarily related to one another but still define the concept. For this reason, Bruner and associates have suggested that disjunctive concepts are more difficult to attain than conjunctive ones. "What is particularly difficult about attaining a disjunctive category is that two of its members, each uniform in terms of an ultimate criterion, may have no defining attributes in common" (Bruner et al., 1956, pp. 156–57). Pain is an example of a disjunctive concept. Attributes that define pain vary but, nevertheless, can be grouped together for use in identifying the concept of pain.

A relational concept is one in which there is a specific relationship between defining attributes. Equation is an example of a relational concept since it expresses a relationship between quantities.

Concept Attainment

Concept attainment involves learning what attributes (or characteristics) are relevant for grouping events or objects into categories and learning the rule to be applied for grouping them. It is the search for defining attributes to distinguish exemplars from nonexemplars of the various concepts (Bruner et al., 1956). Concept attainment, then, is the process of learning a concept invented by someone else. In contrast, concept formation occurs when learners develop concepts of their own.

Nursing diagnosis is an example of a concept attainment task in that the nurse groups attributes, or cues, into a diagnostic category. Nursing diagnoses are disjunctive concepts and are complex because of the number of cues that need to be interpreted and then grouped together, their variability, and their probabilistic nature. Identification of one nursing diagnosis does not necessarily exclude others.

Concepts assist learners in categorizing events and objects they deal with in the practice setting. They enable learners to give meaning to what they perceive. There are many concepts to be learned for effective practice in nursing. To attain these concepts, the learner must identify the relevant attributes for grouping events and objects into the category and rule to be applied.

PROBLEM SOLVING

In the clinical setting, students are continually confronted with problems, either client- or setting-oriented, demanding resolution. Some of these are relatively easy to solve, but most tend to represent difficult tasks for the learner because of the complexity of the problem and solutions or the learner's unfamiliarity with them. Most faculty would acknowledge the importance of the development of problem-solving ability as a critical outcome of a nursing education program. However, Frederickson and Mayer (1977) concluded from a study of associate and baccalaureate nursing students that both groups lacked skill in problem solving, particularly in the evaluation of the solutions proposed. The researchers question if students are actually taught to problem solve and held accountable by faculty for independently solving clinical problems.

Problem-solving Process

The problem-solving process has been viewed as a series of steps commencing with definition of the problem and proceeding through the gathering of data relative to the problem, formulation of solutions, and testing and evaluation of the solutions chosen. It involves developing and then testing hypotheses that represent possible solutions to the problem. Once the hypotheses have been formulated, the learner deduces the logical implications of each. The hypotheses are then tested until the problem is solved:

Parnes (1984) writes that in problem solving:

> The problem-solver goes from an examination of "what is" to an explanation of "what might be" to a judgment of "what should be" to an assessment of "what can be" to a decision of "what will be" to action that becomes a new "what is." (p. 30)

"What is" refers to an understanding of the data relative to the problem; "what might be" implies the development of solutions; "what should be" involves decisions as to the solutions; "what can be" refers to adaptations of approaches into usable solutions; and "what will be" indicates the best plans for solving the problem (Parnes, 1984).

Problem solving is influenced by the learner's knowledge of concepts and theories and past experiences with similar problems. Knowledge is essential for both understanding the problem and arriving at solutions. Past experience with a clinical situation influences a practitioner's perception of the situation and predisposition to act in a certain way. Expert nurses and beginners differ in their problem solving in that the expert perceives the clinical situation as a whole, in comparison with the beginner who tends to focus on pieces of information, and uses past concrete situations as paradigm cases for approaching the present one (Benner, 1984). Individuals facing a problem new to them do not have past situations to refer to and use as a guide for action. They approach problems primarily from a theoretical perspective, which does not take into account the context and variables associated with the specific case, thus limiting their understanding of the situation and ability to identify possible responses. Through experience the learner comes to know what to expect typically in regard to a particular problem and what actions are appropriately taken.

Problem solving is also influenced by the learner's stage of cognitive development, the ability to think and reason. Theories of cognitive development propose that problem-solving abilities and thinking differ according to the stage the learner is at. With advanced stages of development, individuals are able to solve more complex problems (Stonewater & Stonewater, 1984) because they have a greater repertoire of knowledge and ability to manipulate it and have a different perspective about the nature of knowledge and truth.

Theories of Problem Solving

Problem solving has been described according to three theoretical perspectives: (1) stimulus-response theory, (2) cognitive-field theory, and (3) information processing theory.

Stimulus–response Theory. The stimulus–response view of problem solving regards it mostly in terms of covert trial and error behavior. According to this theory, the learner brings to the problem a number of possible habits, or responses, arranged in a hierarchy and varying in strength (Ellis, 1972). Different responses are attempted, in order of their strength, until the correct one is found. Stimulus–response theory does not recognize the process of ideation or thinking. Problem-solving behavior involves trying covertly various solutions until the problem is solved.

Cognitive-field Theory. Cognitive-field theory considers problem solving as a reorganization of one's perception of the world, thereby facilitating achievement of insight into the problem or solution. Problems are approached through the process of reflective thinking in which learners develop new or change existing insights or understandings. Reflective thinking involves recognition of the problem, development of hypotheses (potential solutions in the form of generalizations), and testing of these hypotheses. In cognitive-field theory, the problem is recognized when the learner experiences conflicting goals, an obstacle to goal achievement, or a "newly sensed discrepancy in known data" (Bigge, 1982, p. 105). As the individual continually encounters problems, learnings occur. It is this integration of new learnings into the total cognitive field that provides for transfer to new problem situations. The development of problem-solving skill continues to evolve through repeated experiences with problems.

Information Processing Theory. Information processing theory, a relatively new approach to problem solving, views problem solving in terms of an interaction between the individual, considered an information processing system; and task environment, the task or problem as described by an observer. Problem space is the individual's way of viewing the task environment (Simon, 1978). It is the problem solver's internal representation of the task and serves as the "space" in which the problem-solving activities take place.

In problem-solving, information is extracted from the task environment and used to search for solutions in the problem space. The problem space "contains not only the actual solution but possible solutions that the problem-solver might consider" (Newell & Simon, 1972, p. 809). One way of problem solving involves recognizing the answer which, according to Newell and Simon, indicates the answer "was already in memory and was simply evoked by the act of understanding the question" (p. 94). If the solution is not already in memory and recognized by the learner, then a number of other problem-solving strategies may be used, such as the generate and test method where possible solutions are tested until the problem is resolved.

One of the limitations on the ability to problem solve involves the amount of information the person can process at any given time. This is determined by short- and long-term memory. Short-term memory is used for processing information from the environment which is then either forgotten or stored in long-term memory. There is a limited amount of information that is able to be held in short-term memory, generally between 7 ± 2 two familiar symbols or chunks (Miller, 1956); and information stored there decays in a brief period of time unless rehearsed (Newell & Simon, 1972).

Information is held in long-term memory as sets of associated symbols. There are different theories as to the way knowledge is organized in long-term memory. Biomedical knowledge appears to be "stored in a *hierarchical* manner, wherein abstract concepts are linked with less abstract examples of that concept" (Tanner, 1984b, p. 71). This organization provides sets of concepts and examples for retrieval and use in problem solving.

In complex problem-solving tasks, similar to concept attainment, cognitive strain may be experienced when the individual is faced with extensive information to be assimilated which, in turn, exerts a strain on memory or inference (Bruner et al., 1956). As a result, the individual needs to resort to different cognitive strategies, such as grouping data, to assist in processing the information. In the clinical setting, these strategies help the practitioner deal with the extensive amount of and often complex information with which presented.

Intuition

Not all problem solving involves use of a conscious and logical sequence of steps to identify the problem and arrive at a solution. Problems are also solved through intuition, an understanding in which the individual is unaware of how it occurred. Bruner (1963) views intuition as "the intellectual technique of arriving at plausible but tentative formulations without going through the analytic steps by which such formulations would be found to be valid or invalid conclusions" (p. 13). Intuitive thinking does not follow a careful sequence of steps toward problem solution but instead reflects the process by which an individual arrives at an answer without awareness of how that answer was reached. Bruner emphasizes the importance of intuitive thinking. "Through intuitive thinking the individual may often arrive at solutions to problems which he would not achieve at all, or at best more slowly, through analytic thinking" (p. 58). Problems and solutions arrived at through intuition can often be confirmed later through an analytic approach.

Benner (1984) acknowledges the role of intuition in solving clinical problems and making nursing judgments. Often the nurse begins with vague hunches, not arrived at through a conscious and rational thought process, which then direct the practitioner in obtaining evidence to confirm them. A hunch is not sufficient but leads to confirming data. Benner writes, "Experts dare not stop with vague hunches, but neither do they care to ignore those hunches that could lead to early identification of problems and the search for confirming evidence" (p. xix).

DECISION MAKING

Decisions are made throughout the problem-solving process—decisions as to the nature of the problem, whether or not a solution is necessary, types of data to be collected, potential solutions, and the best one for that particular problem. The very nature of nursing practice requires that nurses make decisions relative to clients, staff, and activities in the clinical setting which are not based on problems but indicate a course of action. For these reasons, decision making represents another essential cognitive skill to be developed in a nursing education program.

Decision making involves choosing among alternatives. This notion of choice is what is important in the process, for in decision making the individual chooses a course of action following consideration of alternatives. Making a choice involves examining different alternatives and the consequences of each and weighing them against criteria to arrive at a judgment as to the best one. Schaefer (1974) identified three phases of decision making:

1. Deliberation: The first phase includes analysis of the situation in which a decision is required, generation of alternatives, and consideration of the possible consequences of each if selected.
2. Judgment: In the second phase, after analysis of each alter-

native and its consequences, the individual is ready to judge
which one is best in terms of its effectiveness in achieving
the goal and efficiency.
3. Choice: The final phase occurs when one of the alternatives,
the best one theoretically, is chosen.

Selection of the best alternative, in terms of its benefits, represents a rational decision. Such a decision requires collection of sufficient relevant information about the situation to render a decision,
generation and examination of as many alternatives as feasible, and
selection of the best one for meeting the related goal (Yeaworth,
1983). In a rational decision, the individual analyzes the situation,
alternatives, and their consequences and then judges which alternative is preferable. "The greater the deliberation and judgment,
the more effective the decision (Schaefer, 1974, p. 1853). Yet, there
are limits to rationality in decision making since rarely does one
make a decision based on knowledge of all possible alternatives and
consequences. Simon (1947) refers to this limitation of complete
objective rationality as "bounded rationality". The effectiveness of
decision making is decreased by inadequate deliberation and judgment which may result in an incomplete analysis of the situation,
the generation of too few alternatives, or not considering important
consequences.
Decisions are affected by one's values and biases and by cultural norms. These influence the individual's perception and analysis
of the situation, alternatives considered, and ultimate choice. What
seems rational to one individual may not be so to someone from a
different cultural group. Decisions are made *with* clients and/or
staff, not *for* them. Participatory decision making is important so
the decision is congruent with the values, beliefs, and culture of the
recipient of the decision and has a greater likelihood of acceptance.
Decisions may be categorized according to the degree of risk
faced in making the choice which is dependent on the extent of
objective knowledge about the possible consequences for a given
alternative action. There is less risk in making a decision when the
person has sufficient knowledge about the actions and consequences.
Radford (1975) identifies four conditions under which decisions
are made: (1) certainty, (2) risk, (3) uncertainty, and (4) competition
or conflict. A decision of certainty is one that is "riskless," not in the
sense of a lack of risk to the client but in terms of the existence of
only one consequence for each alternative. Few decisions as to nursing problems or actions to be taken are made with complete certainty. More commonly, decisions in the clinical setting are made under
conditions of risk or uncertainty. Decisions under conditions of risk
are ones where there is more than one consequence possible, each

with a certain probability of occurring, which is known to the individual. According to Yeaworth (1983), "In real life this happens only when the decision maker has had repeated experience from which he has acquired knowledge about the probability of outcomes" (p. 53). Decisions under conditions of uncertainty are those "when neither the number of possible future states of nature nor their probabilities of occurrence are known to the decision maker" (Radford, 1975, p. 61). Some decisions are also made under conditions of competition or conflict. Yeaworth describes these decisions as "'hot' decisions, which are complex, highly ego involving, and occur under conditions of stress" (p. 54).

In decision making, as with problem solving, the learner's knowledge base is important, for learners must be able to analyze the situation in which a decision is required and know which alternatives to consider and the possible consequences of each. This knowledge refers not only to the substance of the decision but also to factors that will influence its acceptance.

CRITICAL THINKING

Thinking may be creative or critical (Yinger, 1980). Creative thinking results in the development of new ideas and products, whereas critical thinking involves the evaluation of ideas. Critical thinking is rational thinking. It includes ability to (1) evaluate a statement and (2) identify reasons, for instance evidence on which to base that evaluation. "A critical thinker is one who recognizes the importance, and convicting forces, of reasons. When assessing claims, evaluating procedures, or making judgments, the critical thinker seeks reasons on which to base his or her assessment, evaluation, or judgment" (Siegel, 1980, p. 8). Siegel suggests that critical thinking is also principled thinking which entails making judgments that are nonarbitrary, impartial, and objective.

A critical thinker asks questions, seeks evidence, examines carefully different alternatives, and criticizes his or her own ideas and those of others (Scheffler, 1973). Learners who engage in critical thinking do not accept statements outright but instead seek reasons for supporting them. Through evaluation they decide for themselves which ideas to accept and which to reject, and they can provide reasons underlying their decisions. Kitchener (1983) proposes that students at the college level "need more help in actively applying the tools of evaluation and the rules of inquiry to the critical examination of . . . [different perspectives]" (p. 92).

Critical thinking represents the thought process that underlies problem solving and decision making; both intellectual processes require rational thinking. According to Yinger (1980), problem solving and decision making serve as tasks to be accomplished through critical thinking.

Skill in assessing claims and making judgments on the basis of reasons is not sufficient, for critical thinking also requires a certain set of attitudes. A critical thinker is one who is inclined to search for reasons, exhibits a questioning attitude, and avoids judgments that are arbitrary, partial, and subjective. "It is not enough for a student to be able to evaluate claims on the basis of evidence . . . to be a critical thinker, a student must be *disposed* to do so" (Siegel, 1980, p. 9).

Development of critical thinking ability is vital to effective nursing practice, particularly considering the influence of expanding knowledge and technology on health care and political, economic, social, and ethical decisions affecting care delivery. The complexity of nursing practice demands competent and independent judgments. Competent judgments are made on the basis of reasons; such reasoning represents critical thinking.

Cognitive Development

Ability to think and reason develops over time through a series of stages. The developmental stage the student is at in thinking influences the ability to solve clinical problems, make independent decisions and judgments, and deal with ambiguity, as well as the willingness to accept diverse points of view and commitment in personal and professional life. Perry (1970) has developed a theory of cognitive development which postulates how students evolve in their thinking about the nature of knowledge, truth, and values and meaning of commitment.

According to Perry, students move from thinking that is simplistic and categorical to where they recognize and can accept diverse perspectives. Development is represented along a continuum of nine positions, which may be grouped into four categories:

1. Dualism (Positions 1 and 2): At this level students view knowledge and values in terms of absolute and concrete categories. They are unable to deal with multiple points of view. In dualism, the right answer is determined by the teacher and other authorities.
2. Multiplicity (Positions 3 and 4): In this stage of development, learners acknowledge different perspectives to a given problem or situation, although they are unable to evaluate them. There exists an acceptance of uncertainty and, therefore, diversity of opinion.
3. Relativism (Positions 5 and 6): Whereas multiplistic thinkers only acknowledge that different perspectives and solutions to problems exist, relativistic thinkers, in contrast, have acquired the ability to evaluate these perspectives and

solutions. In relativism, learners are able to analyze situations with which they are faced and evaluate their own ideas and judgments and those of others (King, 1978). Decision making often becomes difficult at this point in cognitive development because of the learner's improved understanding of the alternatives and possible outcomes of each if chosen.

4. Commitment in Relativism (Positions 7 to 9): The most advanced stage of cognitive development, representing commitment in personal and professional life, reflects the willingness of learners to act according to their values and beliefs. Instead of indicating further cognitive development, this stage actually focuses on identity development and making personal and professional commitments (King, 1978). At this point, learners have established their own identities. Commitment in relativism "entails a readiness to tolerate paradox, take risks, embrace irony, and identify oneself with chosen notions, even when perfectly plausible alternatives exist and are acknowledged" (Hursh, Hass, & Moore, 1983, p. 46).

Learners do not necessarily progress through these nine positions. Some temporize or remain at a particular position, explicitly hesitating to move on; others escape and stay in relativism to avoid commitment; and still others (Perry, 1970) retreat to dualism and absolute thinking.

The Positions of deflection (Temporizing, Escape, and Retreat) offer alternatives at critical points in the development. A person may have recourse to them whenever he feels unprepared, resentful, alienated or overwhelmed to the degree which his urge to conserve dominant over his urge to progress. (pp. 57–58)

Perry's theory has applicability to nursing education since the learner's stage of development influences the cognitive processes used in practice. It also provides a theoretical framework for interpreting student behavior in response to situations arising in the clinical setting. Dualistic thinkers view knowledge in terms of absolute categories, unable to recognize differing perspectives and solutions to problems. Because of their authoritarian thinking, students at this level depend on the teacher or someone else in authority to tell them the right answer or procedure to follow and make decisions and judgments for them. Complexity in thought and problem solving, acceptance of diverse perspectives, ability to deal with ambiguity, willingness to take risks, independence in practice, and commitment to be responsible, all important in nursing practice, develop at advanced cognitive levels. Valiga (1983) reports, from a study of 123 baccalaureate nursing students, that while students generally increase in cognitive development through their program, they still remain in the category of dualism at graduation. Her research suggests that the learning experiences in which students engage and faculty with whom they work may be ineffective in assisting them to move forward in their cognitive development. Do faculty encourage divergent thinking or do they instead look for one right answer? Are students asked to examine multiple solutions to clinical problems and solve those problems independently? Are they encouraged to take calculated risks and experiment with care? Dualistic thinking is incompatible with professional nursing practice. Nurse educators are challenged to listen to what students say in response to clinical situations and assist them in moving toward a level of cognitive development more compatible with the complexity of nursing practice.

CLINICAL JUDGMENT

In the field, practitioners continually make decisions as to nursing diagnoses and courses of action for these diagnostic problems. Through the process of clinical judgment, the nurse decides on data to be collected about the client, makes an interpretation of the data (an inference) to arrive at the diagnosis, and identifies appropriate nursing actions. Judgment, which emphasizes the evaluation of phenomena, is used throughout the process as are problem-solving, decision-making and critical thinking skills.

Clinical judgment has been viewed according to three theoretical perspectives: (1) information processing theory, (2) decision theory, and (3) phenomenology.

Information Processing Theory

Information processing theory as applied to clinical judgment describes the process by which the practitioner addresses client-oriented problems. The process is similar across health care disciplines although the types of judgments made differ. As described previously, problem solving, within an information processing framework, represents an interaction between the nurse, as the information processing system, and task environment. Initially, the nurse attends to cues, i.e., sensory input, in the clinical situation. Cues include data about the status, responses, and environment of the client and others in the practice setting (Carnevali, 1983). The nurse then associates appropriate diagnostic label with these cues. Students are not as attentive to cues as are expert practitioners because of their lack of knowledge and experience. Tentative hypotheses as to the diagnosis (problem presenting in the clinical situation) are then generated from these cues. Between four and seven hypotheses are considered at any one time (Elstein et al., 1972).

Studies in clinical judgment have indicated that these tentative hypotheses are generated early in the interaction with the client

(Elstein et al., 1972; Elstein, Shulman & Sprafka, 1978). The hypotheses define the problem space of possible diagnoses. Arriving at early hypotheses, it is postulated, limits the size of the space that must be searched. Data can then be gathered in relation to these specific hypotheses, which provides a means of managing the data. Elstein and colleagues (1978) comment that without such a strategy, a diagnostic work-up could never be completed within a reasonable time. This strategy is believed to represent one that all health care practitioners use as a way of coping with the limitations in the amount of information they can process relative to the client.

The finding as to early hypothesis generation in clinical judgment is important since frequently students are taught in the clinical setting not to decide on the diagnosis until all data are collected. Research suggests, however, that practitioners develop hypotheses early in their interaction with the client and then use them to guide further data gathering. It is also important that learners as well as practitioners consider multiple hypotheses to avoid disregarding a diagnosis.

Hypotheses that are related to each other aid retention in short-term memory. (Carnaveli, 1984). Arranging them in a hierarchy, from general to specific, allows for better storage of cues (Elstein et al., 1978). It also directs data collection toward the most general hypotheses, enabling the practitioner to avoid focusing data gathering on specific ones which then may not be accepted. Another way of retaining hypotheses and data in short-term memory relates to the development of competing hypotheses (Carnevali, 1984). Recording data also serves as a way of retaining information in short-term memory.

Generation of hypotheses depends on the possession of an adequate knowledge base stored in long-term memory. With this knowledge, the learner and practitioner alike identify a diagnosis to reflect the cues. The difference between a learner's and an expert's knowledge base is apparent, making it easier for experts to select appropriate diagnoses from long-term memory.

Once early hypotheses are formed, subsequent data gathering focuses on these tentative hypotheses until a diagnosis is made (Elstein et al., 1978; Gordon, 1980; Kassirer & Gorry, 1978). The nurse collects information to evaluate each hypothesis in order to decide which ones to maintain or modify and which to reject. Evaluation involves comparing the new data collected against each hypothesis in terms of its probability of occurrence given these data. Because of their knowledge and experience, expert nurses are more efficient in collecting specific data to accept or reject a hypothesis than are students, who are often nonselective in the data gathered and tend to collect more information before deciding on a hypothesis (Tanner, 1984a). After arriving at the diagnosis, the nurse then decides on an appropriate course of action.

While clinical judgment is conceptualized as following a logical sequence from data collection through identification of the diagnosis, practitioners (particuarly those with expertise in nursing practice) may decide on a client problem without awareness of how they arrived at that problem. Intuition, therefore, enters into the process of clinical judgment.

Decision Theory

Another approach to understanding clinical judgment involves the use of mathematical models for arriving at the diagnosis and course of action. These models attempt to reflect the probabilistic nature of clinical decision making.

Bayesian Model. The Bayesian model is a mathematical formula for determining the probability of a diagnosis following the introduction of new information. In this view of clinical judgment, the decision as to the diagnosis is based on the probability of occurrence of the diagnosis with the addition of a new cue. In making the decision, consideration is given to the prior probability associated with the diagnosis, such as: its incidence; probability of the occurrence of the cue, for example, a symptom; and conditional probability of the occurrence of the cue given the particular diagnosis (Tanner, 1983). Often with the Bayesian model, a decision tree is used, which includes possible diagnostic hypotheses and their probabilities. The nurse moves through the tree to decide if the cues present are associated with a particular diagnosis. Aspinall (1979) examined the effectiveness of a decision tree in improving the accuracy of nurses in making a diagnosis. With a decision tree, accuracy in diagnosis did improve for many of the nurses, although some did not benefit from its use.

Lens Model. The lens model uses correlations to express the relationship between cues and diagnosis. As indicated in Figure 3, cues are viewed as the center of the lens. On the left-hand side is the criterion state, or state of the patient, unknown to the practitioner; and on the right is the judgment or inference made about this state

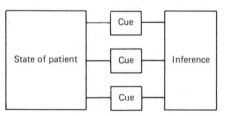

Figure 3. Lens model.

from the cues. The patient state and cues represent the task system or environment. Cues and the inference form the cognitive system. Each cue is individually correlated with the patient state and inference (Elstein et al., 1978). Inferences are made from the cues considering their probabilistic relationships to the patient state. The lens model has been applied to inferential judgment in nursing through studies by Hammond and associates (Hammond, Kelly, Castellan, Schneider, & Vancini, 1966; Hammond, Kelly, Schneider, & Vancini, 1966a, 1966b).

Studies conducted using decision theory as a framework for clinical judgment have indicated that often practitioners do not make the same decisions as prescribed by a mathematical formula (Tanner, 1983). Human error and biases not accounted for in a mathematical model enter into clinical judgment.

Phenomenologic Approach

The phenomenologic approach to clinical judgment views decision making in context. Such an approach emphasizes how judgments are made in real practice and how they are influenced by the clinical situation. Benner (1984) describes five levels of competency in clinical nursing practice, following the Dreyfus model of skill acquisition and development, and characteristics of performance at each level.

Stage 1: Novice—Beginners, i.e. nursing students or practitioners entering a new clinical area, function as novices, using context-free rules learned in the classroom to guide their actions. Because of their lack of practical knowledge and experience, learners at this level have only these principles on which to base their actions which do not reflect the particular clinical situation encountered. Beginners focus on individual pieces of information and lack a unified framework for approaching the situation.

Stage 2: Advanced Beginner—Advanced beginners have had enough clinical experience to identify meaningful characteristics, referred to as aspects, of the clinical situation. Identifying these aspects requires previous experience with related situations.

Stage 3: Competent—The competent level of performance indicates ability to plan in a conscious way considering a projected future situation. Such a plan reflects long-term goals and "is based on considerable conscious, abstract, analytic contemplation of the problem" (Benner, 1984, p. 26). To become competent, the nurse needs at least two years of experience in practice with similar clinical situations.

Stage 4: Proficient—Proficiency represents the ability to view the clinical situation in terms of the gestalt, rather than specific aspects within it. At this level, the nurse, because of prior experience with similar situations, has learned what to expect typically in a particular clinical situation. Benner proposes that this ability to view the clinical situation as a whole promotes clinical judgment because the nurse can more clearly identify which aspects in the present clinical situation are most significant.

Stage 5: Expert—The expert practitioner, because of extensive experience in the clinical field, "has an intuitive grasp of each situation and zeroes in on the accurate region of the problem without wasteful consideration of a large range of unfruitful, alternative diagnoses and solutions" (Benner, 1984, p. 32). Expert nurses have an indepth understanding of the meaning of a clinical situation and actions to be taken. Judgments by proficient and expert nurses are based on a perception of the clinical situation as a whole and the use of past concrete situations as paradigm cases for approaching the present one.

Three major theories represent different perspectives of the process of clinical judgment. In information processing theory, emphasis is placed on how the nurse adapts to limits in the amount of information able to be processed. Clinical judgment within this perspective begins with an identification of cues from which tentative diagnostic hypotheses, generated early in the process, are derived. Data are then collected to test each hypothesis. Decision theory describes through mathematical formulas how the practitioner arrives at a diagnosis or action. In a phenomenologic approach, clinical judgment is viewed as it is actually used in clinical practice. Regardless of the theoretical approach, clinical judgment is recognized as a complex process by which nurses arrive at diagnoses from cues and decide on appropriate courses of action. For an excellent review of research related to clinical judgment, the reader is directed to the reference by Tanner (1983).

TEACHING

The framework for teaching in the cognitive domain is derived from theory and research on how individuals attain concepts, problem solve, make decisions, and arrive at sound clinical judgments as well as the influence of critical thinking and the learner's stage of cognitive development on these processes. An understanding of these cognitive skills provides a basis for teaching them in the clinical field.

Concepts
What is known about concept learning may be used as a framework for teaching concepts in the clinical setting. Principles for teaching are organized in five areas:

   1. Definition of Concept—Teaching concepts begins with a definition of the concept or category to be learned. This defini-

tion specifies the attributes (identifying characteristics of an object or event relevant for grouping it into the category) and the rule (how the attributes are combined). An understanding of these attributes and accompanying rule is critical in learning the concept, for it provides the basis for distinguishing examples from nonexamples of that concept in clinical practice. This knowledge is therefore essential for students to begin to conceptualize in the practice setting.

2. Emphasis on Relevant Characteristics—For instructional purposes, the relevant characteristics of the concept should be emphasized, particularly as they compare with irrelevant ones. Because the number of irrelevant attributes influences the ease with which a concept is learned, a major task of the teacher is to highlight (verbally or through student experience) relevant features of the concept. Asking learners to describe these characteristics in their own words not only promotes learning them but also decreases the chance of memorizing the definition without comprehending the concept. There is evidence that concepts are learned more efficiently and applied more easily to new situations when learners are asked to explain the relevant attributes (Travers, 1972).

3. Use of Examples and Nonexamples—A concept has been attained when the learner can differentiate examples from nonexamples of that concept. In teaching concepts, emphasis should be given to examples of the concept, since individuals learn more efficiently from positive instances than from negative ones, although nonexamples should also be presented for comparison of the two. With all positive examples, the learner has no opportunity to compare the positive and negative instances in terms of the relevant attributes. In teaching the concept narcotics, for instance, if examples only reflect different types of narcotics the learner may not necessarily identify the relevant features of medications for placing them in this category. Comparing examples with ones of nonnarcotic substances assist students in focusing on the relevant features. Differences between examples and nonexamples should be made explicit for learners. In addition, learners should be asked to cite new examples of a concept, which aids in refining their understanding of it and promotes retention.

4. Variety of Examples—Relevant attributes appear to be learned more efficiently with a variety of examples that enable learners to more easily develop inferences about commonalities (Martorella, 1972).

5. Experience with Concept—Concept learning is enhanced

with experiences that enable the learner to become actively involved with an example of that concept. Clinical practice provides these experiences with concepts. For example, students can learn about immobilization through experiences with clients in the immediate postoperative period, in a comatose state, following cerebral vascular accident, or who have a fracture or other problems resulting in immobilization.

Problem Solving

Development of skill in problem solving requires experience in using it with real practice problems. The teacher should be alert to problems, client- or setting-oriented, that relate to the objectives of the experience and are within the level of knowledge and skill of the learner. Principles for teaching problem solving in the field are organized in seven areas:

1. Compatibility with Level of Learner—Solving problems requires ability to use concepts and theories in practice, so the nature of the problems selected for student involvement need to be at an appropriate level in terms of the learner's knowledge base.
2. Identification of Problems—Learners, because of their limited practical knowledge and experience in clinical practice, need assistance in identifying and delimiting problems. The teacher should make explicit for learners aspects of the clinical situation significant in identifying the problem, whether client- or setting-oriented. Students should be asked to describe the problem, reflecting their levels of understanding, and provide supporting data for its identification.
3. Identification of Multiple Solutions—It is vital in teaching problem solving that learners be assisted in identifying multiple solutions for problems. This is important in terms of their cognitive development and promoting divergent thinking. Explanations, verbal or written, by learners as to the solutions considered and a rationale for the decision made provide a means of assessing the thought process used by students and assisting them in identifying other possibilities. Discussions such as this encourage learners to examine own biases and values that may influence problem solving.

   Sometimes the solution proposed may not be part of the accepted practice in the clinical setting, and the teacher may need to assume an advocacy role for the learner so the approach may be implemented. This support on the part of teacher and staff is necessary to provide for experimentation with care and opportunity for calculated risk taking, within the realm of safe practice, in the clinical field.
4. Integrity of Process—Although in reality the problem-

solving process does not always follow a linear sequence of steps from definition of the problem through evaluation of solutions, in developing skill in problem solving, it is important for learners to proceed through these steps so the integrity of the process is maintained.

5. Focus on Process—The emphasis in teaching problem solving is on the *process* by which problems are identified and solutions are proposed and tested, rather than on the outcomes.

6. Use of Intuitive Thinking—Although teaching focuses on the analytic process of solving problems in the field, learners also should be taught the importance of recognizing hunches and searching for evidence to confirm them.

7. Acceptance of Individual Differences Among Learners—The teacher needs to be supportive of differences among learners in their approaches to problem solving. A fundamental difference between field-independent and field-dependent learners, for instance, relates to their analytic ability, which influences problem solving in the field. Field-dependent learners, because they do not readily use a hypothesis testing approach to problem solving, may require additional guidance from the teacher in analyzing clinical situations, identifying problems, and proposing and testing solutions for them.

Decision Making
Similar to problem solving, decisions relative to practice require an adequate knowledge base for analyzing the situation in which a decision is required, generating possible alternatives, determining consequences of each, and making a judgment as to which alternative to select. The decisions students are involved in making need to reflect their levels of understanding.

Consideration of different alternatives and consequences of each is vital to rational decision making in clinical practice. Learners, because of their limited knowledge and experience in the specific area of practice often need assistance in exploring these alternatives.

Discussion of decisions with others provides a means of assessing the thought process used to arrive at the decisions and improving understanding of alternatives that might have been considered. Encouraging learners to examine their own beliefs and values that may influence their decision making and those of the recipient of the decision is also important.

Clinical Judgment
Development of skill in clinical judgment requires: (1) relevant knowledge for application to the clinical situation, (2) skill in data

collection, and (3) knowledge of strategies for effective problem solving with clients. Judgment is influenced by the learner's stage of cognitive development and critical thinking ability. These elements provide direction for faculty as to teaching clinical judgment in the field.

Knowledge Base of Learner. Effective clinical judgment requires an adequate knowledge base for analyzing the clinical situation, gathering and interpreting data, generating tentative hypotheses, considering alternative actions and consequences of each, and deciding on actions to be taken. Clinical judgment cannot proceed without this store of knowledge for retrieval from long-term memory. For this reason, experiences in practice in which the learner is called upon to make a clinical judgment need to reflect the learner's level of knowledge and skill.

Skill in Data Collection. Clinical judgment depends on comprehensive data gathering, for it is from these data that diagnostic hypotheses are generated and then tested and decisions relative to the client and others are made. Teaching for clinical judgment involves assisting students to develop their skill in various means of data collection.

Strategies for Problem Solving. Teaching should be directed toward assisting students to understand the process of clinical judgment and strategies for effective clinical problem solving. Four strategies and related teaching implications are presented:

1. Early Hypothesis Generation—Research has indicated that practitioners generate hypotheses early in their interaction with clients and proceed to gather data to test each hypothesis, thus using a hypothetico-deductive approach. Traditional instruction in nursing, however, often teaches students to complete all of data collection and then analyze the data to determine nursing diagnoses. Teaching, instead, should assist students in identifying tentative diagnostic hypotheses early in assessment of the client and then focusing subsequent data collection on these hypotheses.
2. Multiple Competing Hypotheses—Learners should be assisted in generating multiple competing hypotheses that might be possible given the data, instead of accepting the first diagnosis that comes to mind which may prove to be incorrect. Generating several possible diagnostic hypotheses improves the chance of identifying the correct one.
3. Hypothesis Testing—Students should be taught to search for and evaluate data that assist in eliminating tentative hy-

potheses as well as that which facilitates confirmation. Skill in directing data collection toward specific hypotheses needs to be developed.
4. Relevant and Irrelevant Data—Learners need assistance in distinguishing relevant from irrelevant data.

Cognitive Taxonomy
Important in teaching the cognitive processes inherent in practice is assisting learners in the progressive development of these skills. The taxonomy of the cognitive domain views intellectual abilities within a development perspective and, therefore, is valuable for this teaching.

The taxonomy represents a system for ordering cognitive behaviors from simple recall to the complex processes of analysis, synthesis, and evaluation. The taxonomy is thus organized according to the principle of increasing complexity. Reilly (1980) describes the use of the cognitive taxonomy by Bloom (1956) for the progressive development of intellectual skills in nursing education.

There are six levels in the cognitive taxonomy, each with specific sublevels except for one of the categories, application. The levels in the taxonomy are presented in Table 15.

Use of Taxonomy. The cognitive taxonomy provides a framework for selecting the appropriate level of learning behavior and for writing objectives. The decision as to the level of learning desired is based on the faculty's professional judgment considering the level of the learner, complexity of the phenomenon, and experiences available for achieving the objectives. In using the taxonomy, the teacher first decides on the desired level in the taxonomy, then develops objectives to reflect learning at that level.

Cognitive skill development at the lower levels of the taxonomy, knowledge and comprehension, is oriented toward an understanding of concepts, principles, and theories but not to an ability to use them in practice. Objectives written at the lower levels reflect the student's acquisition of the knowledge base needed for problem solving and decision making in the practice setting. These behaviors are important for development of cognitive skill. Problem solving begins at the comprehension level in which students learn to interpret data and extrapolate meaning.

Objectives written at the application level reflect ability of the learner to problem solve using knowledge that relates to prescriptive solutions. At the analysis level, the learner is able to problem solve and make decisions in a clinical situation through the analytical process. Learning at this level addresses both known and unknown solutions. It reflects ability to analyze data, compare different alternatives and their consequences, search for evidence to

TABLE 15. TAXONOMY OF COGNITIVE DOMAIN

C1.00 **Knowledge**

Knowledge involves the recall of specific facts and information. Learning at this level represents the process of remembering information, not ability to understand its meaning.

1.10 Knowledge of Specifics	Recall of specific pieces of information
1.11 Knowledge of Terminology	Recall of terms
1.12 Knowledge of Specific Facts	Knowledge of dates, events, persons, and other facts
1.20 Knowledge of Ways and Means of Dealing with Specifics	Recall of ways of organizing, judging, and criticizing ideas
1.21 Knowledge of Conventions	Knowledge of ways of presenting ideas
1.22 Knowledge of Trends and Sequences	Knowledge of processes and directions in relation to time
1.23 Knowledge of Classifications and Categories	Recall of classes and divisions considered to be fundamental for a specific discipline, argument, or problem
1.24 Knowledge of Criteria	Recall of specific criteria
1.25 Knowledge of Methodology	Recall of methods of inquiry and techniques employed in a discipline
1.30 Knowledge of the Universals and Abstractions in a Field	Knowledge of major ideas and patterns by which ideas are organized, such as theories
1.31 Knowledge of Principles and Generalizations	Recall of abstractions that summarize observations of phenomena
1.32 Knowledge of Theories and Structures	Recall of a body of principles and generalizations and their interrelationships

C2.00 **Comprehension**

Comprehension indicates understanding, an ability to translate or interpret information and extrapolate beyond that given. Bloom (1956) considers this category as the first level of intellectual skills.

2.10 Translation	Expression of communication in other terms, another language, or another form of communication
2.20 Interpretation	Explanation of a communication reflecting a new perspective of the material
2.30 Extrapolation	Extension of trends beyond given data

C3.00 **Application**

Application, the only category in the cognitive taxonomy without sublevels, refers to *use* of concepts, theories, and other abstractions in concrete situations. Ability to apply requires comprehension of that which is applied.

C4.00 **Analysis**

The fourth level, analysis, pertains to learning that involves a breakdown of material into its constituent parts and determination of the relationships among them.

TABLE 15. *(Continued)*

4.10 Analysis of Elements	Identification of elements of a communication
4.20 Analysis of Relationships	Identification of relationships among elements and parts of a communication
4.30 Analysis of Organizational Principles	Identification of the organization, systematic arrangement, and structure holding a communication together

C5.00 **Synthesis**
Synthesis means the development of a new product through a combination of specific elements and parts. Of the categories in the cognitive taxonomy, this one most clearly provides for creative learning.

5.10 Production of a Unique Communication	Development of a communication reflecting the learner's perspective about some idea
5.20 Production of a Plan or Proposed Set of Operations	Development of a plan of work
5.30 Derivation of a Set of Abstract Relations	Development of a scheme for classifying or explaining certain data or phenomena

C6.00 **Evaluation**
Evaluation, representing the most complex learning behaviors, reflects the ability to make judgments about value in terms of internal and external criteria.

6.10 Judgments in Terms of Internal Evidence	Evaluation of a communication based on its logical accuracy, consistency, and other internal criteria
6.20 Judgments in Terms of External Criteria	Evaluation of a communication with reference to selected criteria, such as comparing a work against known standards in its field (pp. 48–53)

(Modified from Reilly, D. E. (1980). Behavioral objectives—Evaluation in nursing (2nd ed.). New York: Appleton-Century-Crofts, with permission.)

support claims and conclusions, and determine how ideas relate to one another. Problem solving and decision making at this level are needed for professional nursing practice.

Learning at the synthesis level is important in developing new and creative products. At the evaluation level, the learner makes judgments about value based on criteria and standards. "Evaluation represents not only an end process in dealing with cognitive behaviors, but also a major link with the affective behaviors where values, liking, and enjoying . . . are the central processes involved" (Bloom, 1956).

Once faculty determines the cognitive level desired as the outcome of the nursing program and writes objectives to reflect this learning, the outcome objectives for each level in the program are designated to indicate progressive development. There are two ways to level objectives. The cognitive behavior itself may be changed to a higher taxonomic level, thereby representing greater complexity. Ability to *analyze* an interaction is more complex than ability to *use* principles in interacting with clients and others in the clinical field. This leveling may be illustrated as follows:

Level 1
> C3.00 *Uses* principles in interacting with clients and others in the clinical field.
> C4.10 *Analyzes* interactions with clients and others in the clinical field

A second way of leveling involves keeping the cognitive behavior at the same level and making the variables with which the behavior is carried out more complex. Ability to analyze interactions within a *group* is more complex than skill in analyzing interactions with an *individual client*. An example of this leveling is:

Level 1
> C4.10 Analyzes interactions with *clients*

Level 2
> C4.10 Analyzes interactions with *groups of clients*.

In some instances, both the behavior and variables may be changed.

The taxonomy provides a system for ordering cognitive behaviors to be acquired along a continuum of simple to complex. It enables faculty concerned with teaching cognitive skills to plan and sequence instruction to allow for their progressive development.

TEACHING METHODS

There are a variety of clinical teaching methods appropriate for teaching in the cognitive domain. Problem-solving strategies, such as written problem-solving and decision-making situations or ones combined with media, assist learners in applying concepts and theories to a clinical situation; identifying, from their assessment of the situation, problems to be solved or decisions to be made; and examining alternate courses of action and their consequences. They provide for practice in solving simulated problems and improving skill in problem solving and decision making.

Conference represents another teaching method particularly appropriate for cognitive skill development. In relation to concept learning, students can discuss examples of a concept and its relevant characteristics. They can share clinical problems and decisions made, discuss issues and problems affecting nursing practice, and receive immediate feedback on their approaches and underlying rationale.

Conference provides a means for learners to examine data collected, inferences made, and the course of action chosen which assists in the development of clinical judgment skill. It is important that students have an opportunity to discuss the process used in arriving at nursing diagnoses and deciding on actions. A written care plan or other type of written assignment students might complete does not reflect the underlying thought process used by them. Through interaction with others the learner can discuss the diagnostic hypotheses considered, supporting data, and why an inference was made, and can describe the alternate actions considered and consequences of each.

Conferences also provide opportunity for learners to reflect on their decisions and evaluate those of others, important in critical thinking. Group discussion promotes cognitive development in that learners are exposed to multiple perspectives relative to care and diverse points of view. A multidisciplinary conference could also be used to compare approaches of different disciplines to problem solving.

Clinical assignment is particularly valuable in promoting cognitive skill development. Through clinical practice, students experience examples of concepts, important in their attainment of them. They develop skill in problem solving and decision making, learn to accept multiple perspectives, and have an opportunity to experiment with care, make independent judgments, and develop commitment to be responsible in professional practice.

A written assignment, such as a nursing care plan, assists learners in deciding on nursing actions and examining alternate approaches. Case studies, which provide a holistic view of a client's problem, promote problem-solving learning. Simulations, games, and simulation games enable students to practice problem solving and decision making in a safe environment representing a real-life encounter in the field. Role play assists learners in recognizing the value of participatory involvement in problem solving and decision making.

With media, faculty can present client situations similar to ones found in the field for students to identify possible problems and propose different solutions for them. Similar to media, computer-assisted instruction and particularly computer simulations provide a means of presenting a case situation for students to analyze, identify problems or decisions to be made, select approaches, and evaluate outcomes.

There is a wide range of teaching methods appropriate for cognitive skill development. Through real or simulated clinical situations, learners are able to attain concepts and develop skill in solving problems and making decisions relative to practice. Some methods, such as conference and clinical assignment, also are particularly appropriate for promoting critical thinking. The key is how the teacher uses the methods and the standards set relative to the thinking process so the responses of learners represent depth of understanding and consistency in the analytic process.

SUMMARY

Cognitive skill development is a significant goal of clinical practice and must be of major concern to the teacher in the clinical field. It is separate from but interrelated to the affective and psychomotor domains of learning. Cognitive skills essential for nursing practice encompass concept attainment, problem solving, decision making, critical thinking, and clinical judgment.

Concepts provide a means of categorizing information, which reduces the complexity of the environment, enables individuals to identify different events and objects in it, reduces the need for constant learning, gives direction as to actions to be taken, and enables individuals to relate different concepts to one another to form systems. Concept attainment involves learning the characteristics of events or objects relevant for grouping them into categories. A concept has been attained when the learner can differentiate examples from nonexamples of that concept.

Students also need to develop skill in problem solving, decision making, and clinical judgment. Problem solving is viewed as a series of steps commencing with identification of the problem and proceeding through gathering data in relation to the problem, generating solutions, and evaluating the solutions chosen. Problem solving may be viewed according to three theoretical perspectives: (1) stimulus–response theory, (2) cognitive-field theory, and (3) information processing theory.

The very nature of nursing practice requires that nurses make decisions relative to clients, staff, and activities within the clinical field. Decision making involves choosing among alternatives and occurs in three phases: (1) deliberation as to the alternatives and possible consequences of each if selected, (2) judgment of the best one in terms of achieving the goal, and (3) choice.

The decisions and judgments made in clinical practice are influenced by the learner's stage of cognitive development. Complexity of thought and problem solving, aceptance of diverse perspectives, ability to deal with ambiguity, independence in practice, and willingness to assume responsibility, all important in nursing practice, develop at advanced stages of cognitive development. It is important in nursing education that students are moved toward higher levels of cognitive development.

Teaching cognitive skills inherent in practice involves a number of principles. Important in this teaching is providing for the progressive development of skills. The taxonomy of the cognitive domain views intellectual skills within a developmental perspective and, therefore, is valuable as a guide for determining the level of skill development at any particular point in the nursing program.

Methods for promoting cognitive learning in the clinical field include problem-solving strategies, conferences, clinical assignments, written assignments, simulations, games, simulation games, role play, media, and computer-assisted instruction. These strategies provide for student involvement in clinical situations which demand that learners engage in the cognitive processes leading to appropriate decisions and clinical judgment.

Faculty has the responsibility not only to assist learners in attaining and using concepts and theories relevant to practice and in developing skill in clinical judgment, but also to encourage them to accept diverse points of view, challenge and question, and develop commitment as responsible and self-directed learners and professional practitioners. Teachers need to demonstrate these same behaviors themselves—acceptance of diverse points of view among learners and with their own perspective, support for challenging and questioning by learners, and recognition of the self as learner.

REFERENCES

Aspinall, M. J. (1979). Use of a decision tree to improve accuracy of diagnosis. *Nursing Research, 28,* 182–85.

Benner, P. (1984). *From novice to expert: Excellence and power in clinical nursing practice.* Menlo Park, Calif.: Addison-Wesley.

Bigge, M. L. (1982). *Learning theories for teachers* (4th ed.). New York: Harper & Row.

Bloom, B. S. (Ed.). (1956). *Taxonomy of educational objectives: Handbook I: Cognitive domain.* New York: D. McKay.

Bruner, J. S. (1963). *The process of education.* New York: Vintage Books.

Bruner, J. S., Goodnow, J. J., & Austin, G. A. (1956). *A study of thinking.* New York: Wiley.

Carnevali, D. L. (1983). *Nursing care planning: Diagnosis and management* (3rd ed.). Philadelphia: Lippincott.

Carnevali, D. L. (1984). The diagnostic reasoning process. In D. L. Carnevali, P. H. Mitchell, N. F. Woods, & C. A. Tanner (Eds.), *Diagnostic reasoning in nursing.* Philadelphia: Lippincott.

Ellis, H. C. (1972). *Fundamentals of human learning and cognition.* Dubuque, Iowa: Wm. C. Brown.

Elstein, A. S., Kagan, N., Shulman, L. S. et al. (1972). Methods and theory in the study of medical inquiry. *Journal of Medical Education, 47,* 85–92.

Elstein, A. S., Shulman, L. S., & Sprafka, S. A. (1978). *Medical problem-solving.* Cambridge, Mass.: Harvard University Press.

Frederickson, K., & Mayer, G. G. (1977). Problem-solving skills: What effect does education have? *American Journal of Nursing, 77,* 1167–69.

Glaser, R. (1969). Learning. In *Encyclopedia of educational research* (4th ed.). New York: Macmillan.

Gordon, M. (1980). Predictive strategies in diagnostic tasks. *Nursing Research, 29,* 39–45.

Hammond, K. R., Kelly, K. J., Castellan, N. J., Jr., et al. (1966). Clinical inference in nursing: Use of information-seeking strategies by nurses. *Nursing Research, 15,* 330–36.

Hammond, K. R., Kelly, K. J., Schneider, R. J., & Vancini, M. (1966a). Clinical inference in nursing: Analyzing cognitive tasks representative of nursing problems. *Nursing Research, 15,* 134–38.

Hammond, K. R., Kelly, K. J., Schneider, R. J., & Vancini, M. (1966b). Clinical inference in nursing: Information units used. *Nursing Research, 15,* 236–43.

Hursh, B., Haas, P., & Moore, M. (1983). An interdisciplinary model to implement general education. *Journal of Higher Education, 54,* 42–59.

Kassirer, J. P., & Gorry, C. A. (1978). Clinical problem-solving: A behavioral analysis. *Annals of Internal Medicine, 89,* 245–55.

Kim, H. S. (1983). *The nature of theoretical thinking in nursing.* Norwalk, Conn.: Appleton-Century-Crofts.

King, P. M. (1978). William Perry's theory of intellectual and ethical development. *New Directions for Student Services, 4,* 35–51.

Kitchener, K. S. (1983). Educational goals and reflective thinking, *Educational Forum, XLVII* (1), 75–95.

Martorella, P. H. (1972). *Concept learning: Designs for instruction.* San Francisco: INTEXT.

Miller, G. A. (1956). The magical number seven, plus or minus two: Some limits on our capacity for processing information. *Psychological Review, 63,* 81–97.

Newell, A., & Simon, H. A. (1972). *Human problem-solving.* Englewood Cliffs, N.J.: Prentice-Hall.

Norris, C. M. (Ed.). (1982). *Concept clarification in nursing.* Rockville, Md.: Aspen Systems.

Parnes, S. J. (1984). Learning creative behavior: Making the future happen. *The Futurist, 18*(4), 30–32.

Perry, W. G., Jr. (1970). *Forms of intellectual and ethical development in the college years.* New York: Holt, Rinehart & Winston.

Radford, K. J. (1975). *Managerial decision-making.* Reston, Va.: Reston.

Reilly, D. E. (1980). *Behavioral objectives—Evaluation in nursing* (2nd ed.). New York: Appleton-Century-Crofts.

Schaefer, J. (1974). The interrelatedness of decision-making and the nursing process. *American Journal of Nursing, 74,* 1852–55.

Scheffler, I. (1973). *Reason and teaching.* London: Routledge & Kegan Paul.

Siegel, H. (1980). Critical thinking as an educational ideal. *Educational Forum, XLV*(1), 7–23.

Simon, H. A. (1947). *Administrative behavior.* New York: Macmillan.

Simon, H. A. (1978). Information-processing theory of human problem-solving. In W. K. Estes (Ed.), *Handbook of learning and cognitive processes. Volume 5: Human information processing.* New York: Wiley.

Stonewater, J. K., & Stonewater, B. B. (1984). Teaching problem-solving: Implications from cognitive development research. *American Association of Higher Education Bulletin, 36*(6), 7–10.

Tanner, C. A. (1983). Research on clinical judgment. In W. L. Holzemer (Ed.), *Review of research in nursing education.* Thorofare, N.J.: Slack.

Tanner, C. A. (1984a). Diagnostic problem-solving strategies. In D. L. Carnevali, P. H. Mitchell, N. F. Woods, & C. A. Tanner (Eds.), *Diagnostic reasoning in nursing* Philadelphia: Lippincott.

Tanner, C. A. (1984b). Factors influencing the diagnostic process. In D. L. Carnevali, P. H. Mitchell, N. F. Woods, & C. A. Tanner (Eds.), *Diagnostic reasoning in nursing.* Philadelphia: Lippincott.

Travers, R. M. W. (1972). *Essentials of learning* (3rd ed.). New York: Macmillan.

Valiga, T. M. (1983). Cognitive development: A critical component of baccalaureate nursing education. *Image, XV,* 115–19.

Viaud, G. (1960). [*Intelligence: Its evolution and form.*] (A. J. Pomerans, Trans.) New York: Harper & Row.

Yeaworth, R. C. (1983). Decision-making: Political and rational aspects. In M. E. Conway & O. Andruskiw (Eds.), *Administrative theory and practice.* Norwalk, Conn.: Appleton-Century-Crofts.

Yinger, R. J. (1980). Can we really teach them to think? In R. E. Young (Ed.), *Fostering critical thinking.* San Francisco: Jossey-Bass.

BIBLIGRAPHY

Benner, P. (1982). From novice to expert. *American Journal of Nursing, 82,* 402–7.

Benner, P., & Wrubel, J. (1972). Clinical knowledge development: The value of perceptual awareness. *Nurse Educator, 7*(3), 11–17.

Broderick, M. E., & Ammentorp, W. (1979). Information structures: An analysis of nursing performance. *Nursing Research, 28,* 106–10.

Chickering, A. W. (1976). Developmental change as a major outcome. In M. T. Keeton & Associates (Eds.), *Experiential learning.* San Francisco: Jossey-Bass.

DeBack, V. (1982). The relationship between senior nursing students' ability to formulate nursing diagnoses and the curriculum model. In B. J. Brown & P. L. Chinn (Eds.), *Nursing education: Practical methods and models.* Rockville, Md.: Aspen Systems.

Doona, M. E. (1976). The judgment process in nursing. *Image, 8*(2), 27–29.

Dreyfus, H. L. (1979). *What computers can't do: The limits of artificial intelligence.* New York: Harper & Row.

Ennis, R. H. (1962). A concept of critical thinking. *The Harvard Educational Review, 32,* 81–111.

Feinstein, A. R. (1967). *Clinical judgment.* Baltimore: Williams & Wilkins.

Glaser, R. (1968). Concept learning and concept teaching. In R. M. Gagné & W. J. Gephart (Eds.), *Learning research and school subjects.* Itasca, Ill.: F. E. Peacock.

Grier, M. R. (1976). Decision-making about patient care. *Nursing Research, 25,* 105–10.

Kissinger, J. F., & Munjas, B. A. (1981). Nursing process, student attributes, and teaching methodologies. *Nursing Research, 30,* 242–46.

Kitchener, K. S., & King, P. M. (1981). Reflective judgment: Concepts of justification and their relationship to age and education. *Journal of Applied Developmental Psychology, 2,* 89–116.

Marriner, A. (1977). The student's perception of his creativity. *Nursing Research, 26,* 57–60.

Matthews, C. A., & Gaul, A. L. (1979). Nursing diagnosis from the perspective of concept attainment and critical thinking. *Advances in Nursing Science, 2*(1), 17–26.

Nuernberger, P. (1984). Mastering the creative process. *The Futurist, 18*(4), 33–36.

Perry, W. G., Jr. (1981). Cognitive and ethical growth: The making of meaning. In A. Chickering (Ed.), *The modern American college*. San Francisco: Jossey-Bass.

Tanner, C. A. (1981). Instruction in the diagnostic process: An experimental study. In M. J. Kim & D. Mortiz (Eds.), *Proceedings of the third and fourth conferences on classification of nursing diagnoses*. New York: McGraw-Hill.

Tversky, A., & Kahneman, D. (1974). Judgment under uncertainty: Heuristics and biases. *Science, 185*, 1124–31.

Tversky, A., & Kahneman, D. (1981). The framing of decisions and the psychology of choice. *Science, 211*, 453–58.

Widick, C. A. (1977). The Perry scheme: A foundation for developmental practice. *The Counseling Psychologist, 6*, 35–38.

Young, R. E. (Ed.). (1980). *Fostering critical thinking*. San Francisco: Jossey-Bass.

7

Psychomotor Learning in the Clinical Field

Psychomotor skills are an integral part of nursing practice in most settings where nurses participate in the delivery of care. They are found in both the assessment and implementation steps of the nursing process. They constitute a significant portion of nursing interventions. Lack of competency in these skills on the part of new graduates is the subject of much criticism of nursing education, which often is of such vehemence that it takes on a pervasive quality as an indictment of all nursing education.

The teacher of psychomotor skills raises such questions as: How should they be taught? What processes are involved in the learning? What criteria are used in judging the efficiency of a student's performance? A search of current nursing literature provides little assistance in answering these questions. Nursing research in this area, scarce as it is, addresses primarily the comparison of teaching strategies or the scientific rationale underlying the execution of some techniques. A perusal of the indexes of nursing textbooks concerned with teaching or curriculum evidences, in most instances no heading *psychomotor*.

What factors account for this dearth of material in nursing literature on the teaching of psychomotor skills? At an earlier stage in nursing history, excellence in performing psychomotor skills was *nursing,* and the teaching of these skills monopolized much of the curriculum. Other dimensions of care were discussed in classes, but one's expertise in carrying out procedural skills in nursing was the critical evaluative criterion. In one school, students were told by the director of the school, "If your patients tell you that you are a good nurse, don't necessarily believe the praise, for the patient does not know how perfectly you carried out your nursing techniques."

Much has happened since that era as nursing began to redefine its scope of practice and incorporate bodies of knowledge derived from other disciplines' research into its practice. Even more significant changes are underway because nursing is now evolving into a science. For example, remarkable advances in the field of psychiatry during World War II resulted in new directions in the health field where therapeutic use of the self through communication, interpersonal relationships, and other human interactions skills became paramount. Nurses returning to universities through the G.I. Bill developed the knowledge and skills inherent in the behavioral fields and incorporated them in nursing practice. The nurturing role of the nurse moved in new directions and caring took on different meaning with a broader concept of "doing."

The emphasis on the teaching of these new knowledges and skills in nursing programs relegated psychomotor skill teaching to the background. Little concern has been expressed about the teaching processes entailed, in spite of the shift in learning theories from the conditioning and trial-and-error concepts of Thorndyke to the concepts in field theory that emphasize principles and the relationship among phenomena. Today, with emphasis on cognitive skills as inherent in decision making, clinical judgment, and diagnosing, the concern in nursing education relates to the learning and teaching of these skills. Once again, psychomotor skill development is in the background.

CONCEPTS RELEVANT TO PSYCHOMOTOR SKILL DEVELOPMENT

Psychomotor skills in nursing are those dimensions of nursing practice that entail the ability to behave efficiently in an action situation that requires neuromuscular coordination. Singer (1975) states, "Activities that are primarily movement oriented and that emphasize overt physical response bear the label psychomotor" (p. 23). A wide variety of skills is inherent in nursing practice; it is the focus on body or muscular movement patterns which designate psychomotor skills.

Psychomotor skills in nursing are purposeful, complex actions based on principles; they entail cognitive skills in decision making and judgment relative to their use and desired effect. Yet, psychomotor skills are not cognitive skills. They are "doing" skills which result in a performance of a specific act. The teaching of psychomotor skills recognizes skill in practice as an integrated phenomenon comprising cognitive, psychomotor, and affective learning. In teaching, however, emphasis is placed on the performance skill that requires particular teaching, learning, and evaluation strategies. Although the movement component is the focus of the teaching, other cognitive, perceptual, and affective processes interact so that the total act is integrated, meaningful, and successful.

This chapter addresses the teaching of the movement component. It is assumed that relevant cognitive and affective knowledges and skills are being developed concurrently through other strategies. Their synthesis with psychomotor skills will be demonstrated later in the chapter.

Several concepts are essential to understanding the approach to teaching psychomotor skills. Performance and learning are not the same processes. *Performance* is an action, transitory in occurrence, in response to specific cues in the situation. *Learning,* however, is of more permanent nature resulting from practice or past experience, which is stored in the memory of a learner and subject to retrieval on cue. In motor skill learning, the amount of learning is inferred from the performance of the learner, and the process of learning is inferred from the change in learner behavior that is observed as the task is carried out. Kerr (1982) refers to performance as the end product or behavior that we see; learning is represented by an internalized model that allows us to repeat the performance of the skill.

Ability and skill, likewise, are not the same phenomenon. *Skill* relates to a specific task and refers to the ability to execute that task efficiently. *Ability* suggests the notion of a generality of a trait the learner possesses and is influenced by heredity and learning.

Skill is an important concept in this discussion and refers to the ability to carry out efficiently and effectively, in terms of speed and accuracy, muscular or body movements required for the act. Skill is relative; its definition for a specific task is determined by the nature of the task and the circumstances in the situation in which it occurs. Three classifications of skills are noted in the literature:

1. Fine motor skills: muscular coordination involves precision-oriented tasks. Nursing skills include: injections, arterial line manipulation, surgical dressings requiring instrumentation.

2. Manual skills: manipulative tasks that are fairly repetitive and usually involve eye–arm action. Nursing skills include: physical assessment, body hygiene, suctioning, chest drainage, touch.

3. Gross motor skills: involve large muscles and movement of the body. Nursing skills include: cardiopulmonary resuscitation (C.P.R.), ambulation, range of motion, patient positioning.

Singer (1975) proposes the following characteristics of the skilled person:

1. Performance is fairly consistent regardless of factors present that might cause the "average person's" performance to fluctuate.
2. Performance coincides with high degree of spatial precision and timing.

3. Responses to stimuli are set in appropriate sequential order.
4. Performances are executed within certain time limitations.
5. Ability to anticipate quickly is present and there is more time to react.
6. Performance has less variability since there is no need to respond to every potential cue in the environment.
7. Ability to receive maximum information from minimum number of identifiable cues is developed. (p. 29)

Johnson (1961) adds two other behavior characteristics:

1. Form of the activity represents economy of effort.
2. Is adaptable; i.e., performs proficiently under varying and even unpredictable conditions. (p. 163)

The goal of psychomotor skills development is more than the ability to perform; it is the ability to perform in a consistent manner within an appropriate time and spatial context irrespective of environmental variations. In education, it is not only the performance of the skill that is the goal, it is the learning of the skill as reflected in the consistent quality of the skill performance.

One other concept essential to understanding this approach to teaching psychomotor skills is the notion of the word *cognitive*. The word has several different meanings in psychomotor skill learning. Cognitive may refer to the *content* of the skill; i.e., its purpose, principles, and consequences. Cognitive also refers to the *intellectual processes* that the individual goes through between receiving the stimulus from the environment and the response. It is the latter notion of cognitive that is particularly relevant in the learning process entailed in psychomotor skill attainment.

LEARNING PROCESS FRAMEWORK FOR PSYCHOMOTOR SKILL DEVELOPMENT

How does psychomotor skill learning occur? What processes are involved? Until the sixties, this skill learning was primarily perceived within the conditioned or behavioristic paradigm: stimulus–response (S–R) or response–stimulus (R–S), and teaching was directed to this modality. As fields of cybernetic and information processing theory evolved with the advent of computers, many educators, who had been disenchanted with the simplistic mechanistic concept of psychomotor learning, sought answers in these new fields of knowledge. This pursuit has been undertaken by engineers, psychologists, and physical educators and since the 1970s much research has been generated and reported in the literature. Inquiry thus addressed was not limited to the outcome of learning but included the means by which muscles are coordinated and controlled so that accurate and efficient motor behavior results. Questions for educators now address process as well as outcome; the notion of motor-skilled performance as a conditioned reflex is no longer acceptable to many researchers and teachers. As Kerr (1982) states, "the current definition of psychomotor learning says we control with the head, not the muscles" (p. 18).

Theoretical Models

A comprehensive presentation of current research into psychomotor learning process is beyond the purview of this chapter. Selected findings perceived to be particularly relevant to this domain in nursing education are presented. The reader is encouraged to explore the literature in the field of motor learning in greater depth.

Theory development of motor learning is evolving primarily from the perspective of three major models: behavioral cybernetics, information processing, and adaptation.

Behavioral Cybernetic Model. This model is a systems approach to psychomotor behavior that defines a new level of experiential study of body motion and psychologic functions in terms of their variable feedback characteristics and determinants (Smith, 1972). Motor skills are perceived as a closed loop system relying on feedback to make the essential adjustments for efficient motor skill. Sensory input from the motor performance, whose origins may be from proprioceptors, stimuli arising within the organism or sense organs or both, provide feedback to the system controlling the output. In turn, the system makes the modifications in the output as indicated. The feedback system is in essence a detection mechanism which provides for a means of correcting motor performance.

The sensory input signifies the individual's ability to "know about" the status of the performance and thus, through one's own internal mechanism can control errors or make the necessary adaptations to variations in the requirements for motor action in the situation. Singer (1975) notes that all body movements are space structured and that learning is a process of establishing new spatial relationships in patterns of motion. Smith (1972), a researcher in behavioral cybernetics, reminds us that "learning is not determined directly by environmental stimuli, but by self-governed selection and control of all levels of environmental stimuli and psychophysiologic function in energy production and response" (p. 345). Researchers who have pursued the cybernetic model as a basis for understanding motor skill learning include Adams (1968), Keele (1968), Bernstein, (1967) and Smith (1967).

Information Processing Model. This model represents a descriptive communication theory which addresses the mental processes of attention, perception, memory, and decision making involved in the motor act response to environmental stimuli. This model is not un-like the cybernetic one but is concerned additionally with the pro-cesses involved in the transmission of information received by cues in the situation and their resultant response. Of particular concern in this model is the ability of the individual to discriminate among critically relevant and irrelevant cues, select the pertinent and meaningful information, transmit it at a rapid rate, and retrieve desired information from the long-term memory. Each individual has a channel capacity for handling information and any informa-tion above that capacity cannot be transmitted. An overloading of the channel capacity results in motor skill decrement with an in-creasing number of errors.

Singer (1975) identifies three major mechanisms in the infor-mation processing model:

1. Perceptual mechanism—receives and identifies information sent from a sense organ.
2. Translation mechanism—decides choice of action.
3. Effector mechanism—coordinates and phases the action. (p. 3)

It is feedback from the latter mechanism that controls information in the perceptual–transmission process.

Stelmach (1982, pp. 66–67) sees three processing stages that occur from the stimulus to response and notes that each stage is sequential and operates only on the basis of information transmit-ted to it. He diagrams the process as such:

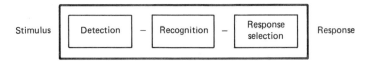

In this paradigm, he identifies two time periods.

1. *Reaction time:* the period between stimulus presentation and the beginning of the response. Keele (1982) found that reaction time is influenced by the number of possible situations that can arise and the number of possible responses that could be made in the situa-tion. The greater the uncertainty, the longer the reaction time to decide upon the response.
2. *Movement time:* refers to psychomotor response, and its efficiency is a function of the speed and precision of the movement. (pp. 70–71)

Schmidt (1976) diagnosed two sources of error in the response process: (1) *Error of response selection* which could result from mis-perceptions of the environment, so that selection of the wrong re-sponse occurs, or the perception and selection seem acceptable. A fluctuation in the environment after the response had been selected, however, could result in an incorrect response; and (2) *Error of response execution* in which the chosen pattern was not followed, possibly due to unexpected environmental fluctuation, fatigue, or "neural noise."

Welford (1968) theorizes that movement is determined more by central processes controlling movement than by factors of muscular effort involved. Researchers involved in pursuing the information processing model in understanding motor skill learning include: Fitts (1964), Stelmach (1969), Schmidt (1976), Keele (1968), and Poulton (1972).

Adaptation Model. This model views motor skill development from a hierarchical perspective with higher and lower operational processes. It is based on the notion that complex motor skills are composites of subskills which must be mastered before the performance goal can be achieved.

In describing this model, Singer (1975) likens it to a computer plan in which man functions with higher order (executive) programs or routines and subroutines or subprograms. Subroutines, which often function in sequential patterns, are perceived as the "foundational building blocks" for the executive routine, and the mastery of each is essential for efficient and effective performance. Singer describes the essence of the model as follows: "The executive program can be thought of as the plan, idea or goal in a situation. The subroutines are the processes, e.g., movements that enable the plan to be executed" (p. 85). The plan in the organism is the basis of human activity.

Psychomotor skill learning is perceived from the perspective of a hierarchical plan of skill development by which goal attainment is achieved through mastery of subacts, each in sequence with increasing complexity as the act gets nearer the ultimate goal. It is the relationship of each of these subacts to each other that is the focus of study in this area. Theorists addressing this model and its saliency to motor learning are Paillard (1960) and Miller, Galantin, and Pribran (1960).

There are areas of similarity in all of these three models, and newer models are evolving from these three classifications. Model development with the intent of psychomotor learning theory development is progressing, as emphasis is placed on the physiologic, psychologic, and cognitive processes that occur within the organism as it responds to cues from the environment with a coordinated and effective performance. To the teacher of psychomotor skills, these movements are of significance, for such learning can no longer be viewed as a mechanistic process in response to environmental stimuli.

PRACTICE

Motor skill learning requires practice; i.e., the opportunity to "try out" and eventually refine all processes essential for a smooth coordinated performance. The nature of practice and its subsequent results are functions of the goal to be achieved, the degree of complexity of the skill to be mastered, the individual characteristics of the learner, and situational variables which have impact on the learning process. Research into the role of practice in motor skill learning has pursued numerous directions and is reported extensively in the literature. Findings of significance to the teaching of psychomotor skills in nursing are presented.

Variations in Individual Response

As with any learning, there is considerable variation in individual response to a practice learning situation and in the ultimate results of such experiences. Singer (1975) suggests that "variations in performance levels between students throughout practice may be due to the relative ease of gaining insight into the problem; the transferability of related learning skills to the task at hand, which might be of special advantage in the early stages of practice; and various psychological, physiological, intellectual, and emotional adjustments" (p. 373).

The readiness factor is an important one as the learner enters into the practice session for new motor skill development. Readiness relates to motivation to learn, the mind set toward the experience, meaningfulness of the new learning to one's own goals, acknowledgment of need for perseverance in pursuit of mastery learning, and a grasp of the goal to be achieved and the processes entailed in achievement. Motivation, although a recognized positive force in responding to demands of new learning of new motor skills, can also be a discordant force if too intense. Research suggests that an excessively intense level of motivation may impede progress in complex skill attainment. The finding that a moderate degree of motivation results in the greatest success suggests that there may be an optimum level of motivation for each skill.

Readiness to achieve mastery in psychomotor skill learning is also a function of the development of integrated neuromuscular and cognitive processes which must result in coordinated movement. Research by Marteniuk (1969) and Henry (1958) indicates that there is no such element as a generalized motor ability, but rather, that motor learning ability is task-specific and dependent upon such factors as innate ability, previous learning, motivation, and other variables. Henry (1958) states, " . . . it is no longer possible to justify the concept of unitary abilities such as coordination and agility, since the evidence shows that these abilities are specific to the test or activity" (p. 126).

Perceptual Variation and Patterns of Practice

A variation in individual response to learning which was previously discussed is the cognitive style of an individual, field-independent or field-dependent. This characteristic is directly related to the perceptual component of motor skill learning as reflected in the current cybernetic and information processing theories which are identified with such learning. The ability to respond to stimuli and select relevant cues from external and internal environments is perceived to be a function of the individual's perceptual style, for sensory input is essential in controlling and regulating motor activity (Fleishman, 1972; Kelso, 1982; Singer, 1975).

Bruton (1976) explored the influence of the perceptual style of learners in using three patterns of practice when learning the fine complex skill of subcutaneous injection. Three patterns of practice were identified: mental (visualizing the task), physical; and a combination of mental and physical. Students were assigned randomly to each of the three groups and then the cognitive style of each student was identified through the Rod and Frame Tests.

Results indicate that field-independent students learn the task, regardless of the pattern used, more readily than do field-dependent students. This is especially true of the physical–mental pattern where it was noted that performance of the field-dependent students deteriorated. Bruton (1976) explains the success of the field-independent student with this pattern. "In learning skills, perceptual awareness of bodily kinesthetic cues and appropriate response to these contributes to mastery of skill regardless of type of practice used" (p. 73). The intelligence variable of the different cognitive styles and its relationship to learning of perceptual motor skills has not been explored sufficiently, but questions are raised to the possible greater intellectual capacity of field-independent persons who are adept at cue selection and hypothesizing problems and solutions. Data from all groups, regardless of cognitive style, suggest that the most effective practice modality is physical practice followed by mental practice.

Length and Frequency of Practice Periods

Lawther (1977) identifies six factors that need to be considered in answering questions as to the length of the practice session and the spacing of rest intervals.

1. Age of learner
2. Complexity and strenuousness of the skill
3. Specific purpose of the particular practice
4. Level of learning already attained
5. Experiential background of the learner
6. Total environmental conditions including other demands and distractions, activity between practices, and other factors. (p. 139)

Distribution of Practice Sessions. Two general classifications of practice sessions are (1) massed and (2) distributed. Massed practice refers to a pattern in which the rest interval is less than the trial length. Distributed practice refers to a pattern in which the rest interval is equal to or greater than the trial length. Practice occurs over a longer period of time, which may include no practice days. The actual practice time may be the same for both patterns; it is the distribution of time that differs. Research studies by Whitley (1970) and Stelmach (1969) noted no difference in the amount of learning between distributed and massed practice, and Stelmach concluded that learning a motor task is a function of the number of trials and is independent of conditions of practice distribution.

Length of Practice Session. Lawther (1977) summarizes the available evidence on the length of practice sessions:

1. In early stages of gross motor skill learning, relatively short practice sessions are more profitable in terms of minutes of practice. Practices can be too long or too short and only experience with the skill and the learner will indicate the most profitable length.
2. Constant lengths of practice sessions have been reported to produce more learning than regular increases and decreases in length in succeeding sessions.
3. Short, interspersed rest periods within the practice session seem to increase the amount of learning.
4. Adults who are in need of acquiring a skill in a short time can practice profitably many hours per day if it is not an activity that demands great physical effort and entails much fatigue. (pp. 141–42)

The short length of time for beginning learners may be based on their shorter attention span, which increases as practice progresses. Keele (1982) notes that "as practice proceeds, not only is decision time less, but some decisions drop out all together as they become redundant when a pattern of movement can be made" (p. 161). The attention of the learner is freed to address more global decisions relative to the task.

Research suggests that gross skills are learned more efficiently and rapidly with more numerous practice periods spaced over a period of time. It is generally acknowledged that a reasonable degree of achievement in most motor skill learning is accomplished with relatively few practice periods.

Overlearning/Repetition
Overlearning refers to any practice, often referred to as drill, which follows one perfect trial, a generally accepted criterion of success. In psychomotor skill learning, overlearning usually results in greater retention. However, there is a point at which overlearning loses its

benefit and actually results in performance decrement. Singer (1975) notes that research indicates a 50 percent overlearning is advantageous. While 100 percent overlearning may produce better performance, the gain is not sufficient to warrant the costs involved in extending practice.

Lawther (1977) sees two significant purposes to be achieved by overlearning: (1) to ensure greater retention over longer periods of time, and (2) to generalize the skill so that its adaptability to innumerable changes in the environment is increased; i.e., automatic response to environmental cues.

The decisions regarding the degree of repetition or drill are dependent upon the purposes to be served by acquiring the psychomotor skill. Too much drill results in no increment in skill performance, possibly due to the onset of fatigue, boredom, or frustration when time might be perceived to be better used in other learning.

Retention and Reminiscence
Retention refers to the persistence of learning over a period of time devoid of overt practice periods. Reminiscence refers to significant improvement in performance after periods of considerable lapse of time in which no practice occurred. The latter may be a function of a low level of learning in the initial period as a result of fatigue, boredom, pressure, or other similar factors; or it may mean that the individual has been mentally practicing the skill even though no overt action was evident.

Retention is closely related to the previously discussed matter of overlearning. Fleishman (1972) reports on a study he conducted which indicated that the most powerful variable operating in a study of retention of a perceptual-motor skill was individual differences in the level of the original learning. Rather than retention being a function of pretask abilities, it is a function of specific habits acquired in the original practice of the task. Singer (1975) postulates that retention of motor skills can be achieved with less practice than verbal skills because of the unique nature of each skill. Its uniqueness means that there are not many other learned skills that can interfere with the originally learned skill.

Transfer of Learning
Closely related to the retention variable is the matter of transfer of one psychomotor skill learning to the new task to be accomplished. The closer the new task or its component parts are perceived by the learner to resemble previous learnings, the more quickly and more efficiently it will be learned. The transfer activity, however, may be primarily evident in the early stages of the motor skill learning. As the skill reaches the complex level, task specificity becomes the focus of the learner, and there is less potential for task similarity.

Singer (1975) suggests four factors which may influence the transfer process:

1. Amount of practice of prior skill
2. Motivation to transfer skill
3. Method of training
4. Intent of transfer (p. 47).

Practice is a process during which the learner has the opportunity to master psychomotor skill learning. In addition to multiple variables, which account for the individuality of each learner response, task specificity is a significant factor in motor skill learning and thus influences the patterning of practice sessions, amount needed, retention for long-term use, and potential for transferability.

TEACHING

The theoretical basis for teaching psychomotor skills finds its roots in theories of learning acknowledged as fundamental to psychomotor skill learning. A teaching model based on the S–R or R–S paradigm differs significantly from one that represents the process as well as the outcome, S–O–R, where "O" signifies processes within the organism that influence response. In the latter model, the teacher becomes more cognizant of what is occurring in the learner during the learning process as well as how the learner is performing and thus is able to assess and direct more effectively the learner's progress during skill development.

The directions that theory development in psychomotor learning are taking have significant implications for nursing education. Periodically, questions are raised about the relevancy of psychomotor learning to professional nursing practice. To some in the profession, the word psychomotor denotes a negative factor in nursing. Yet, nursing involves "hands on" activities whose skills are essential in assuring quality care. The present emphasis on physical assessment skills, touch, and nursing management in a highly technical health care setting suggests that psychomotor skills will continue to be an essential part of the assessment and implementation stages of the nursing process.

The teaching of psychomotor skills is a significant component of the education of nurses. Tisdale (1984) a 1983 baccalaureate graduate nurse affirms this position when she comments on state board examinations and her beliefs about what the new graduate should know. She states:

I have been working since graduation, long enough to see some of the virtues and defects of my education; what I am glad I learned, what I wish I had been offered or listened to more carefully. I'm sorry now that

I let my anxiety about more sophisticated topics and my teachers' nonchalance about practical abilities get in the way of perfecting basic skills. My communication skills are put to use every day, and every situation is unique, but it was skills like I.V. calculations and bladder irrigations that threw me as a new graduate. (p. 166)

Can a nonchalant posture of a faculty member be acceptable in teaching any domain of learning that is pertinent to the practice?

Setting

Two settings are appropriate for teaching psychomotor skills: a learning resource laboratory and the clinical field. The distinguishing characteristics of these two settings were described in Chapter 1 with the significant differential being the matter of focus and control. The other dimension relates to the "realness" quality which a clinical field can provide in terms of client problems and the dynamics of an environment where specific types of nursing care are practiced. Singer (1975) sees a laboratory as an area away from the mainstream of traffic where situations can be controlled fairly effectively. Since realism is likely to be lost, the learner performance observed in this setting may not reflect that which would occur in real-life circumstances.

Learning Resources Laboratory. The laboratory with appropriate equipment provides a setting where the learner can learn to manipulate equipment with a sense of its process and intended outcome. The environment provides the necessary situational cues and enables the student to respond to the cues in a nonthreatening milieu. This environment contains the necessary multimedia, including both hard- and software for use in explaining the process and critical elements of the skill and the models and so forth, essential for practice.

Psychomotor skill learning is an egocentric process. The learner's sense of self as a coordinated being with control over the skill process is essential before one uses the skill in a more public setting. The time necessary to spend in the laboratory is specific to the task and the individual learner. Since no set time can be designated for a particular skill practice, a learning laboratory needs to be available and accessible to learners on their own terms. Such a laboratory might be perceived for psychomotor learning as the library is perceived for cognitive learning an open environment where the learners practice skills according to their own needs to the point of an agreed upon level of achievement. The laboratory, under the direction of a preceptor skilled in the psychomotor domain, provides a milieu where learners can receive formative evaluation as they progress through the practice experience.

Such a laboratory also serves an important testing function, which will be presented in more detail later in this chapter relative to the use of a taxonomy. The use of the laboratory for practice and for monitoring the performance as the learning process proceeds is to facilitate retention, since retention is a function of the effectiveness of the initial learning.

Clinical Field. This setting places the individual in the world where nurses practice, including the hospital, community, nursing home, and client's home. The nature of the milieu has a bearing on skill performance. The concern here is how that milieu is used in teaching psychomotor skills.

The clinical setting for practice needs assessment in relation to the goal of the practice. Whereas earlier periods of nursing education emphasized psychomotor skill development and used the clinical area for such practice, today the clinical field is established on the basis of care of the patient. Infante (1975) challenges us to think about this practice when she says, "We talk about patient selection, instead of selection of the opportunity for learning" (p. 16). Psychomotor skill development should occur without the learner being concerned about the other care activities germaine to the environment. Thus, it is not the setting that determines what the learner will experience, but rather, the needed experience will determine the practice setting.

Teachers will be challenged to reexamine the notion that the learner needs to "know the patient" before performing a psychomotor skill on the patient. Knowledge of the patient is a function of the faculty role. It means that faculty, who are in a setting where there is ample opportunity for practice with a particular skill, may invite their colleagues to send their students to the setting for practice. It also means that when learners reach the predetermined level of skill attainment in the laboratory, they will proceed to the clinical field for immediate practice; for learning of a skill is more meaningful and economical when it is linked to application.

Whole versus Part Approach to Teaching Psychomotor Skills

The decision to teach the skill as a whole or to teach it in terms of its parts is often a reflection of the teacher's belief about how psychomotor skills are learned. For clarification, it is important to define the terms whole and part. Gates and colleagues (1953) offer the following definitions:

> *Whole:* a definitely segregated, independent pattern which possesses
>   unity, coherence and meaning in itself above that implied by
>   its parts.
> *Part:* an element in a total situation which is essential to the meaning

as a whole, but which loses its peculiar meaning when isolated from the whole. (pp. 371–72)

Part teaching is based on a behavioristic mode which considers learning to be additive; i.e., as each part is learned, a new one is introduced and added to the previously learned one once it is mastered. Whole learning is compatible with gestalt or field theory, which views the whole as greater than the sum of its parts and the parts related to each other and to the whole. Learning is integrative.

Naylor and Briggs (1961) identify two aspects of a psychomotor skill that need to be considered in making the decision as to teaching the skill holistically or partially:

Task Complexity: refers to demands made on a person's memory and is a function of information processing.

Task Organization: indicates the nature of interrelationships of several task dimensions or organization.

Their studies and those of others suggest that part practice is more effective in skills that are highly complex and have low organization (few independent components in the task). Whole practice is more effective with high organization where there is an increase in component interaction. Generalization from this notion is still tentative, and analysis of the task to be learned continues to be an essential action.

Singer (1975) poses questions to be asked in relation to the complexity criterion of a skill:

1. How difficult does the learner perceive the task to be?
2. How many things does the learner have to think about; remember from previous related experiences?
3. To what extent is it possible to forget the task over time and therefore pose a challenge for the learner to remember it? (p. 383)

If part teaching is to be used, the units must be large enough to represent a total phenomenon in themselves. Too small a unit fosters boredom and lack of challenge; too large a unit leads to frustration when repeated practice does not produce success and withdrawal results from loss of interest.

In general, the whole approach to learning is more effective because it does enable the learner to see the goal, that is, what the outcome looks like; gain insight into the total process; and see the relationship of the parts to each other and to the goal. It is more economical because the learner can identify those parts that need more practice for an efficient performance of the total and can emphasize their refinement in relation to the whole. Practice is specific to the learner. In additive learning, each step is developed in terms of the selected criteria, but at the conclusion the learner still needs time to learn how the parts are related in order to produce an efficient performance. McGuigan and MacCaslin (1955) add another dimension to the issue of whole versus part teaching when they report their study which indicated that the more intelligent subjects responded more favorably to whole learning. This finding may be a function of their cognitive ability in information processing or their ability to learn more and thus have a greater repertoire of experience to draw upon.

Knowledge of Results
Knowledge of results as the learner progresses through the psychomotor practice is essential if skill development is to occur. Bilodeau and Bilodeau (1961) summarized studies as to the role of knowledge of results in skill development and state: "Studies of feedback or knowledge of results show it to be the strongest, most important variable controlling performance and learning" (p. 250). Singer (1975) refers to the two general types of feedback:

Intrinsic: proprioceptive activity and tactile sense inform learner as to "feel" of the response while visual feedback provides data on accuracy of response.

Augmented: the special cues added to the learning situation such as
(artificial)   verbal cues, supplementary or artificial visual or kinesthetic cues. (p. 47)

Verbal cues are significant factors in adding to skill performance increment, but the learner's reliance on these cues must be avoided, for performance in skill learning is dependent upon the learner's ability to judge his or her own performance. Feedback only on outcome may influence the performance but not facilitate the process of learning. Lawther (1977) notes that "the feedback should be visual and perhaps quantitatively precise in verbal description" (p. 137). In reference to augmented feedback he suggests that it should be as closely adapted to individual learner needs as possible.

Some skill learning can occur without augmented feedback as learners draw upon their own repertoire of knowledge and rely upon intrinsic feedback. Augmented feedback does facilitate the learning process when there is continuity, yet selectivity in terms of the learner's particular needs. When neither intrinsic nor augmented feedback occurs or is discontinued during the learning process, there is a decrement in psychomotor skill performance and learning.

Occurrence of Two Different Learnings Simultaneously
As was noted earlier, psychomotor skill learning is concerned with the three domains of learning: cognitive, affective, and psychomotor. It was suggested that the cognitive element needs to be

viewed from two perspectives: the theory and principles underlying the purpose, process, and outcome of the skill, and the information processes that occur within the individual from the stimulus to the actual performance.

The discussion of the research and concepts pertaining to psychomotor learning indicates that the advancement process from novice to expert requires the coordination of all cognitive processes relative to cue selection, interpretation, and the appropriate response in an efficient manner. The theoretical bases underlying the skill are most important but need to be addressed outside the actual performance so that the learner can focus on the coordination processes essential for a coordinated response.

In nursing education there is a tendency to interject the theoretical component of psychomotor skill learning while the process of cognitive information processing is being developed. For example, as the nursing student is going through the process of learning to administer a drug by injection, the teacher says, "What are the actions of that drug you are going to administer?" The student's psychomotor learning is interfered with because of the need to respond to a "knowledge" question. When learning to drive an automobile, what would be the response of the novice if the instructor interrupted the concentration on the driving activity with the following type of question, "What is the purpose of the sparkplugs in the engine?"

Brown, Tickner and Simmonds (1969) examined this dual activity phenomenon in a study of the interference between concurrent tasks of driving a car through a designated gap and making a telephone call, where the effects of divided attention on judgments of clearance, control skills, and checking auditory messages were explored. Results of this study demonstrated that the driver made reliably more wrong decisions while driving and answering questions than while driving in a controlled condition without questions. Questions were also answered reliably less correctly and took longer for response than in the control situation where questions were asked during the time when the car was not in motion. Poulton (1972) concurs that it is possible to carry out two tasks simultaneously, but in order for a person to accomplish this feat one task must have been practiced sufficiently to the point of being automatic.

In a field study, Cairy (1981) examined the effect of cognitive teaching during nursing students' learning of two skills: intramuscular injection and intravenous insertion. The experimental group received its teaching of the cognitive component of the skill prior to the performance while the control group received its teaching of the cognitive component concurrent with the skill performance. The finding supported the hypothesis that those students who experienced teaching of the cognitive prior to performing the skill carried out the skill with a significantly higher degree of precision. Although the limited sample precludes making generalizations, the findings are in accord with those of Brown and colleagues (1969).

Psychomotor skill learning is a complex activity that requires knowledge of purpose, principles, and anticipated outcome in relation to both the cognitive and affective domains. The knowledge component is discussed in conferences either prior to the actual skill performance or following the performance, where the latter is analyzed and evaluated. It is during the actual performance that the learner needs to be free to follow the sequential pattern of the task without interruption, except in instances where safety is at stake.

TAXONOMY OF PSYCHOMOTOR SKILL PERFORMANCE

During practice of a psychomotor skill, changes occur in the learner's performance that signal movement from novice toward expert practitioner. Fleishman (1972) summarizes studies that deal with practice tasks:

1. As practice continues, changes occur in the particular combinations of the abilities contributing to performance.
2. These changes are progressive, systematic and eventually become stabilized.
3. The contribution of "non motor" abilities (e.g., verbal, spatial) which may play a role in learning decreases systematically with practice relative to "motor abilities."
4. There is an increase in a factor specific in the task itself. (p. 98)

The developments occurring in the process are directed toward a systematic, sequential order of activities accomplished with spatial and temporal reality and reflective of a consistent response pattern. The learner develops selective attention to cues, is able to select relevant information while disregarding other data (thus greatly decreasing decision time between stimulus and response), and is able quickly to anticipate variables entailed in the total performance. An expert performer develops skills that are almost automatic as a result of increased speed, accuracy, and coordination. Schneider and Fish (1982) state that "practice leads to apparently resource-free automatic productions for consistent processing, but does not reduce resources needed for varied processing tasks". (p. 11)

Psychomotor Taxonomy
Several taxonomies, i.e. hierarchies of behavior, have been developed to identify the growth process from novice to expert by practitioners such as Simpson (1966), Harrow (1972), Kibler, Barker, and Miles (1970), and Cratty (1967). Dave (1970) has proposed a tax-

onomy for psychomotor skill performance with an integrating concept of neuromuscular coordination. Reilly (1980) demonstrated the use of this taxonomy in nursing which delineates the skill development to the level of professional competence.

Taxonomy includes five levels of performance but does not identify discrete components of each level. The levels are:

P 1.0 Imitation
Skills are learned in the beginning after they have been demonstrated, whether directly by the teacher or by observation of the process on a film, videotape, or slide tape sequence. The performance lacks neuromuscular coordination or control and, hence, is generally in a crude and imperfect form (i.e., impulse, overt repetition).

P 2.0 Manipulation
In this level, the learner follows a prescription as outlined on a procedure sheet, learning to follow instructions, performing selected actions and fixing performance through necessary practice.

P 3.0 Precision
Performance has reached a level of refinement and can be carried out without a set of directions or a model, and performance is characterized by accuracy, i.e., exactness with reduction in errors.

P 4.0 Articulation
Performance is coordinated in a logical sequence of activities that reflects harmony and consistency among the activities. The time dimension is added here, for speed and time must be within a realistic expectation.

P 5.0 Naturalization
Skill represents a high degree of proficiency, which has become an automatic response to appropriate situational cues. Performance is efficient and meets criteria for professional competence.

Performance Criteria for Each Level of Psychomotor Skill
Specific expected behaviors for each level of the taxonomy can be determined from research findings and theoretical perspectives about learning psychomotor skills. The behaviors can be used as criteria in determining the expected level of performance.

P 1.0 Imitation
Observed actions are followed
Movements are gross
Coordination lacks smoothness

Errors are present
Time and speed are based on learner need

P 2.0 Manipulation
Written instructions are followed
Coordination of movements is variable
Accuracy is in terms of the written prescription
Time and speed are variable

P 3.0 Precision
(3.1)
(3.2)
A logical sequence of actions is carried out
Coordination is at a high level
Errors are minimal and do not involve critical actions
Time and speed are variable

P 4.0 Articulation
A logical sequence of actions is carried out
Coordination is at a high level
Errors are generally limited
Time and speed are within reasonable expectations

P 5.0 Naturalization
Sequence of actions is automatic
Coordination is consistently at a high level
Time and speed are within reality
Performance reflects professional competence

The changes in behavior indicated in this taxonomy reflect the evolution of skilled performance. In the first two levels, behavior is generally gross with the accuracy dimension entering the schema in the second level in terms of following a prescribed format. These two levels may be achieved in a learning laboratory.

Level 3 is divided according to setting: P 3.1 is the learning laboratory and P 3.2 is in the clinical field. In both, the performance behavior is the same. The difference refers to performance in a controlled setting in contrast to performance in an uncontrolled setting with real clients. The attainment of a P 3.0 level in the laboratory does not necessarily indicate that the same behaviors will be exhibited in the clinical field where the skill is performed with less control of environmental cues.

Level 3 also makes a statement relative to the nature of the errors that might occur. Every skill has certain activities that are essential for maintaining its integrity, while other actions can be altered without influencing the general effect of the skill. It is essential that the critical elements of the skill be identified and considered to be nonnegotiable; i.e. they must be error free at this level.

It is noted that a logical sequence of actions as specified in a procedure is not a criterion for skill attainment. The sequence of actions may not necessarily be the same as specified on the procedure sheet, but as long as the learner can rationally support the decisions involved in the sequencing the criterion is met. Too often the actions described in the procedure are so detailed that the critical judgment of the learner is denied and the procedure becomes a sequence of unchallenged actions.

Level 4 adds a significant dimension, the matter of speed and timing in the performance of a skill. One is not skillful if the act is not performed within a reasonable time period. One may be most accurate and skillful in obtaining a blood pressure reading, but if an hour is required for the act one cannot be considered to be skilled.

Questions are often raised as to whether speed or accuracy should be emphasized in psychomotor skill development. The taxonomy described in this chapter suggests that accuracy precedes speed. The nature of the skill to be taught, the speed requirement for its execution, and the particular abilities of the learner determine the response to that question. Early emphasis on speed is appropriate in psychomotor skills momentum, but since that is not a characteristic of many psychomotor skills in nursing, early emphasis on accuracy is preferred. Accuracy is specific to speed in practice.

The speed dimension as it relates to skilled performance is best evaluated in the setting where the actual activity will occur in practice. It is there that the adaptability of the skill is demonstrated and the learner's use of decision time is expedited through selective attention to cues in the situation. Although time can be a factor in skill performance in the laboratory, its significance in relation to skilled behavior is best demonstrated in the practice setting.

Level 5 is the point where the skill most reflects automatic behavior. The learner is no longer concerned about the "how to do" of the skill. It is now an integral part of nursing practice and can be retrieved upon appropriate situational cues. The synthesis of cognitive, affective, and psychomotor domains has occurred and the performance reflects the criterion of professional competence.

USE OF A PERFORMANCE TAXONOMY

Nursing faculty must come to the decision that not all psychomotor skills applicable to nursing practice should be developed to the level of naturalization of professional competency. The quantity of skills is too large and the frequency of use is so variable that faculty need to be more discriminating as to the level at which each psychomotor skill should be performed. Decisions are based upon need, frequency of skill in usual practice in the local geographical region, and the availability of experience for practice.

Essential Decisions

Mastery/Competency. Before identifying the appropriate level, faculty need to clarify the concepts of mastery and competency and decide how the terms will be used. Infante (1975) uses the terms as described previously by Sheffler:

> Competency—Knowing how to do something.
> Proficiency—Knowing how to do it well.
> Mastery—Doing it brilliantly. (p. 34)

Morgan and Irby (1978) define competency as the knowledge and skills necessary for adequate performance in a profession. This definition is more compatible with level P 5.0 being identified as the level of performance competency. Mastery also has a different meaning. In the mastery of learning concept, mastery is defined in terms of objectives to be attained. In this context, mastery relates to the mastery of the learning implied by the designated level to be achieved, not to the ultimate level possible. Because of different meanings attached to these terms, it is important to include the faculty's definition with documents related to psychomotor teaching. In the proposed taxonomy, the ultimate level is considered professional competency with mastery referring to the designated level of achievement.

Skills to Be Included. Decisions as to what skills are to be included are in accord with the overall curriculum plan as it reflects the demands of generic or specialized nursing practice. The decision is best made in joint discussions with faculty and nursing service administrators who employ the graduates. Sweeney and colleagues (1980) report on a study that identified essential skills of baccalaureate graduates from the perspective of education and service. Some programs have such skills identified on a national or state level. All decisions, however, must be based on professional judgment.

The selection of skills must reflect the criterion of motor behavior performance, not cognitive behavior. Recording, although involving some motor action, is in essence a cognitive skill, for the evaluation is based on the substance of the recording, not the actual process of writing. Interviewing is also a cognitive skill although it does involve some muscular activity.

Location of Practice. Another decision affecting the planning for teaching psychomotor skills is the location of the practice; i.e., learning resource laboratory or the clinical field. Preliminary practice in the laboratory for at least the first two levels is generally facilitative, for it affords the student the opportunity to gain a sense of self and the ability to manipulate equipment and coordinate activities in a relatively risk-free environment that does not put patients or others at risk. The student learning a new skill, regardless of the setting, may feel at risk.

When the student enters the clinical field for a first-time performance of a skill in that setting, faculty must recognize the egocentric nature of psychomotor learning. Until the learner feels comfortable and secure in the knowledge that body movements are coordinated in working with equipment and the client, the learner will not be able to focus on other events that occur within the context of the procedure. It is unrealistic to expect the learner performing a skill for the first time in the setting to be able to greet the patient, explain the procedure, and respond to other demands in the situation. At this stage in the learning, the teacher's role is to manage all the other aspects that relate to patient care so that the learner can focus on the performance.

Once the learner is asked to perform a skill in the clinical environment, regardless of the level of skill development, teachers must be cognizant of the impact of the situational variables and needs of the learners on the outcome of the performance. Cleland (1965) studied the impact of stress in a clinical setting on the performance of graduate nurses. Although the study addressed cognitive testing, similar results can be anticipated in psychomotor testing. Increased situational stress interfered negatively with cue utilization. An additional variable reflective of the social nature of the clinical field was studied; the relationship of the need for social approval to performance. A high need for social approval requires a low stress situation; increase in stress brings a performer to a maximum level of motivation quickly and then performance deteriorates. Low level of need for social approval requires a moderate level of stress to bring the performer to an optimum motivation level for maximum performance.

The findings of Cleland relative to social approval needs is reflective of the data on field-independent and field-dependent learners. The field-dependent learner has a high need for social acceptance while the field-independent learner relies more on intrinsic acceptance. Both groups approach psychomotor performance in a dynamic environment differently; a fact that must be acknowledged by the instructor in determining the best strategies to use in teaching.

Outcome Level for Each Skill. The outcome level selected for each skill must be realistic in terms of its potential for attainment by all students. This decision is in essence a contract with the learner; the experiences will be provided that enable the learner to reach the designated level and the evaluation will be in accord with the level. It does not guarantee that the learner will reach the specified level, for much learning is still under the control of the learner.

The designation of a level does not preclude students from advancing further if the opportunity permits. Students should be encouraged to advance in those skills not designated at the professional competency level when experience is available. A faculty may feel that a P 3.2 level is most realistic for skill in catheterization, but if the student is in a clinical setting where there is ample opportunity for experience, the student should be encouraged to proceed to the P 5.0 level. The outcome level specified for any course or the total program reflects perceived reality, not the full potential for any one student.

Methods of Testing. Decisions on the testing of the student's performance, particularly from level P 3.0 through P 5.0, must include considerations relative to timing, strategy, and location. Testing in the laboratory generally is a function of limited availability of experience in the clinical setting. If a faculty feels that some level of achievement of some skills is necessary but the clinical setting does not provide sufficient opportunity, simulation testing in the laboratory may occur. Testing is indicated at the P 3.1 level. In the clinical field, testing may involve direct observation or videotape. Regardless of the setting and method, testing time is designated and extraneous variables are controlled as much as possible. Unlike formative evaluation which addresses what is and what can be, the teacher in summative evaluation, which addresses what is, assumes the posture of a tester not a teacher. Intervention is restricted to evidence of clear and present danger. Skill delineation is not a matter of the number of times a skill has been performed, but rather, the ability of the learner to perform in accordance with predetermined criteria.

Psychomotor Performance Grid
A taxonomy provides a framework for decisions about appropriate levels of performance for each skill and for planning for the teaching of the skill in a nursing program. When using the presented taxonomy in concert with the taxonomy of one or both of the other domains, it is essential to recognize that each domain is discrete, thus there may or may not be consistency in the designated levels among the domains. A P 4.0 level on the psychomotor taxonomy does not mean that the other taxonomies will be so designated. The knowledge level of a skill is not necessarily the same as the performance level.

In the development of a grid, i.e., a mapping of the teaching of psychomotor skills, faculty first make decisions relative to the outcome performance level for each skill that is expected at the conclusion of the educational program. The course in which the skill is introduced is noted and the expected level of achievement is designated. Some skills, such as taking an oral temperature, radial pulse, and respirations, may reach P 5.0 within the first course, while other skills may progress over a longer period.

When a designated skill level is reached by the student, he or she will be held accountable for maintenance of that level in all subsequent courses. Faculty in the subsequent courses are responsible for monitoring students' performance on all psychomotor skills relevant to the practice area. This formative evaluation is essential for skill maintenance and addresses the habitual practice of the students within the context of normal activities.

When faculty in subsequent courses note that the student does not perform at the expected level of psychomotor skill, it is appropriate to refer the student to the laboratory for further practice. It is essential that the laboratory recommendation not be perceived as punitive, but rather as an opportunity to review and refine performance. This is another example of viewing the learning resource laboratory from the same perspective for psychomotor learning as the library is viewed for cognitive learning. Cognitive and psychomotor skills must be differentiated during these formative evaluation periods. If the student performs the skill at the appropriate level but is unable to answer questions relative to the theory basis of the skill, the problem is cognitive, not psychomotor, and must be addressed accordingly. A return to the learning resource laboratory would not be an appropriate resolution of the problem.

An example of a grid for teaching psychomotor skills is demonstrated in Table 17. The grid represents four terms in which students would be in a clinical field practicing their skills with real clients. The format of the nursing program (Table 16) is intended to be general rather than representative of any specific nursing theory so that its potential can be demonstrated, regardless of the curriculum framework. In a school setting, faculty would develop its own curriculum and plan the sequence in accord with whatever theoretical framework it chose. The grid would relate to the program sequencing and may well differ from the grid proposed here. The program presented is not necessarily meant to depict a total program. Some programs may include an introductory course in which basic skill development is highlighted. Others may have an additional term that provides for synthesizing practice skills and practice in some of the leadership activities of nursing.

The skills used in the grid are derived primarily from the study of Sweeney and colleagues (1980), which listed the skills upon which there was agreement by faculty and nursing service personnel as expected behaviors of graduates (Table 17).

Once faculty have developed a psychomotor grid, there exists a

TABLE 16. NURSING PROGRAM

	Term I	Term II	Term III	Term IV
	Nursing Care of Clients with Minimal Health Care Needs	*Nursing Care of Clients with Moderate Health Care Needs*	*Nursing Care of Clients with Acute Health Care Needs*	*Nursing Care of Clients with Long-term Health Care Needs*
Role of Nurse	Supportive Monitoring Maintenance Educative	Supportive Supplementary Educative Palliative	Compensatory Monitoring Protective Consultative Educative	Supplementary Monitoring Educative Protective Consultative
Setting	Ambulatory care setting Convalescent home Nursing home	Hospital Client's home Ambulatory care setting	Hospital Intensive care Acute care Psychiatric hospital	Long-term care facilities Rehabilitation facilities Home for mentally retarded Community agencies Client's home

master plan which designates what skills are to be taught, where in the total program they are to be taught, and the desired levels of achievement to be reached at any point throughout the curriculum. Such a plan is not static and needs to be subjected to periodic reviews in relation to its relevance to current nursing practices and to the accuracy of faculty judgments in level determination.

Psychomotor Grid and Accountability
The grid has built into it a system for assigning accountability. Faculty in each course are accountable to assure that students are at the designated level of mastery before proceeding to the next course. Although there is provision for the unexpected that interferes with a student's achievement of the goal, subsequent faculty have the right to expect that students have met the expectations so that the new learning demands of the next course can proceed. When changes in practice require alterations in expected accomplishment, this is a matter for faculty deliberation.

Student accountability is also prescribed. If students are given a copy of the grid and informed that the completion of the skills at the designated level is a requirement for the course grade and advancement to the next course, they will need to assume responsibility for obtaining the necessary experience. This demand fosters the development of a self-directed learner and facilitates the establishment of a systematic plan for one's own learning.

TABLE 17. PSYCHOMOTOR GRID

Skill	Outcome	Minimal *Term I*	Moderate *Term II*	Acute *Term III*	Long-Term *Term IV*
Fundamental					
Mobilization	P 5.0	P 3.2	P 5.0		
Range of motion	P 5.0	P 3.2	P 4.0	P 4.0	P 5.0
Bed bath	P 5.0	P 3.1	P 5.0		
Mouth care—general	P 5.0	P 3.1	P 5.0		
special	P 3.2	P 2.0	P 3.1	P 3.2	
Hair care	P 5.0	P 3.2	P 5.0		
Back rub	P 5.0	P 3.1	P 5.0		
Positioning	P 5.0	P 3.1	P 5.0		
Feeding a patient	P 5.0	P 2.0	P 3.2	P 5.0	
Occupied bed	P 5.0	P 3.1	P 5.0		
Temperature—oral, rectal	P 5.0	P 5.0			
Pulse—radial	P 5.0	P 5.0			
apical	P 5.0	P 3.1	P 5.0		
carotid	P 5.0	P 5.0			
Blood pressure	P 5.0	P 3.2	P 5.0		
Weight/height	P 5.0	P 5.0			
Assist with bed- pan/urinal	P 5.0	P 3.1	P 5.0		
Body mechanics	P 5.0	P 3.2	P 5.0		
General Therapeutic and Diagnostic Procedures					
Auscultation					
Heart sounds	P 5.0	P 3.1	P 4.0	P 5.0	
Respiratory sounds	P 5.0	P 3.1	P 4.0	P 5.0	
Neurologic—reflex, etc.	P 5.0	P 3.1	P 3.2	P 4.0	P 5.0
Ear/nose/throat exam	P 5.0	P 3.1	P 3.2	P 4.0	P 5.0
Specimen collection	P 5.0	P 3.2	P 5.0		
Palpation	P 5.0	P 3.1	P 4.0	P 5.0	
Care of skin—Pre- vention	P 5.0	P 3.2	P 5.0		
Sterile dressings	P 5.0	P 3.2	P 5.0		
Bandage application	P 5.0	P 3.2	P 5.0		
Sterile gloving	P 5.0	P 3.1	P 3.2	P 5.0	
Use of instruments in a sterile field	P 5.0	P 3.2	P 5.0		
Precaution technique (isolation)	P 4.0	P 2.0	P 3.2	P 4.0	
Wound irrigation	P 3.2		P 3.2		
Change IV bottles	P 5.0		P 3.2	P 5.0	
Remove IV needles	P 5.0	P 3.1	P 3.2	P 5.0	
Administration of medications					
Oral	P 5.0	P 3.2	P 5.0		
Topical	P 5.0	P 3.2	P 5.0		

(Continued)

TABLE 17. (*Continued*)

Skill	Outcome	Minimal *Term I*	Moderate *Term II*	Acute *Term III*	Long-Term *Term IV*
Subcutaneous	P 5.0	P 3.2	P 4.0	P 5.0	
Intramuscular	P 5.0	P 3.2	P 4.0	P 5.0	
Draping a patient	P 5.0	P 3.1	P 5.0		
Cleansing enema	P 5.0	P 3.1	P 5.0		
Assist with cough- ing/deep breathing	P 5.0	P 3.1	P 5.0		
Catheterization	P 3.2			P 3.1	P 3.2
Urine tests	P 5.0	P 5.0			

Specialized
  Therapeutic and
  Diagnostic Mea-
  sures					

Bottle feeding	P 3.2		P 3.2		
Fetal heart reading	P 3.2	P 3.1	P 3.2		
Assist with postural drainage	P 3.1		P 3.1		
Respiratory suction	P 4.0		P 3.1	P 3.2	P 4.0
Tracheostomy suction	P 4.0		P 3.1	P 3.2	P 4.0
Nasogastric	P 4.0		P 3.1	P 3.2	P 4.0
Ileostomy care	P 3.2		P 3.1		P 3.2
Colostomy care	P 3.2		P 3.1		P 3.2
Traction	P 3.1		P 3.1		
Oxygen therapy	P 3.2		P 3.1	P 3.2	
Maintenance of chest drainage	P 3.2		P 3.1	P 3.2	
Vision testing	P 3.1	P 3.1			
Eye drops	P 3.1	P 3.1			
Measure central ve- nous pressure	P 3.2		P 3.1	P 3.2	
Change total parent- eral nutrition lines through volumetric pump	P 3.2		P 3.1	P 3.2	

Procrastination in scheduling experience obligations may result in student inability to secure faculty assessment time. The lesson is learned. It is not meant to imply that the total responsibility lies with the student; a shared accountability is in order. Periodic formative evaluation conferences with students to determine what performance experiences have been achieved and to propose plans for the remaining skills assist the planning process for both the teacher and learner.

The grid also prescribes accountability for the school when it is used as a communication for future employers of the graduates. Since it identifies the quantity and quality of psychomotor skill attainment at the conclusion of the program, employers have a framework of expectations relative to the new graduate's abilities and future learning needs. Each service area in a health care agency might develop a grid of skills appropriate to nursing care in that area, which would be informative to new employees and provide a basis for monitoring performance of the nursing staff at periodic intervals.

In essence, a psychomotor grid provides a framework for ordering the process of skill development within the context of the total program, for designating persons accountable for the learning attainment, and for assuring the place of psychomotor skill learning in a nursing program.

TEACHING METHODS

Methodology for teaching psychomotor skill from the performance perspective includes demonstration, whether by the presence of the individual in the setting or by single concept films or videotapes. The visual component enables the learner to obtain a general idea of the action pattern and supports the notion of whole learning. Playbacks of videotapes of the learner's performance fosters self-knowledge of the action and facilitates correction of errors or unprofitable actions. The principles for using these methods are described in Chapter 5.

Computer-assisted instruction is being developed in this area of teaching. Combinations of verbal and visual cues enable the learner to participate in the process cognitively. Computer instructions can facilitate the learner's grasp of the theoretical basis of the skill and anticipate its use under varying environmental situations.

Whatever the methods used in the demonstration stage, practice is essential in the development of a coordinated, efficient performance. Cognitive learning, which provides for the knowledge of principles and processes, does not develop the body movements responsive to situational cues.

Some psychomotor skills may be approached from a problem-solving or discovery methodology. However, since many nursing skills have been formalized into a procedure, it is more efficient to use the procedure for initial learning. Because nursing has many psychomotor skills that have been "adopted" from other disciplines, there is a great need for nursing research to establish the validity of present procedures or offer modifications as indicated. Newer developments in nursing and science disciplines might well influence current approaches to some of the skills.

The use of client problem situations in the learning of psychomotor skills is best when the learner has obtained a reasonable degree of self-confidence in skill performance. The student is then in a better position to see the skill within the context of patient care and to hypothesize modifications indicated by specific cues in the patient situation. Once the cognitive information processing has been developed for the skill, the learner is ready to deal with the cognitive processes of judgment, inferential reasoning, and decision making.

SUMMARY

Psychomotor skill learning is a significant domain in nursing, separate from but closely related to the cognitive and affective domain. There is a difference between psychomotor performance, the visible evidence of learning and psychomotor learning, the ability to retrieve the skill upon pertinent situational cues.

Skilled performance is characterized by an efficient coordinated behavior pattern within a realistic time, motion, and speed context which is generally consistent in quality whenever it occurs. Practice enables the individual to develop cognitive informational processes which facilitate the skill through selective attention to cues, thus decreasing decision-making time. Use of practice sessions requires consideration of their frequency, distribution, and length and must address the notions of overlearning, retention, feedback, and transfer of learning.

Psychomotor skills are practiced and learned in two practice settings: the learning resource laboratory and the clinical field, which provide a reality context to the learning. Each setting contributes to the skill development, but it is in the clinical field where the evidence of skill learning, especially in relation to the time dimension, is most persuasive.

Not all psychomotor skills in nursing need to or should be developed to a level of professional competency. A psychomotor taxonomy of performance provides a framework for designating a level of achievement for each skill and for sequencing of psychomotor skill learning in a nursing program. The grid that is developed facilitates accountability by all involved.

Psychomotor learning is an egocentric process and requires that the learner feel comfortable with him- or herself in the performance before the skill can be related on a more sophisticated level to the greater sphere of nursing practice.

REFERENCES

Adams, J. A. (1968). Response feedback and learning. *Psychological Bulletin, 70,* 486–504.
Bernstein, N. (1967). *The coordination and regulation of movements.* Elmsford, N.J.: Pergamon Press.

Bilodeau, E. A., & Bilodeau, I. (1961). Motor skills learning. *Annual Review of Psychology, 12,* 250.

Brown, I. D., Tickner, H., & Simmonds, D. C. (1969). Interference between concurrent tasks of driving and telephoning. *Journal of Applied Psychology, 55,* 419–24.

Bruton, M. R. (1976). *The influence of perceptual style and various combinations of mental and physical practice in facilitating the learning of a novel, fine, complex perceptual-motor skill.* Unpublished doctoral dissertation, New York University.

Cairy, M. (1981). *The timing of cognitive teaching as it affects the performance of psychomotor skills.* Unpublished field study, Wayne State University, Detroit, Mich.

Cleland, V. (1965). The effect of stress on performance. *Nursing Research, 14,* 292–98.

Cratty, B. J. (1967). Movement behavior and motor learning (2nd ed.). Philadelphia: Lea & Febiger.

Dave, R. H. (1970). *Psychomotor levels in developing and writing objectives.* Tucson, Ariz.: Educational Innovators Press.

Fitts, P. M. (1964). Perceptual and motor skill learning. In A. Melton (Ed.), *Categories of human learning.* New York: Academic Press.

Fleishman, E. A. (1972). A structure and measurement of psychomotor abilities. In R. Singer (Ed.), *The psychomotor domain: Movement behavior.* Philadelphia: Lea & Febiger.

Gates, A. I., Jersild, A. T., McConnell, T. R., & Challman, R. C. (1953). *Educational psychology,* (2nd ed.). New York: Macmillan.

Harrow, A. J. (1972). *A taxonomy of the psychomotor domain: A guide for developing behavioral objectives.* New York: D. McKay.

Henry, F. M. (1958). Specificity vs generality in learning motor skills. *Proceedings of College Physical Education Association, 61,* 126–28.

Infante, M. S. (1975). *The clinical laboratory in nursing education.* New York: Wiley.

Johnson, H. W. (1961). Skill = speed × accuracy × form × adaptability. *Perceptual and Motor Skills, 13,* 163–70.

Keele, S. W. (1968). Movement control in skilled motor performance. *Psychological Bulletin, 70,* 387–403.

Keele, S. (1982). Learning and control of coordinated motor patterns: The programming perspective. In J. A. Kelso (Ed.), *Human motor behavior: An introduction.* Hillsdale, N. J.: Lawrence Erlbaum Assoc.

Kelso, J. A. (Ed.). (1982). *Human motor behavior: An introduction.* Hillsdale, N. J.: Lawrence Erlbaum Assoc.

Kerr, R. (1982). *Psychomotor learning.* Philadelphia: Saunders.

Kibler, R. J., Barker, L. L., & Miles, D. T. (1970). *Behavioral objectives and instruction.* Boston: Allyn & Bacon.

Lawther, J. D. (1977). *The learning and performance of physical skills* (2nd ed). Englewood Cliffs, N. J.: Prentice-Hall.

Marteniuk, R. G. (1969). Generality and specificity of learning and performance of two similar speed tasks. *Research Quarterly, 40,* 552.

McGuigan, F. J., & MacCaslin, E. F. (1955). Whole and part methods in learning a perceptual motor skill. *American Journal of Psychology, 48,* 658–61.

Miller, G., Galantin, E., & Pribran, K. (1960). *Plans and the structure of behavior*. New York: Holt, Rinehart & Winston.

Morgan, M. K., & Irby, D. (1978). *Evaluating clinical competence in the health professions*. St. Louis: C. V. Mosby.

Naylor, J., & Briggs, G. (1961). Long term retention of learned skills: A review of the literature. *Academy of Education Development Technical Report, U.S. Department of Commerce, 61,* 390.

Paillard, J. (1960). The patterning of skilled movement. In J. Field, (Ed.), *Handbook of psychology: Neurophysiology, 3*. Baltimore: Williams & Wilkins.

Poulton, E. C. (1972). Skilled performance. In R. Singer (Ed.), *The psychomotor domain: Movement behavior*. Philadelphia: Lea & Febiger.

Reilly, D. E. (1980). *Behavioral objectives—evaluation in nursing* (2nd ed.). New York: Appleton-Century-Crofts.

Schmidt, R. A. (1976). Control processes in motor skills. In J. Koegh, & R. S. Hutton (Eds.), *Exercise and Sport Sciences Review*. Santa Barbara, Calif.: Journal Publishing Affiliates.

Schneider, W., & Fish, A. (1982). Attention theory and mechanisms for skilled performance. *ERIC Reports*, Champaign, Ill.: Illinois University.

Simpson, E. J. (1966). *The classification of educational objectives: Psychomotor domain*. Urbana, Ill.: University of Illinois Press.

Singer, R. (Ed.). (1975). *Motor learning and human performance*. New York: Macmillan.

Smith, K. U. (1967). Cybernetic foundations of physical behavioral science. *Quest, 8,* 26–82.

Smith, K. U. (1972). Cybernetic psychology. In R. Singer (Ed.), *The psychomotor domain: Movement behavior*. Philadelphia: Lea & Febiger.

Stelmach, G. E. (1969). Efficiency of motor learning as a function of intertrial rest. *Research Quarterly, 40,* 198–202.

Stelmach, G. E. (1982). Information processing framework for understanding human motor behavior. In J. A. Kelso (Ed.), *Human motor behavior: An introduction*. Hillsdale, N. J.: Lawrence Erlbaum Assoc.

Sweeney, M. A., Regan, P., O'Malley, M. & Hedstrom, B. (1980). Essential skills for baccalaureate graduates: Perspectives of education and service. *Journal of Nursing Administration, 10,* 37–44.

Tisdale, S. (1984). Reflections: The nouveau boards. *American Journal of Nursing, 84,* 166.

Welford, A. T. (1968). *Fundamentals of skill*. London: Metheun & Co., Ltd.

Whitley, J. D. (1970). Effects of practice distribution on learning a fine motor task. *Research Quarterly, 40,* 577–82.

BIBLIOGRAPHY

Baker, N. C., Cerone, S. B., Gaza, N., & Knapp, T. R. (1984). The effect of type of thermometer and length of time inserted in oral temperature measurement of afebrile subjects. *Nursing Research, 33,* 109–11.

Barsevick, A. M., & Llewellyn, J. L. (1982). A comparison of the anxiety-reducing potential of two techniques of bathing. *Nursing Research, 31,* 22–27.

Bates, B. (1983). *A guide to physical exam* (2nd ed.). Philadelphia: Lippincott.

Corbin, C. (1967). Effects of mental practice in skill development after controlled practice. *Research Quarterly, 38*, 534–38.

Corbin, C. (1967). The effects of covert rehearsal in development of a complex motor skill. *Journal of General Psychology, 76*, 143–50.

DeRusney, E. A., & Fitch, E. (1972). Field dependent–field independent as related to college curricula. *Perceptual and Motor Skills, 33*, 1235–37.

Dressler, D. K., Smejkal, C., & Ruffolo, M. L. (1983). A comparison of oral and rectal temperature measurement of patients receiving oxygen by mask. *Nursing Research, 32*, 373–75.

Dunn, M. A. (1970). Development of an instrument to measure nursing performance. *Nursing Research, 19*, 502–10.

Feldman, H. (1969). Learning transfer from programmed instruction to clinical performance. *Nursing Research, 18*, 51–54.

Fowler, W., & Leithwood, K. (1971). Cognition and movement: Theoretical, pedagogical and measurement consideration. *Perceptual and Motor Skills, 32*, 523–32.

Harris, R. B. (1984). Clean vs sterile tracheostomy care and level of pulmonary infection. *Nursing Research, 33*, 80–91.

Hoding, D. H. (Ed.). (1981). *Human skills.* New York: John Wesley.

Jarvis, L. (1967). Effects of self-instructional materials in learning selected motor skills. *Research Quarterly, 38*, 623–29.

Jones, D. A., Lepley, M. F., & Baker, B. A. (1984). *Health assessment across life span.* New York: McGraw-Hill.

Kieffer, J. S. (1984). Selecting technical skills to teach for competency. *Journal of Nursing Education, 23*(5), 198–203.

Larsen, D. (1983). *Computerized nursing skills simulations.* Philadelphia: Lippincott.

Lewis, E. (1971). Secure in her skills. *Nursing Outlook, 19*, 519.

Lewis, L. (1984). *Fundamental skills in patient care.* Philadelphia: Lippincott.

Lindberg, J. B., Hunter, M. L., & Kruszewski, A. Z. (1983). *Skills manual for person-centered nursing care.* Philadelphia: Lippincott.

Manderino, M. A., Hollerbach, A. D., & Brooks, C. P. (1984). Clinical evaluation of three techniques for administering low dose heparin. *Nursing Research, 33*, 15–19.

McCormick, K. A. (1983). Preparing nurses for the technologic future. *Nursing & Health Care, 5*, 379–82.

McGill, S. L., & Smith, J. R. (1983). *I V therapy.* Bowie, Md.: Robert J. Brady.

Millen, H. (1974). *Body mechanics and safe transfer techniques.* Detroit: Aronsson.

Nelson, E. J., Morton, E. A., & Hunter, P. M. (1983). *Critical care respiratory therapy: A laboratory and clinical manual.* Boston: Little, Brown.

Norris, S., Campbell, L., & Brenkert, S. (1982). Nursing procedures and alterations in transcutaneous oxygen tension in premature infants. *Nursing Research, 31*, 330–36.

Oxendine, J. B. (1969). Effects of mental and physical practice on the learning of three motor skills. *Research Quarterly, 40*, 755–78.

Oxendine, J. B. (1984). *Psychology of motor learning* (2nd ed.). Englewood Cliffs, N.J.: Prentice-Hall.

Phipps, S. J., & Morehouse, C. A. (1969). Effect of mental practice on acquisition of motor skills of varied difficulty. *Research Quarterly, 40,* 773–78.

Quiring, J. (1972). The autotutorial approach. *Nursing Research, 21* 332–37.

Randolph, G. L. (1984). Therapeutic touch and physical touch: Physiological response to stressful stimuli. *Nursing Research, 33,* 33–36.

Schmidt, R. A. (1982). *Motor control and learning.* Champaign, Ill.: Herman Kinelus Publ.

Singer, R. (Ed.). (1972). *Psychomotor domain: Movement behavior.* Philadelphia: Lea & Febiger.

Smith, S. F., & Duell, D. (1982). *Nursing skills and evaluation: A nursing process approach.* St. Louis: C. V. Mosby.

Sorenson, K. C., & Luckman, J. (1979). *Basic nursing: A psychophysiologic approach.* Philadelphia: Saunders.

Stelmach, G. E. (1978). *Information processing and motor control learning.* New York: Academic Press.

Takacs, K. M., & Valenti, W. M. (1982). Temperature measurement in a clinical setting. *Nursing Research, 31,* 368–70.

Wachtel, P. L. (1972). Field dependence and psychological differentiation. Reexamination. *Perceptual and Motor Skills, 34,* 179–81.

Weiss, S. J. (1979). The language of touch. *Nursing Research, 28,* 76–79.

Welford, A. T. (1976). *Skilled performance: Perceptual and motor skills.* Glenview, Ill.: Scott, Foresman & Co.

Yonkoma, C. A. (1982). Cool and heated aerosol and the measurement of oral temperature. *Nursing Research, 31,* 354–57.

8

Affective Learning in the Clinical Field

Affective competencies, moral reasoning, and value based behavior, are essential elements in skilled nursing practice. They represent those dimensions of nursing that characterize it as a humanistic discipline whose practice is noted for its quality of caring. They transcend all aspects of nursing. Competencies, so critical to a practice discipline, must be taught in preparatory programs, and opportunities for their development must be provided. The development of affective competencies must be subject to the same rigor and pedagogy as are competencies in the other two domains, cognitive and psychomotor.

The notion of teaching the affective domain in a nursing program is surrounded with mythology and confusion, reflective of a lack of understanding of the nature of the affective domain and its relationship to personhood and the profession. Some faculty see the affective domain as primarily concerned with problems of attitude or behavior, especially in relation to students or staff. Others perceive affective behavior to be based on values that are personal and not subject to questioning. Some equate the teaching of values with indoctrination, a practice antithetical to a free society. For many, the idea of teaching values conjures up the image of a teacher "imposing" values on captive students. Interestingly, one never hears fears expressed as to the danger of the teacher imposing cognition or psychomotor skills on the student. Affective competencies, like the competencies in the other two domains, are developed within the same framework of the teaching–learning process, and the levels of competence are delineated in terms of expected behaviors that are subject to appropriate evaluation processes.

Affective competencies have a more positive connotation than is often associated with them. They relate to the individual's ability to use moral reasoning in decisions for the management of moral and ethical dilemmas and to the development of a value system that guides decisions and activities compatible with the individual's and society's notion of what is good and what is right. Affective competency is more than the affirmation of personal beliefs. It requires cognitive skills of choice and decision making and a pattern of behavior reflective of commitment to the choice made.

The Talmud says:

Let not thy learning
exceed thy deeds
Mere knowledge is not the goal, but action

James Turro (1972) elaborates on this theme:

How laughable
some persons in our midst
make themselves by talking
so glibly of love
and being so obviously
unloving.
Think of
their expressed attitudes
toward established authority
too often
gratuitously hostile.
How incredible
they make themselves
by their incessant chatter
about community
while being so intolerant
of differing tastes and personality.
We must learn from their failures.
Let it not be said
of us
as, I believe
it can be said
of them
vox, vox, et praeteria nihil
words, words, and nothing else. (p. 63)

There is no place in nursing for "words, words, and nothing else." It is the fostering of integrity between the nurse's verbal affirmations on positions and beliefs compatible with nursing as a helping profession and the behaviors exhibited in moral and value conflicts that become the charge to teachers of nursing.

The need for affective competencies is particularly evident in contemporary society. The ever-changing technologic world in which nurses practice and live is forcing them to seek those humanistic qualities inherent in their practice which enables them to minister to clients in a manner that is satisfying and fulfilling to the clients and to themselves.

Nursing practice is value laden; indeed it is an ethical enterprise. What do the terms, "value-based practice" and "ethical enterprise" mean to the professional nurse, educators, practitioners, and researchers? The notion that nursing, like other health professions, is scientifically based is acknowledged. What are the implications of stating that they are also value based? Are the two ideas compatible or are they sources of conflict? Can a practice be both scientific and value based?

H. Tristan Englehardt, Jr. (1977) says, "The Holy Grail of modern western thought has been objective truth untouched by uncertainty or value judgment, along with a secular account of values" (p. 1). What has this Holy Grail search meant to educators, practitioners, and researchers in nursing? Does nursing perceive the world of facts as the only world of truth and reality while designating the world of values as primarily one of emotion devoid of truth?

Science implies impersonality and objectivity and is empirical and descriptive. It is perceived to be value free; although this perception is open to challenge. But science is not all of health care. Nurses care for and about people. This component of practice is personal and value based. Is it considered to be unscientific? Ayer (1946) supports this position when he says: "In so far as statements of values are significant, they are ordinary scientific statements and in so far as they are not scientific, they are not in the literal sense significant, but are simply expressions of emotions which can be neither true nor false" (pp. 102–3). The fact that the affective domain has not been addressed with the same intensity of teaching as the other domains suggests that Ayer's position may be supported by some nurse educators and practitioners.

Historically in nursing education programs, caring about the patient was stressed as a worthy goal in practice. However, the teaching of this goal was more by fiat and precept. One more or less "caught" the skills pertinent to the *caring about* action of nursing. Professional adjustment was the thrust of the time. Emphasis was on the decorum of the professional nurse in matters of dress, appearance, and actions that reflected the "image of the nurse." Ethical and moral decisions were examined more from a legalistic than an ethical or moral framework.

It is important to recognize that in an earlier period, the necessity for developing other strategies for teaching the affective skills was not present, for a simpler society existed where differences were limited, hidden, or ignored. Many nurses went to school and practiced nursing in their own communities where the same beliefs and value systems were accepted at least tacitly by the majority of the residents of that community. One's patients were of the community and they often attended the same school, church, or community functions as the nurse. These institutions were strong enforcers of community values. Limitation of knowledge presented few challenges to nursing, medicine, and other disciplines. Decisions as to when life began and ended were simplistic and accepted by all; e.g., the failure to obtain an apical pulse was sufficient for the physician to declare a person dead. The advent of mass media and mass travel exposed persons to differing beliefs, values and life styles. The relative homogeneity and absolutism of beliefs and values held by members of a community were displaced and the handling of divergent and contradictory claims became a necessity.

Contemporary world and the portents for the future world indicate an increasingly complex society where moral decisions will be more numerous and intricate and where value conflicts will be more evident. Differences are now more overt, although the institutionalizing of some prejudices (unsubstantiated beliefs) still persists. Knowledge and mechanisms for using that knowledge continue to expand, thus providing society and individuals with extraordinary power to control lives of persons in that society. The very nature of our society and the political processes by which it is governed are regarded with cynicism by many whose trust is shattered by the unethical behavior of leaders they chose to direct the society toward its potential. A democratic society that values individual freedom and rights yet makes decisions more reflective of materialistic values than humanistic ones serves only to confuse its body politic. Dewey (1962), a democratic philosopher, raised the question: "Can a materialistic industrial civilization be converted into a distinctive agency for liberalizing the minds and refining the emotions of all?" (p. 28).

American society is now in the postindustrial era, embarked on an information society overwhelmed by technology. This technology has improved instrumentation, but its use may or may not contribute to the improvement in the quality of life, society, or the care provided by health professionals. Dewey's question becomes even more significant in relation to a materialistic technologic civilization. There are some positive responses to the question as citizens' voices are being heard in the political arena. They are saying "No" to decisions that threaten the quality of the environment, health of a community, or quality of life. The voices of minority groups; i.e., women, elderly, and those of various ethnic persuasions are now raising the issue of justice as decisions not in their interest are being proposed. Political power no longer has a negative value. Justice for the less fortunate, however, is an unstable factor influenced by mood swings of the populace from a humanistic view, which sees these individuals as victims of societal pressures, to a derogatory view, which blames them for their inability to keep pace with society's movements.

Allocation of resources is developing as a major concern of government and citizens with much potential for generating moral and ethical dilemmas. Financial resources are of particular relevance to those in the health field as the realization that there are limits to moneys for health care becomes more apparent. Efforts toward cost-effective health care limit the hospitalization options for individuals receiving Medicare through the use of diagnostic categories as a basis for prospective payment to hospitals. What conflicts will nurses encounter when decisions for early discharge of patients are not congruent with the nurse's judgment? Decisions will need to be made indicating who should receive care, especially the costly diagnostic and treatment modalities. Will some individuals not be eligible because of age, lack of money, or importance to society? As care becomes more costly and financial resources become more restricted, a period of hard moral choices awaits nurses and other health care providers.

Nurses will be challenged to abet humanistic values and to be ever sensitive to the changes instigated by technology and societal decisions that threaten the rights of the individual. The advent of computers challenges the notion of the client's right to privacy in a way never anticipated by those who saw gossip, for example in elevators, public transportation, and other similar situations, as the primary means of violating this right. Although the legalistic approach to problems will be ever present, decisions for action must also be on the basis of moral reasoning in terms of the ethical or moral concepts inherent in the dilemma.

The question today is not should the affective competencies of moral reasoning and value development be taught, but rather the question is in terms of how they should be taught. Of particular concern is how one uses the rich resources of the clinical practice field in fostering the development of those affective skills so central to the evolution of the individual from a novice to an expert practitioner.

CONCEPTS RELEVANT TO AFFECTIVE SKILL DEVELOPMENT

There are several significant concepts encompassed under the rubric *affective domain,* whose understanding is essential for those teaching in this area.

Beliefs
The terms "beliefs" and "values" are often used interchangeably, but there is a significant difference in their interpretation. Beliefs respond to questions of fact, irrespective of the actual reality of the fact. Beliefs are perceptions of reality that have significant meaning to the individual. Beliefs may be supported by valid and reliable data or they may be unsubstantiated, as occurs in prejudice, which

is often a reflection of ignorance due to lack of contact or exposure to the substance of the fact or due to fear of change in behavior necessitated by alterations in belief.

Some individuals maintain beliefs in spite of new information that disputes the claim for the original belief that guided the actions of the individual. Scheibe (1970, p. 91) relates this rigidity of beliefs to the common information tendencies of human beings which act as mechanism of conservation in mind whereby the interpretation of incoming information is in relation to its congruence with the original belief. He cites two ways information is distorted:

> Assimilation—give more support to an entrenched belief than it should
>
> Contrast—deny the relevance of information to the belief if it is sufficiently incompatible with it.

Stated beliefs are not always reliable because of an individual's proclivity for stating one thing while inwardly accepting a very different belief. Statements of belief are particularly vulnerable to social forces operating in a situation at any one particular time. Beliefs, like values, serve as a guiding influence in behavior, but unlike values, the commitment based on rational choice is not apparent. A belief becomes a value when it is rationally examined, freely chosen, and a commitment is made to support the belief in action.

Values

Values are judgments about the worth of an object, person, group, belief, or event. They connote a preference for something, as exhibited in behavior, on a selective basis. Values are viewed contextually within a group or society standard, which may or may not reflect what is good for the total society. Moral values are those that are in accord with ethical and moral standards which refer to the good of the greater society with protection of the individual's rights within that society.

Scheibe (1970) notes that the statement of values refers to what is wanted, what is best, what is desirable, and what ought to be. He supports the contextual nature of values in that they depend upon a variety of internal conditions, external stimulus configuration, and response option. Morrill (1980) defines values as standards and patterns of choice that guide persons and groups toward satisfaction, fulfillment, and meaning. Davis and Aroskar (1983) describe their concept of values thusly: "Values may be considered to be a set of beliefs and attitudes for which logical reasons can be given. Values are significant as they influence perception, guide our actions and have consequences" (p. 197). Steele and Harmon (1983) perceive a value as an affective disposition toward a person, object, or idea. Values represent a way of life.

Carl Rogers (1983) supports the classification of values by Charles Morris:

Operative—tendency of living things to show preference in their actions for one kind of object or objective. No cognitive activity is involved.

Conceived—preference of the individual for a symbolized object. In choice there is anticipation or foresight of the outcome of behavior directed toward such a symbolized object.

Objective—objectivity preferable, whether or not it is sensed or conceived as desirable.

Raths and colleagues (1966) define values as those elements that show how a person has decided to use his or her life. They note that values are learned through experience and must meet the criteria of choice, commitment, and action. They introduce the notion of valuing, a process that suggests the action dimension of values and the interrelationship between knowing and doing. The three processes as defined by Raths and colleagues (1966, pp. 28–30) are:

Choosing (1) freely
          (2) from alternatives
          (3) after thoughtful consideration of the consequences of each alternative
Prizing   (4) cherishing, being happy with choice
          (5) willing to affirm the choice publically
Action   (6) doing something with the choice
          (7) repeatedly in some pattern of life. (pp. 28–30)

Raths and colleagues contend that unless these three processes are involved, a value is not present. Interests, aspirations, or attitudes (perhaps operative values described by Rogers) are seen as value indicators. One may affirm an interest or a belief but be unwilling to act in accord with that interest or belief. Likewise, one may act in a pattern reflective of a belief but be unwilling to make the choice that leads to commitment. The general consensus of most authorities is that values are important motivators of actions that are selective and the result of rational choice and commitment.

Attitudes
Attitudes, often confused with values, represent a feeling for or against a person, object, belief, or event. The rationale for the feeling may or may not be understood by the individual, but the responses generated by the feeling greatly influence the individual's ability to maximize the potential from the relationship with the object, person, or event. Positive attitude may be a value indicator and present a signal to the teacher to help the student move through

the valuing process toward transforming it into a value. Negative attitudes may be a reflection of ignorance, fear of an unfulfilled need. One must recognize that all behavior is not value based, for needs are powerful forces for action. In general, a need, for example, love, must be fulfilled before one can value love. Reilly (1978, p. 38) drawing from the work of Raths and colleagues differentiates between the characteristics of value and need.

Needs	Values
1. Start with life	1. Start when child becomes conscious that he is different from what he was
2. Push one into action	2. Pull one toward action
3. Ashamed of	3. Cherish
4. Pervasive	4. Selective
5. Strong visceral component	5. Strong intellectual component
6. Met by others	6. Met by self
7. Deficiency behaviors: aggression, withdrawal, submission, psychosomatic illness symptoms	7. Deficiency behaviors: apathy, flighty, inconsistency, hesitancy, overconforming, overdissenting role playing

Knox (1977) refers to attitudes as the residue of past experiences in the form of inclination or feelings that predispose a person to the choice of activities, companions, and locations. Because attitudes lack the rational choice and commitment, they are vulnerable to external and internal forces in a situation and may shift as the individual interacts with these forces.

Moral Reasoning
Moral reasoning implies the cognitive processes of analysis and interpretation of a moral dilemma as a basis for determining some course of action. Moral reasoning, according to Kohlberg (1981), does not involve knowing or deriving specific ethical rules of conduct; rather, it concerns the structure through which reflection and experience in the moral sphere are first processed and organized. Moral reasoning, dependent upon skills of critical thinking, is called into play when a moral situation is evident for which the usual rules of conduct are not sufficient. Davis and Aroskar (1983) refer to this situation as a dilemma, a difficult situation incapable of satisfactory solution. They further define such a situation as a moral claim conflict when a choice or situation involving choice between equally unsatisfactory alternatives exists. Moral reasoning is a fundamental process in making choices but does not guarantee that moral behavior will result.

Kohlberg (1981) is one of the most noted theorists in the area of cognitive development as it pertains to moral reasoning. He sees justice as the highest moral condition and has developed a cognitive hierarchical schema which moves from the lowest to the highest type of moral reasoning. Basing his work on that of Piaget and Dewey, he identifies three moral levels individuals pass through en route to principled action. Each level encompasses two stages. The literature contains many references to this theory and the characteristics of the stages. A brief summary of the levels is included here.

Preconventional Level. Two stages are included: obedience–punishment orientation and personal interest orientation. Behavior at this level is determined by cultural roles and notions of what is considered good or bad as defined by superior power consequences, punishment, reward, or exchange of favors.

Conventional Level. Two stages are: interpersonal concordance ("Good Boy, Nice Girl") orientation and law and order orientation. Behavior at this level is in terms of maintaining expectations of the individual's family, group, or nation, regardless of immediate or obvious consequences. Attitude is one of loyalty to the prevailing order and conformity to the rules and expectations held by those who are significant.

Postconventional Level. Two stages are: social contract, legalistic orientation and universal, ethical principled orientation. Behavior at this level is internally controlled; the standards conformed to have an internal source and the decision to act is based on an inner process of thought and judgment concerning right and wrong. The universal principles of justice, reciprocity, and equality of human rights and the respect for the dignity of human beings as individuals become the basis for moral decisions.

For purposes of viewing this theory in relation to the development of affective competencies, its assumptions are significant. This theory proposes that there are patterns of moral reasoning behavior associated with each level and that individuals with appropriate stimuli can move to a higher level. The stimulus of moral disequilibrium at the next highest level for the student enables the individual to seek out a more sophisticated level of reasoning. The theory operates on the findings that most people function at one level of moral reasoning most of the time but some regression can occur at intervals. Smith (1978) summarized some of the research in the use of Kohlberg's theory and found general support for it, especially for individuals who complete high school and go on to college.

Holstein (1976) and Gilligan (1977) found evidence of sex bias in the test scoring which favors men. This is a concern since nurses are primarily women. Some questions are raised in relation to the cultural bias of the questions and scoring, although Kohlberg asserts that the theory has no cultural boundaries. Other questions are raised about the emphasis on moral rationality through patterns of thinking to the exclusion of any concern about conduct resulting from these cognitive processes. Morrill (1980) reminds the reader that Kohlberg argues that moral rationality is a precondition for moral action, for one can scarcely choose a good that one does not know.

Perry (1970), another cognitive development theorist, has also developed a hierarchy of stages of ethical development toward the highest level of moral commitment. These stages, previously discussed, are based on the assumption about the way students perceive the nature and characteristics of truth, values, and life goals. The scheme of the stages of development describes the steps by which students move from a simplistic, categorical view of the world to a realization of the contingent nature of knowledge, relative values, and the formation and affirmation of their own commitments.

Ethics
Ethics refers to standards of conduct or "right" behavior based on moral judgment. Scheibe (1970) sees ethics concerned with questions of value, the importance of emotions, the nature of value judgments, and standards and criteria for morality (p. 5). Churchill (1982) considers ethics as a systematic reflection of moral behavior; morality as the practical activity; ethics as the theoretical and reflective one (p. 305). Stent (1977), in developing his theory of structural ethics, supports Gustafson's notion of ethics "as a human intellectual discipline which develops the principles which account for morality and moral action and the normative principles and values that guide human action" (p. 243).

Morrill (1980) differentiates between the traditional study of ethics, *metaethics*, which concerns itself with logical, epistemologic, and semantic issues addressed to the question of what *ought* to be done in situations, not the actions themselves, and the current study of ethics, *normative*, which is concerned with classification, analysis, and critique of moral arguments and issues at hand (pp. 44–45). It is normative ethics that relate to the exploration of ethical dilemmas in nursing practice that is the focus in teaching for the development of affective competencies.

Morality
Morality, although concerned with moral judgment and right behavior, is perceived within a social context. It is a system of moral conduct. Societies, whether communities, cultural groups, nations, professions, and even schools of nursing, determine the ethical standards and values to be respected and supported by its membership.

Exemplars serve as models of the accepted code of behavior and can be most effective in teaching the behaviors that a group accepts. Sanctions are instituted less by the legal route than by verbal or nonverbal responses of the group members. These sanctions serve to bring the errant or potentially errant individuals into accord with the group's idea of morality. Societies have often attempted to legislate morality, for example, prohibition in the United States in the 1920s, but have generally been less successful than when group pressure is exerted.

CHOICE

One concept that is fundamental to the other concepts in affective learning and critical in teaching is that of choice. Choice entails making decisions for or about something. In the affective domain, it refers to decisions based on values and moral beliefs. René Dubos (1981) associates choice making with the quality of humanness when he states: "We are human beings, not so much because of our appearance, but because of what we do, the way we do it, and more importantly, because of what we elect to do or not do" (p. 9). He further states: "Intentionality and freedom of choice are at least as important in human life as is biological determination, whether genetic or environmental" (p. 15).

Frankl (1963) attests to the value of choice in maintaining the human quality of persons. He vividly describes his life in a concentration camp where any semblance of value of human life and human dignity was nonexistent and where individuals were robbed of their will and served only as objects to be manipulated by their captors. Frankl raised the question: Does man have no choice of action in the face of such circumstances? He affirms from experience as well as principle that man does have a choice of action. He states: "There is sufficient proof that everything can be taken from a man, but one thing—the last of the human freedoms—to choose one's attitude in any given set of circumstances to choose one's way" (p. 105). Referring to human beings' ability to preserve even a trace of spiritual freedom and independence of mind under such circumstances as he encountered, he concludes that people can decide what will become of them spiritually and mentally and that each individual has the freedom to make a choice between accepting or rejecting an offer.

Both Dubos and Frankl affirm that choice making is essential to the very human nature of the person and is a characteristic of one's freedom. Podeschi (1976) interprets William James' concept of freedom and its meaning in choice making as: "Human freedom does not mean any choice that tempts us, but choices that lead to maturation of our human capacities" (p. 228). He further notes that free choices come in the form of forced options. McBee (1978) refers to self-imposed limitations on freedom of action—a choice among options open to free people. Freedom within this context is not perceived as license where one "does one's own thing." Freedom does not mean freedom from structure, but rather freedom within the structure. It means the individual is free from coercion in making choices.

The making of choices within the concept of the affective domain involves more than expressing a preference, which is often transitory. Competency in choice making is the ability to ponder evidence, examine assumptions, make judgments, and evaluate. When one makes a choice, one takes a position which has been logically and rationally determined. It tells what one will stand up for. Podeschi, drawing upon Wild's (1969) interpretation of James' view of freedom, suggests James' position about the substance of choice making. "The individual who believes that choices really matter will take life seriously. What we freely choose to do makes a difference; real issues are at stake. This means the willingness to live with energy, though energy brings pain" (p. 228). The making of choices can be an uncomfortable experience because it involves dealing with alternatives and then assuming responsibility for the choice made. Dubos (1981) suggests: "The greater freedom of an organism to select where it goes and what it does and how it responds to stimuli, the more complex and creative is the living experience" (p. 31).

Skill in the selection of choices is a critical component in affective learning, but it is only one part of the learning. In teaching, faculty must be concerned not only with the process of choice making, but also with the pattern of behavior that reflects that choice.

AFFECTIVE COMPONENT IN NURSING

The discussion thus far has addressed the processes of affective skill development. What about the content of these competencies? Are there certain values that all nurses must accept as their own? The answer must be in the affirmative if, as stated earlier, the affective domain must be subjected to the same pedagogy as the other domains of learning; i.e., objectives are written, learning experiences provided, and evaluation carried out. This response may be disturbing to those who perceive values only from the personal perspective. The concern of teachers is not the personal values held by students, but rather, those values inherent in the nursing profession. Levine (1977), who sees ethical responsibility in every dimension of nursing practice, notes that the very nature of nursing practice precludes the individual nurse from standing aside from the experience of interacting with human beings (pp. 8–9).

Conflict Sources

Much of the emphasis in the nursing literature that refers to moral, ethical, or value issues relates to those entailed in the interactions of the nurse with the client or with the physician, often reflective of medical ethics. A much broader perspective is needed, for these issues transcend all aspects of nursing practice.

In 1972, the Carnegie Commission on Higher Education published a report on professional education. The challenge to educators addressed their failure to see in this time of rapid social change that new clients and new client systems were evolving that markedly influence the need for greater balance of science and humanism in educational programs. Recognizing that health problems are now too complex for the purview of one health profession, there is a plea for more realistic analysis of health problems and the involvement of multidiscipline approaches.

In the report, Schein (1972) notes that the professional of the future will need to have a different set of skills, a different set of images, and a different set of attitudes from the professional today. According to Schein, six factors of particular significance to nursing are identified as influencing these changes:

1. Change in work setting within which professionals operate
2. Change in fee structure
3. New concept of who is the client
4. Multiple client systems with which professionals must work
5. Availability to client of more basic knowledge and sophisticated technology
6. Change in social values calling for the professional to be an advocate, to improve not just serve society, and to be more an initiator than a responder.

All helping professionals need to think in terms of multiple client systems arising from the increasing bureaucratization of health professionals and thus prepare to work with values and goals of organizations. A concern of this matter was expressed in the Carnegie Report by Schein (1972) as:

> . . . client systems become more differentiated and as clients become more resourceful and powerful, the professions have a less clear concept of what standards and ethics should govern client relationships and are therefore more vulnerable to a variety of attacks and pressures both from their employers and their intermediate and ultimate clients. (p. 31)

Nagel (1977) identifies five fundamental types of values that give rise to basic conflict, especially in a practice field:

> 1. Specific obligations to other people or institutions: to patients, one's family, hospital or university at which one works, one's community, or one's country.

2. Constraints on action deriving from general rights that everyone has either to do certain things or not to be treated in certain ways.
3. Utility: the effect of what one does on everyone's welfare and includes all aspects of benefit and harm to all people, not just the recipient.
4. Perfectionist ends or values: the intrinsic value of certain achievements or creations apart from the value *to* the person.
5. Commitment to one's own projects or undertakings. (pp. 281–283)

The determination of the stance of a profession, such as nursing, must take into account the world in which it practices and the social and political values that motivate the decision makers, especially as they impact on the quality, quantity, and delivery of health care. MacIntyre (1979) sees the overt moral stance of our culture as characterized by a temporary and fragile nature. The indignation expressed over a perceived immoral act is short lived. There is no real endeavor to explore in depth the substance of the indignation as a basis for resolution of the problem. MacIntyre feels that the central feature of contemporary moral debates is that they are unsettlable and interminable. This characterization is derived from the cultural plurality in our society with each group proclaiming a particular moral tradition.

The plurality of citizenry in a society means a plurality of value systems represented in cultural norms, values, and behavior. The loss of significance of the melting pot theory means the acknowledgment of varied culture groups. Since each group has its own value system and seeks to maintain it while bringing it into accord with that of the larger society, nurses are finding that their practice is taking on different meanings. Recognition that concepts of health, illness, and sick role have particular meanings to each group requires that nurses respect these diversities as they provide care. Nursing process, the methodology of practice, facilitates the nurse in providing for these diversities, but the nurse is continually challenged to avoid biases from influencing the assessments or interventions on the basis of the nurse's own value system.

Bonaparte (1979) found in her study of 300 nurses a significant relationship between closemindedness and attitude toward culturally different patients. She depicted the closeminded nurse as unconsciously avoiding culturally different patients with incongruous health-related beliefs and practices that tended to be seen as a conflict with a rational scientific approach and anxiety producing and threatening to the nurse's professional image. Patients received less care. The open minded nurse readily sought out information about culturally different clients relative to their diet, language, inter- and intragroup social patterns, value concepts of health and illness, and other factors helpful in planning care.

Saunders (1954) refers to biases and misconceptions of health workers. These include (1) assuming a universal human nature which presumably leads all normal people to respond in certain uniform ways in a given situation; (2) exaggerating the extent to which reason determines human behavior to the exclusion of tastes, customs, and cultural norms; and (3) accepting the notion of ethnocentrism, which is the tendency to think that the person's way of acting and behaving are the only correct way and regard beliefs and practices of others, especially when different, as strange, bizarre, and unenlightened.

As nursing operates within the society where multiple sources of ethical, moral, and value conflicts exist, it must also deal with these conflicts within itself. The pursuit of a value system by which it functions as a discipline and a practice profession is confronted with ambiguity and uncertainty. Gardner (1978) responds to the present decision-making state when he states: "The heart of our problem is not that betrayal of values is more vivid and more acknowledged today. The trouble runs deeper. The disintegration of traditions, customs, and communities has shaken our confidence. Our standards and guiding ideas are in disarray" (p. 23). Nursing has also lost some of its traditions, customs, and sense of community. The charge to nursing educators and practitioners is to clarify the concept of standards and ethics governing nursing practice. A paraphrase of Gardner's statement regarding obligations of society by inserting the word *nursing* for the word *society* would read: The whole structure of values, beliefs, laws, and standards by which *nursing* lives must be continuously restored or they will degenerate. They will survive and flourish only if people continuously renew their values and reinterpret traditions to make them serve contemporary needs.

Gardner calls upon nursing to rebuild. It is not necessary to develop a new set of values. Inherent in nursing are values reflective of the dignity and worth of each human being. The fundamental values have been there, although their interpretation and expression differed in accord with the society's values at any particular time.

Sources of Values

Bill of Rights. What is the source of values that must be accepted by professional nursing? One source would be the Bill of Rights of the Constitution (Figure 4) which clearly states those dimensions of an individual's life that must be respected if justice is to prevail. These rights are based on a moralistic premise about the individual in society and reflect the acceptance of the worth and dignity of the individual.

Throughout history, the concept of human rights has been challenged; sometimes resulting in an era of denial, sometimes one of indifference, and sometimes in an era of acknowledgment. Cranston

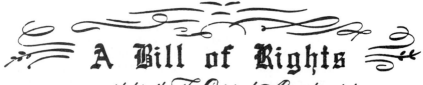

A Bill of Rights

as provided in the Ten Original Amendments to

The Constitution of the United States

in force December 15, 1791.

Article I

Congress shall make no law respecting an establishment of religion, or prohibiting the free exercise thereof; or abridging the freedom of speech, or of the press; or the right of the people peaceably to assemble, and to petition the Government for a redress of grievances.

Article II

A well regulated Militia, being necessary to the security of a free State, the right of the people to keep and bear Arms, shall not be infringed.

Article III

No Soldier shall, in time of peace be quartered in any house, without the consent of the Owner, nor in time of war, but in a manner to be prescribed by law.

Article IV

The right of the people to be secure in their persons, houses, papers, and effects, against unreasonable searches and seizures, shall not be violated, and no Warrants shall issue, but upon probable cause, supported by Oath or affirmation, and particularly describing the place to be searched, and the persons or things to be seized.

Article V

No person shall be held to answer for a capital, or otherwise infamous crime, unless on a presentment or indictment of a Grand Jury, except in cases arising in the land or naval forces, or in the Militia, when in actual service in time of War or public danger; nor shall any person be subject for the same offences to be twice put in jeopardy of life or limb; nor shall be compelled in any Criminal Case to be a witness against himself, nor be deprived of life, liberty, or property, without due process

of law; nor shall private property be taken for public use, without just compensation.

Article VI

In all criminal prosecutions, the accused shall enjoy the right to a speedy and public trial, by an impartial jury of the State and district wherein the crime shall have been committed, which district shall have been previously ascertained by law, and to be informed of the nature and cause of the accusation; to be confronted with the witnesses against him; to have compulsory process for obtaining Witnesses in his favor, and to have the Assistance of Counsel for his defence.

Article VII

In Suits at common law, where the value in controversy shall exceed twenty dollars, the right of trial by jury shall be preserved, and no fact tried by a jury shall be otherwise re-examined in any Court of the United States, than according to the rules of the common law.

Article VIII

Excessive bail shall not be required, nor excessive fines imposed, nor cruel and unusual punishments inflicted.

Article IX

The enumeration in the Constitution, of certain rights, shall not be construed to deny or disparage others retained by the people.

Article X

The powers not delegated to the United States by the Constitution, nor prohibited by it to the States, are reserved to the States respectively, or to the people.

Figure 4. A Bill of Rights. (*Reprinted with permission from American Civil Liberties Union, New York.*)

(1983) presents the various historical swings regarding the acceptance of human rights as society policy when he raises the question: Are there any human rights? He defines human rights as ". . . something that everybody has. They are not rights a man acquires by doing certain work, enacting a certain role, or discharging certain duties; they belong to him simply because he is a human being" (p. 11). In response to those who believe that rights are earned, Cranston identifies three tests that confirm the existence of universal rights:

1. It is something that no one, anywhere, may be deprived of without a grave affront to justice.
2. It must be a universal right, one that pertains to every human being as such.
3. It must be of paramount importance. It is something that can and from a moral point of view *should* be respected here and now. If it is violated, justice itself is abused.

The significance of these rights was recently rediscovered, so that there are now many movements in society of groups seeking to redress the wrongs caused by violations of these rights. The individual in the health care system is also asserting these rights through active consumer movements. How quickly are these rights taken away from individuals who enter health care agencies? Of particular concern are the rights to know, to participate in decisions about one's own care, and the right to privacy and protection from unwarranted search. The American Hospital Association has published a Bill of Rights for Patients, which is designed to protect the rights of patients while in the hospital. The nurse has a responsibility to see that these rights are implemented in the care setting.

Code for Nursing. The source of values particularly relevant to nursing is the body of professional documents that arise from the professional organization. The Code for Nurses (Table 18) is one such document. The first Code for Nurses was endorsed in 1950, and, characteristic of that era, it provided prescriptions for appropriate personal conduct of nurses. As the rebuilding process occurred in revisions of the Code, emphasis moved from the nurse to broader ethical values which are applicable to a variety of situations. The latest revision of the Code, adopted in 1976, provides a guide for the resolution of ethical dilemmas with an underlying theme of moralistic concept of the dignity and worth of each individual. It also addresses issues of accountability of the nurse to the efforts of the profession as it assumes its role in promoting the health and well-being of society.

It is important, however, to recognize the limitations of such a document. Toulmin (1977) recognizes that there is no conflict-free code, for individuals wear many hats and often their obligations are at variance. He says: "Professions organize their procedures and frame their codes of professional responsibility to minimize the risk of recurrent conflicts of obligation" (p. 261). Intraprofessional conflicts are of three types; accountability to group loyalty, accountabil-

TABLE 18. CODE FOR NURSES

1. The nurse provides services with respect for human dignity and the uniqueness of the client unrestricted by consideration of social or economic status, personal attributes, or the nature of health problems.
2. The nurse safeguards the client's right to privacy by judiciously protecting information of a confidential nature.
3. The nurse acts to safeguard the client and the public when health care and safety are affected by the incompetent, unethical, or illegal practice of any person.
4. The nurse assumes responsibility and accountability for individual nursing judgments and actions.
5. The nurse maintains competence in nursing.
6. The nurse exercises informed judgment and uses individual competence and qualifications as criteria in seeking consultation, accepting responsibilities, and delegating nursing activities to others.
7. The nurse participates in activities that contribute to the ongoing development of the profession's body of knowledge.
8. The nurse participates in the profession's efforts to implement and improve standards of nursing.
9. The nurse participates in the profession's efforts to establish and maintain conditions of employment conducive to high-quality nursing care.
10. The nurse participates in the profession's effort to protect the public from misinformation and misrepresentation and to maintain the integrity of nursing.
11. The nurse collaborates with members of the health professions and other citizens in promoting community and national efforts to meet the health needs of the public.

(Reprinted from the American Nurses Association. *Code for Nurses with Interpretive Statements, Kansas City, Mo., 1976, with permission.)*

ity for competence, and accountability for respectability. The conflicts nurses face in their practice may cause them to choose one of these accountabilities as a priority. The Code for Nurses guides nurses in their decisions, but it does not provide a means of establishing priorities when ethical or value conflicts arise. The nurse must ultimately make the choice for his or her own self.

Standards of Practice. The American Nurses Association has published a set of standards for nursing care in many of the specialty areas of practice as well as general standards which transcend all nursing. These standards, as is true of other documents, reflect the belief in the rights of clients in maintaining their dignity and control in matters affecting them. The meaning and implications of these standards are appropriate subjects for analysis as the learner or practitioner identifies the moral and ethical components of their practice. The reader is referred to these standards for a more detailed presentation.

One standard to be examined refers to rights of patients to appropriate knowledge for making decisions.

The client/patient and family are provided with the information needed to make decisions and choices about:
Promoting, maintaining, and restoring health
Seeking and utilizing appropriate health care personnel
Maintaining and using health care resources. (ANA, 1973, p. 5)

This standard relates to the teaching function of nursing. Consider the dilemma of a nurse whose professional standards require the nurse to teach, yet a physician states that his or her patient is not to be taught by the nurse? If the nurse follows the command of the physician, then teaching is a delegated task, not a professional activity. Of even greater concern is the fact that if the nurse does not teach the client, the nurse is vulnerable both ethically and legally. The issues raised in this dilemma concern the patients' right to know and the nurses' right to tell. This standard, like the others, is a statement of accountability and demands careful analysis.

Social Policy Statement. A significant document was published by the American Nurses Association in 1980. *Nursing, A Social Policy Statement* was prepared by a task force of the Congress of Nursing Practice and addresses three main themes: the social context of nursing, the scope of nursing practice, and the role of specialization in nursing. The document reflects the rebuilding process advocated by Gardner.

The social context statement notes: "Nursing can be said to be *owned* by society in the sense that nursing's professional interest must be perceived as serving the interest of the larger whole of which it is a part" (ANA, 1980, p. 7). The concept of *society ownership* needs to be pondered more fully for it suggests rights that society can proclaim from those it has licensed as practitioners.

The statement of the nature and scope of nursing practice includes the following:

Nurses have the highest regard for self-determination, independence and choice in decision-making in matters of health. Nurses are committed to respecting human beings because of a profound regard to humanity. Basic commitment is unaltered by social, educational, economic, cultural, racial, religious, or other specific attributes of human beings receiving care, including nature and duration of disease and illness. (ANA, 1980, p. 18)

This document clearly states commitment and responsibilities of nurses to those they serve, individuals, and the larger society. It demands that nurses be open-minded and care about those who place trust in them for quality care.

All three professional documents have a common theme, i.e., a commitment to the dignity and worth of each person and accountability to society for a quality performance. There is a danger that the content of these pronouncements will sound familiar and not receive the careful analysis required. The basic premise is not new; but the interpretation and expression is new within the context of present society. The four documents referred to provide the subject matter of teaching in the affective domain. They provide the subject for objectives to be developed and attained.

APPROACHES TO TEACHING

Two general approaches are entailed in teaching the affective domain. One addresses the valuing process toward the end of developing an integrated value system and the other addresses the skills of moral reasoning when encountering moral or ethical dilemmas.

Values Clarification
Raths and colleagues (1966) and Simon and associates (1972) have developed the values clarification strategy which enables people to identify for themselves the values that guide their own actions. Numerous types of activities, such as games, questionnaires, and role playing, are designed to aid the student through the valuing process. Examples of strategies are found in the previously mentioned two references and those that are relevant to nursing are in Steele and Harmon (1983) and Reilly (1978).

This approach is process oriented and does not concern itself with content, the *what* to value. An unfortunate outcome of the activity is that expressed conscious awareness may be perceived as the goal without any examination of the validity of the expressed belief and the potential consequences. Choices may be superficial and lack the rigorous discipline of intellectual inquiry and commitment. Speaking of the limitations of this approach and its emphasis on personal values, Morrill (1980) states: "The obligatory and normative dimensions of the experience of values are given virtually no direct attention nor does the technique adress as ends in themselves the values that inhere in the social and political dimensions of life" (p. 17).

Values Inquiry
This is a process that speaks to some of the weakness in the values clarification method. Its aim is to explore the meanings and possibilities of a human situation by discovering the values that motivate choice and decisions by individuals (Morrill, 1980). Values inquiry is an intellectual activity which is descriptive and seeks to assist the individual in discovering the value and moral connotations in activities or situations encountered.

Although process is an essential component of this method, the content, i.e. values, is also significant. Value choices identified in the inquiry process are examined from a normative perspective in accord with social and moral standards. Morrill (1980) notes two limitations in the value inquiry method when he raises these questions:

> If one's analysis has depicted a set of competing and conflicting values—as it usually does—is that the final word? To what extent does a full and clear analysis of values affect the development of a student's own values and the exercise of choice? (p. 23)

In the first question the issue of principles for selecting from competing values is addressed. The second question raises the critical issue of the internalization of the value so that it is an integral part of the student's value system and is exemplified in actions.

Moral Reasoning
The theories of Kohlberg (1972), Perry (1970) and others have been presented as viable approaches to moral development. Kohlberg's work involves moral reasoning relative to hypothetical moral dilemmas. That may have been a factor in the criticism of the method as being biased against women and cultural groups. Nursing offers numerous examples of dilemmas to which students can relate. Examples may be found in Davis and Aroskar (1983), Steele and Harmon (1983), and Reilly (1978).

The use of this method requires disciplined critical thinking and that inquiry be substantive and methodic. Ketefian (1981) studied 79 practicing nurses relative to their educational preparation, skill in critical thinking, and score on moral reasoning. Higher scores were more evident in nurses with professional preparation in contrast to those with technical preparation. Munhall (1980), using Rest's Defining Issue Test (DIT) based on Kohlberg's theory, found that the average baccalaureate student functioned at the conventional level while faculty were primarily at the principled level. There was no difference according to level of student, but it was noted that students with the higher grade point average scored higher in the levels of moral reasoning. These studies indicate that moral reasoning is a cognitive skill activity dependent upon knowledge and reflective thinking. It is a legitimate concern for faculty teaching the affective domain.

Experience
It must be noted that all of the described methods rely primarily on the cognitive processes of judgment and choice making and do not provide for experiential sequences where the learner develops a pattern of behavior consistent with stated values or moral decisions. The methods can be used appropriately in teaching students providing that the faculty understand the purpose for each and the limitations in terms of outcome.

Provision for experiential learning in dealing with ethical, moral and value conflicts is essential if affective skills are to be acquired. However, experiential methods without disciplined cognitive skills are not sufficient. Cross (1975), who sees *reasoning* as the heart of the educational process no less in areas of morality than in other fields of learning, refers to the need of practice when she states: "Just as we do not expect the student in mathematics to become proficient without practice in solving problems; so we should not expect students to develop skills in moral reasoning without practice in thinking about moral dilemmas" (p. 627).

CLINICAL FIELD FOR EXPERIENTIAL AFFECTIVE LEARNING

Much discussion surrounds the teaching of the affective domain in nursing programs. Some proposals include such formal courses as ethics and logic, while other proposals suggest integrating concepts into all nursing courses. Aroskar and Veatch (1977), in a study of baccalaureate nursing programs found six nursing programs with a formal course in ethics while two thirds of the respondents stated that ethical aspects were integrated in the curriculum.

Whether or not there is a formal course, provision must be made for the student to deal with the issues that are real in practice. Most of that experience is obtained in the clinical field where issues are directly related to nurse–client interactions, nurse–nurse interactions, nurse–other-discipline interactions, or nurse–bureaucratic conflict. Although these conflicts occur within the practice setting, many have much broader implications that incorporate issues of the larger society. Inquiry and analysis need to include all significant dimensions of the issue so that the student's data are qualitatively and quantitatively sufficient for making choices. Once the choice is made, students need to experience the choice in action and evaluate the action. Experiences need to be repeated, for consistency in response pattern is the desired goal.

The clinical field is replete with affective learning experiences. The setting in which students are asked to effect behavior change is a complex one where values and expectations of participants are shared, competitive, or contradictory. The teacher comes to the setting with his or her own perceptions, values, and convictions about the world of nursing, student learning behavior in a practice setting, and how health care "ought" to be delivered in that setting. Likewise, the student brings to the setting his or her own ideas and values, some of which will be altered in the process of learning. Marshall (1973) reminds teachers that they "are working with learners who are plagued with questions about self, own worth and the meaning of this experience and things that are happening to him or her in the immediate environment" (p. 9). Adult learners in the program bring a more stabilized value system and decision-making process yet may be threatened when alteration is indicated. Regardless of the age of the student and life experiences, there is a need for a supportive, trustworthy, and authentic environment where mistakes or trying out of new selves will occur within a learning rather than a punitive context.

PREPARATION OF OBJECTIVES

As with the other domains, planning for experience is required. Objectives must be prepared, relevant learning experiences and teaching strategies devised, and evaluative methods selected. As with the other domains, affective learning must be a developmental process, proceeding from simple to complex. The student does not enter the practice setting with a *tabulae rasa;* some values inherent in nursing are developed, some are still at the value indicator stage, and some have not been recognized. For those values that have been developed, their expression in nursing may be different from what the students have experienced in their life encounters. This situation is no different from what occurs with the other domains; there are various levels of achievement among students.

Taxonomy
In preparing objectives for the field experience, the level of achievement needs to be identified. Behaviors to be demonstrated in the clinical field must arise out of course objectives. In some instances they may be the same ones, with the cognitive component taught and evaluated in the classroom and the use of the cognitive behavior in a consistent pattern of behavior taught and evaluated in the clinical field.

A taxonomy serves the purpose of identifying the increasingly complex level of value development. Krathwohl and associates (1964) developed a taxonomy of the affective domain which Reilly (1980) applied to nursing. The essence of affective learning is internalization, continuity between knowing and doing in a consistent pattern. Internalization is the integrating principle of the taxonomy.

The first two levels relate to the value indicators that Raths and colleagues (1966) mention. It is at the third level where choosing occurs and internalization begins. The levels in the taxonomy are described in Table 19.

Use of Taxonomy
Like the other taxonomies, the affective taxonomy provides a framework for selecting the appropriate level of learning behavior and for writing objectives. The desired level is selected in terms of the learner's status in the program, the complexity of the phenomenon, and

TABLE 19. TAXONOMY OF AFFECTIVE DOMAIN

Taxonomy	Behavior
A 1.0 Receiving (attending)	
1.1 Awareness	Knows about, no response offered
1.2 Willingness to receive	Interested in giving attention; may or may not act
1.3 Controlled or selected attention	Differentiates stimuli; selects ones of personal interest
A 2.0 Responding	
2.1 Acquiescence in responding	Responds to authority's command
2.2 Willingness to respond	Voluntary action; likes idea
2.3 Satisfaction in response	Enjoys act; still no commitment
A 3.0 Valuing	
3.1 Acceptance of value	Reasonably certain about belief
3.2 Preference for value	Attaches worth to belief and acts accordingly
3.3 Commitment	High degree of certainty; usually consistent in action
A 4.0 Organization	
4.1 Conceptualization of value	Conceptualization gives value stability; action is consistent
A 5.0 Characterization by a value or value complex	
5.1 Generalized set	Internalization provides means of ordering complex world and acting consistently and effectively
5.2 Characterization	Integration so complete that actions are consistent and compatible

(Adapted from Reilly, D. E. Behavioral objectives—evaluation in nursing. New York: Appleton-Century-Crofts, 1980, pp. 57–58, with permission.)

experiences available for achieving the objective. Preparation of objectives in terms of the taxonomy follows using the nursing standard cited earlier.

> Standard V: Nursing action provides for client/patient participation in health promotion, maintenance, and restoration.
> 2. The client/patient and family are provided with the information needed to make decisions and choices about: promoting, maintaining and restoring health, seeking and utilizing appropriate health care personnel, maintaining and using health care resources. (ANA, 1973, p. 5)

A 1.0 Receiving
> 1.1 The student acknowledges that nurses provide information for client/family.
> 1.2 The student listens to client/family express concerns and need for knowledge.

1.3 The student listens to comments by client/family which indicate areas where they wish information before making decisions.

A 2.0 Responding

2.1 The student provides information to client/family according to requirements of the care plan.

2.2 The student seeks opportunity to provide client/family with information needed for making decisions.

2.3 The student responds willingly in meeting information needs of client/family.

A 3.0 Valuing

3.1 The student assists client/family in obtaining data relevant to decisions to be made.

3.2 The student supports the right of client/family to be informed about all matters relevant to decisions affecting them.

3.3 The student assumes responsibility for informing client/family on matters pertinent to decisions involving them.

A 4.0 Organization

4.1 The student formulates a position relative to the client/family right to information and the nurse's responsibility to that end.

4.2 The student formulates a plan of action which assures advocacy of client/family rights to be knowledgeable in making decisions irrespective of circumstances.

A 5.0 Characterization

5.1 The student acts consistently both in protecting the information rights of client/family and assuring that they possess sufficient knowledge for making decisions relative to their health needs.

5.2 The student develops a philosophy of life and nursing which manifests itself in practice as a consistent advocacy for the value of client/family knowledge in maintaining control of decisions affecting their lives.

The level of affective competency to be achieved at the end of the program or at any point in the curriculum is a professional judgment decision of the faculty. On any one objective, one must recognize the time it takes to integrate knowing and doing. The upper two levels require considerable commitment and may be beyond the purview of some undergraduate programs. Professional schools may bring the students to the first stage in level four. Graduate programs should seek the upper levels for their students.

When the program outcome is determined, the level for each year of the program and courses are designated to show development. As with the other taxonomies, leveling may occur by increasing the taxonomy level, increasing complexity of the variables with which a behavioral level interacts, or by both processes at the same time. An illustration of the use of the taxonomy with the above objectives might appear in a baccalaureate program thusly:

End of program (senior year)	A 4.1
Junior Year	A 3.3
Sophomore Year	A 2.3

A technical program might expect level A 3.3

Reilly (1978) notes that many courses direct evaluation of cognitive learning at the three lower levels (knowledge, comprehension, application) while expectations of affective learning are directed to the complex level of consistency in behavior. She states:

> . . . for both domains, the lower levels of learning can be evidenced within a reasonable space of time and can be evaluated with rather easily developed appraisal strategies. In both domains, the complex learning behaviors require an extended period of development and require sophisticated appraisal techniques. (pp. 51–52)

TEACHING STRATEGIES

The principal criterion in selecting teaching strategies in the affective domain is involvement; experiential involvement, cognitive involvement. Hypothetical situations involving ethical, moral, and value conflicts are useful for teaching, but they often lack the reality; i.e., the student can remain outside the conflict. Situations drawn from actual practice enable the student to identify with the individuals dealing with the conflict. Teaching in the clinical field then provides not only the experiential and cognitive learning, but it also adds the reality dimension.

Some strategies are directed at the affective domain specifically; some strategies are an added dimension to other ongoing methods. A teacher attuned to affective teaching keeps an "antenna" focused on all activities in which the student is engaged in the search for affective learning experiences.

Analysis and Confrontation

Decision making is often considered primarily in the cognitive domain, yet almost every decision has an affective component reflective of a belief, value, or moral stance. Examination of the student's decision from a value, ethical, or moral perspective as well as from a cognitive one helps the students to know their own frame of reference. When this analysis of a decision occurs in clinical conferences, then affective questions are explored with input of differing perspectives as viewed by the members of the group. Through divergent thinking, various alternatives are explored and the potential consequence of each is noted.

The reliance on cognitive analysis only of students' decisions and actions in the practice setting impedes the development of the students toward an advocacy role in matters of health and welfare for a pluralistic society. The exploration of values, which often means confrontation, can raise consciousness of disharmony and inconsistency of values that are often quiescent. Confrontation is an important strategy for use by the teacher; for with no challenge to one's beliefs no growth will occur. Confrontation can be difficult, even painful for students and teachers. Churchill (1982) sees confrontation as essential and states: "The refusal of a teacher to challenge and even critically evaluate the values of a student, however benevolently motivated, undermines appreciation of the moral life and handicaps the development of students into self-affirming and self-critical moral agents" (p. 302). Shinn (1979) recognizes the disarming effects that may accompany value confrontation as self-images are threatened, but he sees positive results from the experience. "It may also lead a person to confront conflict and to recognize values more coherently. It may be a social and personal healing experience" (p. 30).

Clinical Assignment

In the National Geographic Society's publication *Journey into China,* the following statement occurs: "The Wall (Great) stood for the proposition that unbridgeable cultural differences exist among people, differences so profound that they could be dealt with only by separation" (Smith, 1982, p. 84). Does such a wall exist in nursing practice, whether within a person or within a system? Teaching in the affective domain requires that such a wall be dismantled if it exists, for the respect for the dignity and worth of each person, as stated thematically through all nursing documents, does not mean "persons like me." The ANA Social Policy Statement previously cited declares that nursing's concern is for all individuals, regardless of life style, value system, or appearance.

Confrontation is once again called upon as a method, this time in terms of the clients or situations to which students are assigned. Augmentation of the care component of "different" clients with study of particular mores, values, or behavior patterns of the client's group will help students place the client in the client's own perspective, not in that of the students. Conferences, which are exploratory not only in terms of the client's behavioral responses but also the student's, will foster the student's growth in serving and living in a pluralistic society. Emphasis must be placed on the client's right to his or her own life style and values with the recognition that the acceptance of this right does not mean that the nurse accepts the life style and values for himself or herself.

Teachers' biases in making these assignments must be scrutinized so that assignments are compatible with growth needs of students. In urban schools of nursing, faculty are often concerned that suburban students obtain community health nursing experience with city clients in order to broaden their perspective of how nursing care needs are influenced by socioeconomic and cultural factors. However, seldom do they see the need for city students to gain experience with clients in suburban areas on the same premise.

Hands-on Care

Hands-on care is usually taught from the psychomotor perspective with recognition of the student's need to know the underlying principles. The affective domain has much to contribute to expert performance. The domain refers to the nonverbal message the student brings to the client in the process of carrying out a procedure.

Nursing is one of the few professions in which society permits the touching of individuals on any part of their body. How is that touch administered? Literature in nursing is now addressing the therapeutic value of touch. The concern in the affective domain is the way the nurse touches and carries out the procedures so as to connote the message: "I care. I respect your dignity and worth."

Baths can be stimulating and refreshing or they can be uncomfortable and wearisome, resembling more of a dry cleaning. Careless tossing of limbs, ignoring of privacy needs of patients through failure to keep covered those parts of the body not involved in the treatment and/or failure to explain to the client the processes involved in a procedure all reflect a communication that ignores the dignity of the client. Nurses are particularly challenged when caring for clients with body drainage or inability to control bodily functions. At that time, clients already distressed with loss of control and disturbed body image are particularly sensitive to the nurse's response to them and to the nurse's manner in caring for them.

Faculty observing students in carrying out psychomotor skills need to note the affective component of the skill. Acceptable performance incorporates not only the quality of the technique and knowledge but also the quality of the touch and caring.

Examination of Verbal Expressions

The human proclivity to use a generalized word to convey a complicated phenomenon is particularly relevant in teaching the affective domain. The word is generally a way of categorizing information and beliefs to simplify the handling of large amounts of data. The teacher in the affective domain listens carefully to the labels the learner uses when referring to clients or others in the practice setting. Such words as uncooperative, culturally deprived, basket case, or lazy may be heard.

Labels do two things. To the one labeled, the label signifies that since what others say is the way it is, there is nothing the person can do about it. To the labeler, the nurse, it means one accepts the fact and need do nothing about it. It is the latter interpretation that is of concern, for there is no attempt on the part of the nurse to seek the cause of the client's behavior and address the cause. One group of students sought data about a group of patients which the nursing staff labeled as uncooperative. Most of these patients were over 50 years of age with a terminal illness and had few visitors. The patients were exhibiting fear of dying alone, but the label accepted by the nursing staff prevented them from recognizing the patients' behavior as need behavior. One might suggest here that teachers need to examine labels they use in referring to students.

In addition to learner use of labels, the teacher needs to note also the way students present their ideas regarding patients in clinical happenings. The frequent or habitual use of global words such as, all, every, or never suggest the student is failing to accept individual difference among people, events, situations, or phenomena. Some students couch their ideas with expressions that take the onus of owner responsibility away from themselves, such as, "the other nurses say," "the doctor says," "the author says," "the teacher says." Concern here is that the students do not take a position and accept the inherent responsibility, an essential behavior in the role of advocate.

Other students will not make a statement that reflects a position for or against anything or anyone. If the student is to be able to make decisions in ethical, moral, or value conflicts, the student must be able to clarify his or her own thinking and be prepared to take a stand and accept the consequences. Faculty noting the communication patterns described that reflect avoidance or inadequate inquiry need to confront the students and select experiences in the clinical field that will foster the students' examination of their own behavioral responses and ability to communicate with confidence decisions rationally made.

Model Learning

Modeling, a method of formal learning whereby the learner seeks to imitate a behavioral pattern of another individual who exemplifies an ideal to the student, is often referred to as essential for learning in a practice discipline. It is often noted in reference to affective learning.

Teaching is not value free, regardless of what the teacher thinks or desires. The very approach the teacher uses in teaching within the practice field, selection of learning experiences, interactions with students, interactions with clients and participants in the delivery of care in the setting, and expected performance standards of all students all reflect in some way the moral beliefs and values of the teacher.

What should be the position of a teacher in discussions of moral, value, and ethical issues? Should the teacher remain neutral? Baumgarten (1982) supports a neutral advocacy stance for liberal arts teachers, for he feels that the declaration of a position by a teacher will stifle inquiry by students' unquestioning acceptance of that position and deprive them of creative anguish that comes with thinking through an issue without knowing the ultimate result.

Other authors support the notion that neutrality is not possible and that, indeed, the teacher may in essence only be feigning neutrality (Casement, 1984; Churchill, 1982; Robertson & Grant, 1982). Even though a verbal statement of a position may not be made, nonverbal messages, e.g., facial and body cues given in directing the discussion, convey the teacher's real beliefs or values. Robertson and Grant (1982) state, "Teachers who are trying to persuade rationally their students should rely on presentation of arguments to accomplish goals rather than on personal charisma in emotional appeals" (p. 349). Shinn (1979) sees exhortation as the least effective way of inculcating values. The suggestions of these two authors are particularly relevant to a professional program such as in nursing, where persuasion for accepting a particular set of professional values is in order.

Robertson and Grant see educational value to the teacher's declaration of a position on an issue when the teacher encourages students to criticize and question the position. When the teacher tells students how that position was originated, what processes the teacher went through in developing the position, what alternatives were considered, and what doubts or questions still persist the teacher is demonstrating a model of rational and emotional self-searching in preparation for a declared position with which the person can live.

The emphasis in the use of modeling as a teaching strategy entails leading the student through thought and experiences to one's own conclusions. There is danger in the use of models. Adelson (1962) differentiates between the teacher's style and the teacher's skill. He is concerned that the student may imitate the teacher's style, i.e., way of responding to a conflict, rather than the teacher's skill, i.e., process by which the teacher achieved the responses. Imitation may be a form of flattery, but it is dangerous if the student does not examine the teacher's response in relation to its rationale and appropriateness for self. Style follows skill; the imitation of the skill does not mean that the student's style will be the same as the teacher's. Style is personal.

SUMMARY

Affective learning occurs in the clinical field and must be subject to the same pedagogic demands as the other domains in learning. The goals of affective learning are the development of skill in moral reasoning for managing ethical and moral dilemmas and the development of a value system which incorporates those values espoused by the profession of nursing through its documents, namely the Code of Nursing, Standards of Nursing Practice, and the Social Policy Statement.

Affective skills are becoming increasingly essential for practitioners of all disciplines as they are faced with complex decisions where values representing quality of life, justice, and conservation are in conflict with values associated with profit, expediency, and technology. Although professional documents provide guidelines for the responses of practitioners to conflict situations, they do not suggest priorities in competing values nor the means by which values are expressed. It is the individual who ultimately must resolve the question of what response to make in a conflict situation.

Affective learning entails such concepts as: ethics—standards of conduct; morality—systems of moral conduct; belief—individual perceptions of reality; value—judgment of worth arising from choice and demonstrated in action; attitude—feeling for or against; and moral reasoning—cognitive process of analysis and interpretation of moral issues.

Skills in making rational decisions are not sufficient, for affective competency also requires action consistent with stated beliefs or positions. The clinical field provides an excellent environment, for by its very nature it represents many of the types of conflicts that nurses encounter in practice. The opportunity to experience conflicts, both through cognition and action, enables learners to explore and test out their own choices.

Value clarification, value inquiry, and exercises in moral reasoning where the substance of each is generated by the practice environment are appropriate methods for teaching the affective domain. Clinical conferences or written issue papers are vehicles for addressing the cognitive component implied by these methods. Behaviors of students connoting action of beliefs, values, and moral stances can also be subject to confrontation and examination. Action is evident in the words students use in expressions about people, events, and situations and in the way they carry out their psychomotor skills. The use of clinical conference, selective client or activity assignment, and field placement as well as the use of modeling are appropriate for teaching the affective domain from a clinical perspective.

The ethical and moral values inherent in nursing practice have a significant bearing on the value orientation of nursing and direct the affective behavior of its practitioners as they serve their clients. Donaldson and Crowley (1978) address themselves to the goal of nursing in fostering self-care behavior which leads to individual health and well-being and to nursing's accountability for social needs. "As a result of this value orientation, knowledge of the basis of human choices and of methods for fostering individual independence are sought, rather than knowledge of interventions that control and directly manipulate the person per se into a societally determined state of health" (p. 117). The charge is made to the faculty teaching the affective domain in the clinical field.

REFERENCES

Adelson, J. (1962). The teacher as a model. In N. Sanford (Ed.), *American College*. New York: Wiley.

American Nurses Association. (1973). *Standards: Nursing practice*. Kansas City, Mo.: American Nurses Association.

American Nurses Association. (1976). *Code for nurses with interpretive statements*. Kansas City, Mo.: American Nurses Association.

American Nurses Association. (1980). *Nursing: A social policy statement*. Kansas City, Mo.: American Nurses Association.

Aroskar, M., & Veatch, R. (1977). Ethics teaching in schools of nursing. *The Hastings Report, 7*(4), 23–26.

Ayer, A. J. (1946). *Language, truth, and logic*. New York: Davis.

Baumgarten, E. (1982). Ethics in the academic profession: A socratic view. *Journal of Higher Education, 53*, 282–95.

Bonaparte, B. (1979). Ego defensiveness, open-closed mindedness and nurses' attitude toward culturally different patients. *Nursing Research, 28*, 166–71.

Casement, W. (1984). Moral education: Form without content? *Educational Forum, 48*, 177–78.

Churchill, L. (1982). The teaching of ethics and moral values in teaching: Some contemporary confusions. *Journal of Higher Education, 53*, 296–306.

Cranston, M. (1983). Are there any human rights? *Daedalus, 112* (4), 1–18.

Cross, K. P. (1975). Learner centered curriculi. In D. Vermilye (Ed.), *Learner centered reform: Current issues in higher education*. San Francisco: Jossey-Bass.

Davis, A. J., & Aroskar, M. A. (1983). *Ethical dilemmas and nursing practice* (2nd ed.). Norwalk, Conn.: Appleton-Century-Crofts.

Dewey, J. (1962). *Individualism, old and new*. New York: Capricorn Books.

Donaldson, S. K., & Crowley, D. (1978). The discipline of nursing. *Nursing Outlook, 26*, 113–20.

Dubos, R. (1981). *Celebration of life*. New York: McGraw-Hill.

Englehardt, H. T., Jr. (1977). Knowledge, value, and belief. In H. T. Englehardt, & D. Callahan (Eds.), *The foundations of ethics and its relationship to science: Vol. 2. Knowledge, value and belief*. Hastings-on-Hudson, N.Y.: Institute of Society, Ethics and Life Sciences.

Frankl, V. E. (1963). *Man's search for meaning*. New York: Washington Square Press.

Gardner, J. W. (1978). *Morale*. New York: W. W. Norton & Co., Inc.

Gilligan, C. (1977). In a different voice: Women's conceptions of self and of morality. *Harvard Education Review, 47,* 481–517.

Holstein, C. B. (1976). Irreversible stepwise sequence in the development of moral judgment: A longitudinal study of males and females. *Child Development, 47,* 51–61.

Ketefian, S. (1981). Critical thinking, educational preparation, and development of moral judgment among selected groups of practicing nurses. *Nursing Research, 30,* 98–103.

Knox, A. B. (1977). *Adult development in learning.* San Francisco: Jossey-Bass.

Kohlberg, L. (1972). The cognitive–development approach to moral education. *The Humanists, 32,* 12–18.

Kohlberg, L. (1981). *The philosophy of moral development.* New York: Harper & Row.

Krathwohl, D. R., Bloom, B. S., & Masia, B. (1964). *Taxonomy of educational objectives, Handbook 2, Affective domain.* New York: D. McKay.

Levine, M. (1977). Nursing ethics and the ethical nurse. *American Journal of Nursing, 77,* 845–47.

MacIntyre, A. (1979). Why is the search for foundations of ethics so frustrating? *Hastings Center Report, 9,* 8–11.

Marshall, J. P. (1973). *The teacher and his philosophy.* Lincoln, Neb.: Professional Educators Pub.

McBee, M. L. (1978). Higher education: Its responsibility for moral development. *Phi Kappa Phi Journal, 58,* 30–33.

Morrill, R. L. (1980). *Teaching values in college.* San Francisco: Jossey-Bass.

Munhall, P. (1980). Moral reasoning of nursing students and faculty in a baccalaureate program. Image, *12*(3), 57–61.

Nagel, T. (1977). The fragmentation of values. In H. T. Englehardt, & D. Callahan (Eds.), *The foundations of ethics and its relationship to science: Vol. 2. Knowledge, value and belief.* Hastings-on-Hudson, N.Y.: Institute of Society, Ethics, and Life Sciences.

Perry, W. G., Jr. (1970). *Forms of intellectual and ethical development in the college years.* New York: Holt, Rinehart & Winston.

Podeschi, R. L. (1976). William James and education. *The Educational Forum, 40,* 223–29.

Raths, L. E., Harmin, M., & Simon, S. (1966). *Values and teaching.* Columbus, Ohio: Chas. E. Merrill.

Reilly, D. E. (Ed.). (1978). *Teaching and evaluating the affective domain in nursing programs.* Thorofare, N.J.: Charles B. Slack.

Reilly, D. E. (1980). *Behavioral objectives—evaluation in nursing.* 2nd ed. New York: Appleton-Century-Crofts.

Robertson, E., & Grant, G. (1982). Teaching and ethics: An epilogue. *The Journal of Higher Education, 53,* 345–57.

Rogers, C. (1983). *Freedom to learn in the 80's.* Columbus, Ohio: Chas. E. Merrill.

Saunders, L. (1954). *Cultural differences and medical care: The case of Spanish-speaking people in the Southwest.* New York: Russell Sage Foundation.

Scheibe, K. E. (1970). *Beliefs and values.* New York: Holt, Rinehart & Winston.

Schein, E. H. (1972). *Professional education: Some new directions.* New York: McGraw-Hill.

Shinn, R. L. (1979). An educational impossibility: The value-free classroom. *Columbia,* 26–30.

Simon, S., Howe, I., & Kirschenbaum, H. (1972). *Values clarification.* New York: Hart.

Smith, A. F. (1978). Lawrence Kohlberg's cognitive stage theory of the development of moral judgment. *New Directions for Student Services, 4,* 53–66.

Smith, G., Jr. (1982). On the trail of the long stone serpent. In *Journey to China.* Washington, D.C.: National Geographic Society.

Steele, S. M., & Harmon, V. M. (1983). *Values clarification in nursing* (2nd ed.). Norwalk, Conn.: Appleton-Century-Crofts.

Stent, G. S. (1977). The poverty of scientism and the promise of structuralist ethics. In H. T. Englehardt, & D. Callahan (Eds.), *The foundations of ethics and its relationship to science: Vol. 2. Knowledge, value and belief.* Hastings-on-Hudson, N.Y.: Institute of Society, Ethics, and Life Sciences.

Toulmin, S. (1977). The meaning of professionalism: Doctors, ethics and biomedical science. In H. T. Englehardt, & D. Callahan (Eds.), *The foundation of ethics and its relationship to science, Vol. 2. Knowledge, value and belief.* Hastings-on-Hudson, N.Y.: Institute of Society, Ethics, and Life Sciences.

Turro, J. (1972). *Reflections.* Paramus, N.J.: Paulist Press.

Wild, J. (1969). *The radical imperialism of William James.* New York: Doubleday.

BIBLIOGRAPHY

Beiter, C. (1978). Morality and moral education. *The Hastings Report, 8*(2), 20–24.

Benoliel, J. Q. (1983). Ethics in nursing practice and education. *Nursing Outlook, 31,* 210–15.

Bok, D. (1976). Can ethics be taught?. *Change, 8*(9), 26–30.

Bowen, H. (1977). Values, the dilemmas of our times and education. In D. Vermilye (Ed.), *Relating work and education: Current issues in higher education.* San Francisco: Jossey-Bass.

Brink, P. (1984). Value orientation as an assessment tool in cultural diversity. *Nursing Research, 33,* 198–203.

Brummer, J. J. (1984). Moralizing and value education. *Educational Forum, 48,* 263–76.

Callahan, D., & Boks, S. (1979). The role of applied ethics. *Change, 2*(6), 23–27.

Cannon, R. B., Gilead, M. P., Haun, E. B., et al. (1984). A values clarification approach to cultural diversity. *Nursing & Health Care, 5,* 160–64.

Caws, P. (1978). Teaching ethics in a pluralistic society. *The Hastings Report, 8*(5), 32–37.

Chickering, A. W. (1974). *Commuting vs resident students.* San Francisco: Jossey-Bass.

Cotanch, P. H. (1981). Self-actualization and professional socialization of nursing students in clinical laboratory experience. *Journal of Nursing Education, 20*(8), 4–14.

Davis, A. J. (1979). Ethics rounds with intensive care nurses. *Nursing Clinics of North America, 12,* 9–13.

Davis, A. J. (1982). Helping your staff address ethical dilemmas. *Journal of Nursing Administration, 9,* 9–13.

Delattre, E. J., & Bennet, W. (1979). Where the values movement goes wrong. *Change, 8*(9), 26–30.

Dewey, J. (1975). *Moral principles in education.* Carbondale and Edwardsville, Ill.: Southern Illinois Press.

Englehardt, H. T., & Callahan, D. (Eds.). (1978). *The foundation of ethics and its relationship to science, Vol. 3. Morals, Science and Society.* Hastings-on-Hudson: Institute of Society, Ethics, and Life Sciences.

Ethics in the academic profession. (1982). *Journal of Higher Education, 53.*

Ethical dilemmas in nursing. (1977) *American Journal of Nursing, 77,* 845–76.

Eble, K. (1972). *Professors as teachers.* San Francisco: Jossey-Bass.

Felsmesser, R. A., & Cline, H. F. (1982). To be or not to be: Moral education in the schools. *New York University Education Quarterly, 13,* 11–20.

Fromer, M. J. (1980). Teaching ethics by case conflicts. *Nursing Outlook, 28,* 604–8.

Gaylor, W. (1973). Editorial: The patients' bill of rights, *Saturday Review, 1,* 22.

Hawks, J. H. (1984). Should nurses give moral advice? Image, *16*(1), 14–16.

Human rights. (1983). *Daedalus, 112*(4).

Illich, I. (1975). *Medical Nemesis.* New York: Pantheon Books.

James, W. (1962). *Talks to teachers.* New York: Dover.

Jameston, A. (1977). The nurse when roles, rules conflict. *The Hastings Report, 7*(4), 22–23.

Johnson, D. W. (1984). *Computer ethics: A guide for the new age.* Elgin, Ill.: Brethen Press.

Keasey, C. B. (1979). Cognitive stages in developmental phases: A critique of Kohlberg's stage–structural theory of moral reasoning. *Journal of Moral Education, 8,* 168–81.

Kelly, L. (1976). The patient's right to know. *Nursing Outlook, 24,* 27.

Ketefian, S. (1981). Moral reasoning and moral behavior among selected groups of practicing nurses. *Nursing Research, 30,* 55–58.

King, V., & Gerwig, N. (1981). *Humanizing nursing education: A confluent approach through group process.* Rockland, Md.: Aspen.

Kohlberg, L. (1978). The cognitive-development approach to moral education. In P. Scharf (Ed.), *Readings in moral education.* Minneapolis: Winston Press.

Levine, A. (1980). *When dreams and heroes died: A portrait of today's college student.* San Francisco: Jossey-Bass.

Lockwood, A. (1975). A critical view of values clarification. *Teachers College Record, 77,* 35–50.

Mooney, M. N. (1980). The ethical component of nursing theory: An analysis of ethical components in four nursing theories. *Image, 12*(1), 7–12.

Murphy, C. P., & Hunter, H. (1983). *Ethical problems in nurse–patient relationships.* Boston: Allyn & Bacon.

O'Rourke, K. V. (1983). Moral considerations in nursing curricula *Journal of Nursing Education, 22,* 108–13.

Piaget, J. (1965). *The moral judgment of the child.* New York: Free Press.
Rest, J. (1976). New approaches in assessment of moral judgment. In T. Lickona (Ed.), *Moral development and behavior: Theory, research and social issues.* New York: Holt, Rinehart & Winston.
Revez, M. C. (1981). Open-closed mindedness, intolerance of ambiguity and nurse faculty attitude toward culturally different patients. *Nursing Research, 30,* 177–81.
Smith, S. P., & Davis, A. J. (1980). Ethical dilemmas: Conflicts among rights, duties, and obligations. *American Journal of Nursing, 80,* 1463–66.
Sredl, D. (1983). The head nurse as ethical and legal leader. *Nursing Management, 14*(11), 55–58.
Steinfels, M. (1977). Ethics, education and nursing practice. *The Hastings Report, 7*(4), 20–21.
Summing up: The ethical and legal problems in medicine and biomedical and behavioral research. (1983). President's Commission for study of ethical problems in Medicine, Biomedical, Behavioral Research. Washington, D.C.: U.S. Government Printing Office.
Thompson, K. S. (1981). Changes in the values and life styles preferences of university students. *Journal of Higher Education, 52,* 506–18.
Toulmin, S. (1979). Can science and ethics be reconnected? *The Hastings Report, 9*(3), 27–34.
Trow, M. (1976). Higher education and moral development. *American Association of University Professors Bulletin, 62,* 20–27.
Williams, M. A., Bloch, D. W., & Blair, E. M. (1978). Values and value changes of graduate nursing students: Their relationship to faculty values and to selected educational factors. *Nursing Research, 27,* 181–89.

9

Place of Clinical Practice within a Nursing Curriculum

Competency in clinical practice develops over a period of time as a result of planned sequential experiences in the field. In practice professions, experiential learning in selected clinical fields is essential if the requisite skills are to be achieved by the student. Each practice experience is dependent upon a specified body of knowledge concerned not only with the theoretical basis of the experience but also the processes entailed and the anticipated outcomes.

Some practice disciplines view clinical practice as the culminating experience in a program, often designating the last term as a period of concentrated practice. Others view clinical practice as a concurrent experience offered throughout a program which evolves in complexity as the program itself addresses more complex phenomena. Some nursing programs subscribe to the latter, while others modify the latter by requiring a period of concentrated academic study to provide the knowledge necessary for building the discipline's basis for practice.

The selection of an educational model that provides a concurrent field practice component denotes the belief that the acquisition of knowledge and its use in developing practice competencies requires a carefully thought out plan of instruction which demonstrates the integration of learning experiences in both the classroom and clinical field. This plan of instruction is the curriculum of a school. Its development entails continuous attention not only to requisite classroom learning as specified in the outcomes of the program but also to the practice experiences which enable the student to integrate this learning in the evolution of one's own theory of practice. This synthesis process occurs not only at the program level, but occurs each time a clinical course or unit in that course is planned.

CONCEPT OF CURRICULUM

There are varying conceptions of curriculum, although in most instances it refers to some type of educational plan. Beauchamp (1975) writes that "a curriculum is a written document which may contain many ingredients, but basically it is a plan for the education of pupils during their enrollment in a given school" (p. 7). Bevis (1978) views curriculum as "the learning activities that are designed to achieve specific educational goals" (p. 8). The key phrase in this definition is *learning activites or experiences.* Most definitions of curriculum refer to this notion of learning experience, which originated with Dewey's (1944) philosophic concept of experience.

Curriculum development entails the determination of behavioral outcomes to be attained by students at the conclusion of the program, selection and organization of learning experiences directed toward achievement of these behaviors, and provision for formative and summative evaluation strategies to ascertain their fulfillment. These activities in curriculum development are the responsibility of the faculty; thus, faculty must be held accountable for their execution.

COMPONENTS OF THE CURRICULUM

A curriculum in nursing includes a conceptual framework of nursing, a philosophy, a statement of purpose, program and level objectives, and a sequence of courses.

Conceptual Framework of Nursing

The first step in the development of a nursing curriculum is the identification of a conceptual framework of nursing. This action precedes the development of a philosophy of the educational program and its purposes and objectives, for the entire curriculum is influenced by the concept of nursing practice, which is its core. The framework delineates concepts about human beings, environment, health, and nursing and their interrelationships and provides an overall structure for the curriculum. Conceptual framework has been defined by Santora (1980) as a "a cohesive, supporting linkage of selected, interrelated multidimensional concepts" (p. 3). The conceptual framework describes the practice of nursing and serves as the basis for the selection and organization of content to be taught in the curriculum. It is the source of what nursing to teach. The conceptual framework also provides a rationale for the selection of learning experiences and direction for evaluation.

Reilly (1975) classified conceptual frameworks for nursing as: (1) systems, (2) developmental or longitudinal, or (3) life processes.

Each framework has a unifying concept, such as stress adaptation, to which other components are related. The unifying concept, giving direction to the curriculum, is evident in every nursing course with a practice component. If stress adaptation is the unifying element, then students learn nursing assessment in relation to data gathering about stress and the nature of the client's adaptation to these stressors. Intervention strategies are directed toward promoting adaptation. The conceptual framework provides a way of viewing nursing practice and the focus of the teaching of that practice to learners.

Philosophy
A nursing school's philosophy represents a statement of beliefs to be honored in the nursing program congruent with those of the parent institution. Such a document usually includes beliefs about the individual, health, society, the concept of nursing, nursing education (including the relationship of academic and professional disciplines), the teaching–learning process, evaluation, and personal and professional development of the learner. The philosophy influences the other curriculum components, and it guides the teacher in planning for and carrying out the educational process. Beliefs about the roles of the teacher in terms of teaching, research, and service (also expressed in this document) are reflective of faculty responsibilities in the educational setting.

Purpose
The purposes of the nursing program are reflected in broad statements of program goals. These goals are usually few in number and include: (1) preparing a practitioner who is able to deliver nursing care to clients in multiple settings, (2) preparing a practitioner who will contribute to society, and (3) providing the basis for further development and continued learning. In advanced nursing programs, other goals pertain to contributing to the body of nursing knowledge and development of nursing theory.

Program Objectives
Program objectives as outcomes of the nursing program are derived from the conceptual framework, philosophy, and purpose and in turn provide the basis for determining objectives at other levels of the curriculum. Torres and Stanton (1982) have referred to the program objectives as characteristics of the graduate since they reflect the "behaviors which are expected of the graduate at the end of the program of study" (p. 47). The program objectives represent the senior year objectives since it is assumed that the learner will achieve these at the completion of the program.

TABLE 20. EXAMPLES OF PROGRAM OBJECTIVES

Theory framework:
The learner relates Orem's self-care model to nursing management of individuals, families, and groups throughout the life cycle and in varying health states.
Nursing process:
The learner uses the nursing process in promoting self-care of individuals, families, and groups.
Inherent worth and dignity of client:
The learner formulates judgments which reflect respect for the inherent worth and dignity of the client.
Interrelationships:
The learner assumes responsibility for developing working relationships with clients, families, colleagues, and members of other health care disciplines.
Development of learner:
The learner assumes responsibility for self-growth and development.
Profession:
The learner identifies the accountability of the nurse and profession in meeting the health care needs of society.

Program objectives are broadly stated and encompass behaviors in the cognitive, psychomotor, and affective domains. According to Reilly (1980), these objectives generally reflect six areas:

1. Theory framework for nursing
2. Nursing's methodology: nursing process
3. Concept of inherent worth and dignity of the individual
4. Interrelationships, including interactions with clients and intra- and interdisciplinary interactions
5. Development of the learner
6. Profession, relating to the responsibility and accountability of the learner to the client, the nursing profession, and society. (pp. 81–82)

Examples of program objectives in each of these areas are presented in Table 20. The taxonomic level at which the objectives are written is determined by faculty in accordance with the nature of the educational program involved. In an advanced nursing program, an additional objective may be needed relating to the competency expected of the learner in terms of research.

Level Objectives
The curriculum provides for progressive development of the learner in terms of knowledge, skills, and values. A level is a point in this developmental process at which certain competencies are to be demonstrated. Level objectives represent the behaviors expected, in relation to each of the program objectives, at a particular point in time in the nursing curriculum. This time dimension is often defined in terms of years in the curriculum but also may reflect the achieve-

ment expected upon completion of a group of courses or modules. The level needs to represent an adequate period of time for a learning change to occur.

Leveling of Objectives. As previously described, objectives may be leveled by changing the behavior to a higher taxonomic level, changing the variables with which the behavior is carried out or altering both of these. Leveling begins with determination of the program objectives, reflecting the six areas the objectives address, which indicate the outcomes expected at the end of the curriculum. Based on the number of levels in the curriculum, objectives are written to reflect behaviors to be achieved in relation to these six areas, at the completion of each level. Course objectives, more specific than level objectives, represent the outcomes expected at the conclusion of a course. Some courses are divided into units and spec-

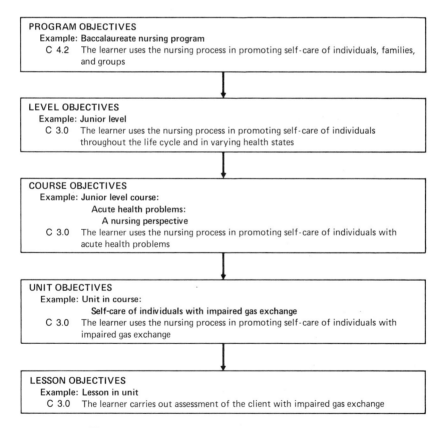

Figure 5. Leveling of objectives in a nursing curriculum.

ify objectives for achievement at the completion of the unit. For nursing faculty who develop lesson plans, objectives, derived from the unit objectives, may be written to indicate the learning outcomes at the end of a particular lesson. Objectives can also be developed for individual learning experiences. The developmental process of deriving objectives for instruction and examples of objectives at each level are illustrated in Figure 5. Objectives at any point in the curriculum are leveled according to the process described previously.

Courses

The courses in the nursing curriculum provide the means through which the conceptual framework, philosophy, and objectives become operationalized. Each course contains objectives, content, teaching methods, learning experiences, and an evaluation component.

The content of a course, identified from the objectives, represents the subject matter (cognitive, psychomotor, and affective) to be learned. An objective specifies the *learner, behavior* the learner is to demonstrate to indicate competence and *content* to which the behavior relates. The level of behavioral competency is determined by the taxonomic level deemed appropriate by faculty. These three components are identified in the following objective:

The nursing student	describes	steps of the nursing process.
Learner	**Behavior**	**Content**

An analysis of the objectives reveals broad content areas to be included in the course, which are then organized logically. Instruction proceeds according to the way in which the content is sequenced.

Development of a course involves the selection of teaching methods and learning experiences directed toward attainment of the course objectives in the classroom, learning laboratory, and clinical setting. One other component of a course plan is the development of an evaluation protocol for assessing the process and outcomes of the course. Evaluation includes strategies for measuring learning in the classroom, learning laboratory, and clinical setting and addresses the need for both formative and summative evaluation.

PLANNING THE CLINICAL COMPONENT

Clinical practice is an integral part of the total nursing curriculum. Experiences in the field provide for the development of the learner in terms of the knowledge, skills, and values inherent in the profession's practice. Not all nursing courses in the program require a clinical component, for they contribute experiences in analyzing theoretical knowledge and developing cognitive skills which affect the broader sphere of nursing as a practice discipline.

Clinical Objectives

Each clinical nursing course includes objectives for clinical practice and a systematic plan for learning in the field. Rather than preparing separate objectives denoting competencies to be achieved in the practice setting, clinical objectives are those course objectives and behaviors for which clinical practice is required for attainment. An objective represents a composite of behaviors that must be accomplished to demonstrate achievement of the objective. These behaviors often involve two or more domains of learning. To identify the clinical objectives, faculty determine which behaviors are to be accomplished in class, in the clinical setting, or in both class and the clinical setting. Some behaviors may also be identified for attainment in the learning laboratory.

Table 21 identifies this process for a unit on chronic pain management. The unit is presented in Tables 22 A and B where the objectives and behaviors are coded according to the taxonomies. Table 21 demonstrates the process by which these six unit objectives with their specified behaviors are designated according to the locus of activities for attainment. There are 58 behaviors: 7 are allocated only to classroom experience; 40 only to clinical experience; while 11 are attainable in both classroom and clinical settings. For this unit, there is a total of 51 behaviors that have the potential for achievement in the clinical field.

The decision as to the designation of behaviors of a course or unit as outcomes of the class or clinical experience represents a professional judgment on the part of faculty. Decisions may be altered at any time when indicated, with the consensus of faculty involved.

The objectives for clinical practice provide the framework for teaching in the field since they specify the learning outcomes to be achieved and give direction to faculty in the selection of teaching methods and learning experiences. They also serve as the basis for evaluating learning, for evaluation focuses on the learner's progress in meeting and attaining these objectives.

Some of the objectives represent learning outcomes achieved in previous courses but are now being taught within the context of the new course plan. Students are held accountable for competency in using these previously learned skills but may need assistance with their application to a new set of variables in a different clinical context.

Planning for Clinical Practice Experience

Since the objectives for clinical practice are already stated when the course or unit objectives are developed, it can be concluded that planning for the clinical field experience should occur concurrently with the classroom experience. Once the content for the course or unit is extrapolated from the objectives and arranged in a logical

**TABLE 21. CLASSIFICATION OF OBJECTIVES AND BEHAVIORS FOR A UNIT
ON CHRONIC PAIN MANAGEMENT**

Unit Objectives and Behaviors	Class	Clinical
I. Relate Orem's self-care model to nursing management of patients with chronic pain		
A. Analyzes the relationship between theories of pain and Orem's model of self-care	X	
B. Evaluates the biopsychosocial and cultural influences on the individual's ability to manage one's own pain	X	X
C. Identifies the impact of chronic pain on the developmental tasks of an individual	X	X
D. Analyzes the impact of chronic pain on family relationships and dynamics	X	X
E. Identifies criteria for distinguishing between the use of traditional and nontraditional methods of pain management	X	
F. Analyzes the various nontraditional pain management techniques in terms of the individual's and family's learning needs and self-care potential	X	X
G. Evaluates critically scientific rationale for implementing traditional and nontraditional methods of chronic pain management	X	
II. Use the nursing process in promoting self-care of patients with chronic pain *Assessment:*		
A. Carries out a systematic pain assessment of patient		X
B. Evaluates impact of chronic pain on patient's life style		X
C. Identifies patient's strategies for coping with pain		X
D. Appraises the impact of biopsychosocial and cultural factors on the patient's response to pain		X
E. Identifies developmental level of patient and family		X
F. Analyzes the influence of support systems on patient's ability to manage chronic pain	X	X
G. Assumes responsibility for identifying one's own values and biases that may affect the assessment		X
H. Integrates pain assessment data in calculation of therapeutic self-care demand		X
I. Identifies the nature and reasons for the existence of self-care deficits in relation to managing chronic pain		X
J. Analyzes the learning needs of patient and family in relation to chronic pain management		X
K. Formulates nursing diagnoses based on identified self-care deficits		X

TABLE 21. (*Continued*)

Unit Objectives and Behaviors	Class	Clinical
Planning:		
L. Develops with patient goals of care congruent with nursing diagnoses		X
M. Plans nursing management related to self-care deficits of patient and family		X
N. Supports the patient in decision making relative to options for pain management		X
O. Selects appropriate traditional and nontraditional methods of pain management		X
P. Provides for use of appropriate resources to assist patient and family		X
Implementation:		
Q. Implements nursing interventions congruent with a scientific rationale, research, and the mutually established plan of care		X
R. Is competent in the use of traditional pain management techniques		X
S. Demonstrates skill in the use of nontraditional pain management techniques		X
T. Initiates referrals to health care providers and/or agencies essential in assisting patient to meet optimum self-care agency		X
U. Encourages patient in use of his or her own potential and resources in addressing self-care limitations		X
V. Protects patient's self-care abilities as a means of preventing new self-care limitations		X
W. Documents pertinent nursing observations and interventions		X
Evaluation:		
X. Develops criteria for evaluating the effectiveness of the plan toward a decrease in self-care deficit and increase in self-care agency		X
Y. Uses criteria in evaluating patient and family outcomes of care in terms of stated goals		X
Z. Uses professional nursing standards as a framework for evaluating the process of the delivery of nursing care		X
AA. Modifies plan of care as indicated by the evaluation results		X
III. Formulate judgments which reflect respect for the inherent worth and dignity of the patient with chronic pain		
A. Defends the patient's right to be informed regarding traditional and nontraditional methods of chronic pain management relative to their expected outcomes and inherent risks		X

(*Continued*)

256

TABLE 21. (*Continued*)

Unit Objectives and Behaviors	Class	Clinical
B. Supports the patient's choice regarding the selection of pain control methods		X
C. Is consistent in respecting the patient's expressed perception of the degree of self-care deficit		X
D. Provides care reflective of the patient's own sociocultural preferences, psychologic needs, and health beliefs		X
E. Protects the patient's rights to privacy and confidentiality		X
F. Assumes responsibility for assessing one's own biases and values that may interfere with effective determination of the patient's self-care requisites	X	X
G. Acts as advocate for patient and/or family when individuals or situations appear to impede progress toward goal attainment		X
IV. Foster facilitative relationships with patients with chronic pain, families and colleagues		
A. Analyzes one's own interactive behavior within a therapeutic or collegial relationship	X	X
B. Assumes a liaison role between patient and other persons who have an impact upon the health care of the individual		X
C. Contributes readily to discussions and decisions that have an impact on matters concerning the patient's pain management		X
D. Serves as clarifier to patient, family, and other health team members in situations where misunderstanding or lack of knowledge is evident		X
E. Maintains ongoing communication with appropriate health providers regarding the plans, implementation, and evaluation of care		X
V. Assume responsibility for continued development of the knowledge base and competencies essential for promoting self-care agency in the presence of chronic pain		
A. Assumes responsibility for expanding one's own knowledge base regarding care of the patient with chronic pain	X	X
B. Maintains knowledge of current research findings which address the phenomenon of pain and its management	X	X
C. Examines one's own beliefs about health, illness, and an individual's potential as a self-care agent in formulating a philosophy of chronic pain management	X	X

TABLE 21. (*Continued*)

Unit Objectives and Behaviors	Class	Clinical
D. Is accountable for seeking out those learning experiences that enhance the development of requisite competencies		X
E. Analyzes research on chronic pain management	X	
F. Identifies researchable problems in care of patients which lend themselves to exploration within nursing's body of knowledge		X
VI. Affirm the accountability of nurses and the nursing profession to contribute to the development of a theory of practice for patients with chronic pain		
A. Takes a position on the responsibility of nurses and nursing to protect a vulnerable public against quackery and other kinds of deceptive methods purported to alleviate chronic pain		X
B. Analyzes societal, political, economic, legal, and ethical factors affecting management of the patient with chronic pain	X	
C. Takes a position on issues related to care of the patient with chronic pain	X	
D. Evaluates the role of the nurse as a significant health team member in the research and practice domains that address pain management	X	
E. Identifies the responsibility of nursing to generate knowledge pertinent to nursing actions in helping the patient with chronic pain meet self-care demands	X	X
F. Declares a position on nursing's ethical and moral responsibilities in the various pain management methods used in practice		X

sequence for presentation, both the class and clinical activities are planned concurrently. Some content will be addressed in the classroom and further developed in the clinical setting. Other content will be the purview of only the class experience or only the clinical experience. The plan, however, should demonstrate the locus and related learning and teaching activities, whatever they may be, in terms of the objectives to be achieved.

The proposal being made here considers the theory and clinical components of a practice course as one holistic phenomenon. It is recognized that some curricula separate these components into two courses, which may or may not have the prerequisite of integrated experiences in both settings.

The ideal of maintaining the integrity of the relationship of class and clinical experience may be challenged when the numbers of students and availability of clinical settings preclude all students from receiving experience in the same type of setting at the same time. A conceptually developed curriculum with an emphasis on concepts and theories rather than specific entities, such as diseases, enables faculty to plan more effectively for concurrent theory and clinical experiences under these circumstances. In some courses students may be in a variety of clinical settings; some of the experiences may be with children and others with adults. In situations in which students are in varied clinical placements, all learners may be involved in the same classroom instruction that addresses overall concepts and theories. Specific application of these concepts and theories to the populations in the different clinical settings may be taught separately in these settings and then repeated as new learners enter them. For instance, if three credits of a course are allocated for classroom instruction, two of these credits may involve all students in learning about the concepts and theories. The third credit would be allotted to teaching relevant specifics about the populations with whom the students are currently engaged in practice.

As an illustration, in a course that addresses the chronic illness phenomenon, students at any point in time in the course may be with clients in an outpatient service, acute care facility, or community setting. The concepts of chronic illness from the biopsychosocial, economic, and political perspective constitute the general core of classroom activity. In each setting, these concepts are explored in relation to the specifics as they pertain to the population with whom the students are involved. In addition to the classroom credits, there are clinical credits that provide for conferences and experiences which augment both the general and specific classroom discussions. The distribution of credit between the general and specific for any particular course is a function of faculty judgment.

Many concepts can be addressed with a wide variety of clients. It is important that when diverse client populations are required, the selection is based on relevancy to the concepts rather than to a geographical setting.

Planning for clinical learning experiences requires consideration of the taxonomic level of the objectives, for the teaching methods and learning activities need to promote learning at the level indicated by the objectives. For example, an objective at the application level requires methods and learning activities that enable the student to use concepts and theories in practice. An experience in which the learner merely describes the meaning of the concept is inappropriate for this taxonomic level in which the experience needs to focus on how the concept may be applied in the clinical situation.

In planning the clinical component, consideration should also be given to the types of clinical settings in which students practice and kinds of activities in which they engage throughout the nursing program. The settings and experiences should reflect the scope of nursing practice within the health care system. Clinical experiences in only an acute care setting are not representative of the health care problems learners will encounter in practice. Without variety in clinical settings and experiences throughout the curriculum, it would be difficult for learners to meet many of the clinical objectives in a nursing program.

MODEL FOR A UNIT OF A CLINICAL COURSE

A design for a unit of a clinical course is proposed in Tables 22 A and B to demonstrate the interrelationship of class and clinical practice experiences as they relate to specific objectives. The unit illustrated here is one of five units in a senior level nursing course, in a baccalaureate program, on Chronic Health Problems: A Nursing Perspective. The overview describes the purpose of the course, prerequisites, credit allotment, units in the course, teaching personnel, teaching methods, and evaluation strategies.

Course objectives indicate expected achievement at the completion of the course. Unit objectives and related behaviors represent the learning outcomes at the completion of Unit IV: Chronic Pain Management. The objectives are coded as to taxonomic level.

The components of the model shown in Table 22B include:

1. Objectives: This column includes the designated number and letter of the objectives and behaviors to which the content and activities relate. It is recognized that an experience may incorporate one or many behaviors, so the same objective and behavior will often be designated at varied points in the unit plan.
2. Content: Derived from the substance of the objectives, the content is organized in a logical sequence within the time constraints of the unit.
3. Teaching Methods: These columns include the activities used by the teacher in addressing the content. One set of activities takes place in the classroom; the other set of activities in the clinical setting.
4. Learning Activities: The experiences in which the learner is involved are noted in the learning activities columns, one within the classroom and the other within the clinical setting.

Overview

Course: Chronic Health Problems: A Nursing Perspective

Purpose: This course is designed for senior students to enable them to acquire the knowledge, skills, and values necessary for care of patients with chronic health problems. The course focuses on promoting self-care within this patient poulation.

Prerequisites: Senior standing. Competency in use of Orem's self-care model of nursing practice.

Course plan: This is a six credit course with three credits for classroom instruction, three hours per week, and three credits for clinical practice, nine hours per week, over a 15-week period. A 1:3 ratio is used for determining the number of clock hours per week for each credit of clinical experience.

Units in course:
Unit I: Socioeconomic and Political Dimensions (2 weeks) of Chronic Health Problems
Unit II: Nursing Management of Chronic Health (3 weeks) Problems in Children
Unit III: Nursing Management of Chronic Health (4 weeks) Problems in Adults and the Elderly
Unit IV: Chronic Pain Management (3 weeks)
Unit V: Nursing Management of Chronic Grief (3 weeks) and Depression

Teaching personnel: Teaching of the course is a collaborative effort of faculty with expertise in the biophysical and psychosocial dimensions of care of children and adults with chronic health problems.

Teaching methods: Lecture, discussion, media, self-paced module, computer simulation, handouts, readings, small group activities, written assignments, clinical assignments, conferences, role play, demonstrations, observation, nursing rounds.

Evaluation: Evaluation is based on achievement of the objectives. Evaluation strategies include midterm and final examinations, term paper, observation in clinical setting, patient care conference, two nursing care plans, case study, and log. Students also will complete a self and course evaluation.

Course Objectives[a]

At the completion of the course the learner will:

C 4.2 I. Relate Orem's self-care model to nursing management of patients with chronic health problems

C 4.2 II. Use the nursing process in promoting self-care of patients with chronic health problems

A 4.1 III. Formulate judgments which reflect respect for the inherent worth and dignity of patients with chronic health problems

A 4.1 IV. Foster facilitative relationships with patients with chronic health problems, their families, colleagues, and health team members

A 4.1 V. Assume responsibility for continued development of the knowledge base and competencies essential for promoting self-care of patients with chronic health problems

A 4.1 VI. Affirm the accountability of nurses and the nursing profession to contribute to the development of a theory of practice for patients with chronic health problems

Unit IV: Chronic Pain Management Unit Objectives

At the completion of the unit the learner will:

C 4.2 I. Relate Orem's self-care model to nursing management of patient with chronic pain

C 4.2	II.	Use the nursing process in promoting self-care of patients with chronic pain
A 4.1	III.	Formulate judgments which reflect respect for the inherent worth and dignity of the patient with chronic pain
A 4.1	IV.	Foster facilitative relationships with patients with chronic pain, families, and colleagues
A 4.1	V.	Assume responsibility for continued development of the knowledge base and competencies essential for promoting self-care agency in the presence of chronic pain
A 4.1	VI.	Affirm the accountability of nurses and the nursing profession to contribute to the development of a theory of practice for patients with chronic pain

Unit Objectives and Behaviors

C 4.2	I.	Relate Orem's self-care model to nursing management of patients with chronic pain
C 4.2		A. Analyzes the relationship between theories of pain and Orem's model of self-care
C 4.2		B. Evaluates the biopsychosocial and cultural influences on the individual's ability to manage one's own pain
C 4.2		C. Identifies the impact of chronic pain on the developmental tasks of an individual
C 4.2		D. Analyzes the impact of chronic pain on family relationships and dynamics
C 4.2		E. Identifies criteria for distinguishing between the use of traditional and nontraditional methods of pain management
C 4.2		F. Analyzes the various nontraditional pain management techniques in terms of the individual's and family's learning needs and self-care potential
C 4.2		G. Evaluates critically scientific rationale for implementing traditional and nontraditional methods of chronic pain management
C 4.2	II.	Use the nursing process in promoting self-care of patients with chronic pain

Assessment:

C 4.2		A. Carries out a systematic pain assessment of patient
C 4.2		B. Evaluate impact of chronic pain on patient's life style
C 4.2		C. Identifies patient's strategies for coping with pain
C 4.2		D. Appraises the impact of biopsychosocial and cultural factors on the patient's response to pain
C 4.2		E. Identifies developmental level of patient and family
C 4.2		F. Analyzes the influence of support systems on patient's ability to manage chronic pain
A 3.3		G. Assumes responsibility for identifying one's own values and biases that may affect the assessment
C 4.2		H. Integrates pain assessment data in calculation of therapeutic self-care demand
C 4.2		I. Identifies the nature and reasons for the existence of self-care deficits in relation to managing chronic pain
C 4.2		J. Analyzes the learning needs of patient and family in relation to chronic pain management
C 4.2		K. Formulates nursing diagnoses based on identified self-care deficits

(*Continued*)

TABLE 22A. (Continued)

Planning:

C 4.2 | L. Develops with patient goals of care congruent with nursing diagnoses

C 4.2 | M. Plans nursing management related to self-care deficits of patient and family

A 3.3 | N. Supports the patient in decision making relative to options for pain management

C 4.2 | O. Selects appropriate traditional and nontraditional methods of pain management

C 4.2 | P. Provides for use of appropriate resources to assist patient and family

Implementation:

C 4.2 | Q. Implements nursing interventions congruent with a scientific rationale, research, and the mutually established plan of care

P 5.0 | R. Is competent in the use of traditional pain management techniques

P 3.0 | S. Demonstrates skill in the use of nontraditional pain management techniques

C 4.2 | T. Initiates referrals to health care providers and/or agencies essential in assisting patient to meet optimum self-care agency

A 4.1 | U. Encourages patient in use of his or her own potential and resources in addressing self-care limitations

A 4.1 | V. Protects patient's self-care abilities as a means of preventing new self-care limitations

C 4.2 | W. Documents pertinent nursing observations and interventions

Evaluation:

C 4.2 | X. Develops criteria for evaluating the effectiveness of the plan toward a decrease in self-care deficit and increase in self-care agency

C 4.2 | Y. Uses criteria in evaluating patient and family outcomes of care in terms of stated goals

C 4.2 | Z. Uses professional nursing standards as a framework for evaluating the process of the delivery of nursing care

C 4.2 | AA. Modifies plan of care as indicated by the evaluation results

A 4.1 | III. Formulate judgments which reflect respect for the inherent worth and dignity of the patient with chronic pain

A 4.1 | A. Defends the patient's right to be informed regarding traditional and nontraditional methods of chronic pain management relative to their expected outcomes and inherent risks

A 4.1 | B. Supports the patient's choice regarding the selection of pain control methods

A 4.1 | C. Is consistent in respecting the patient's expressed perception of the degree of self-care deficit

C 4.1 | D. Provides care reflective of the patient's own socio-cultural preferences, psychologic needs, and health beliefs

A 4.1 | E. Protects the patient's rights to privacy and confidentiality

A 4.1 | F. Assumes responsibility for assessing one's own biases and values that may interfere with effective determination of the patient's self-care requisites

A 4.1 | G. Acts as advocate for patient and/or family when individuals or situations appear to impede progress toward goal attainment

TABLE 22A. (*Continued*)

A 4.1	IV.	Foster facilitative relationships with patients with chronic pain, families, and colleagues
C 4.2		A. Analyzes one's own interactive behavior within a therapeutic or collegial relationship
A 4.1		B. Assumes a liaison role between patient and other persons who have an impact upon the health care of the individual
A 4.1		C. Contributes readily to discussions and decisions that have an impact on matters concerning the patient's pain management
A 4.1		D. Serves as clarifier to patient, family, and other health team members in situations where misunderstanding or lack of knowledge is evident
A 4.1		E. Maintains ongoing communication with appropriate health providers regarding the plans, implementation and evaluation of care
A 4.1	V.	Assume responsibility for continued development of the knowledge base and competencies essential for promoting self-care agency in the presence of chronic pain
A 4.1		A. Assumes responsibility for expanding one's own knowledge base regarding care of the patient with chronic pain
A 4.1		B. Maintains knowledge of current research findings which address the phenomenon of pain and its management
A 4.1		C. Examines one's own beliefs about health, illness, and an individual's potential as a self-care agent in formulating a philosophy of chronic pain management
A 4.1		D. Is accountable for seeking out those learning experiences that enhance the development of requisite competencies
C 4.1		E. Analyzes research on chronic pain management
C 4.1		F. Identifies researchable problems in care of patients which lend themselves to exploration within nursing's body of knowledge
A 4.1	VI.	Affirm the accountability of nurses and the nursing profession to contribute to the development of a theory of practice for patients with chronic pain
A 4.1		A. Takes a position on the responsibility of nurses and nursing to protect a vulnerable public against quackery and other kinds of deceptive methods purported to alleviate chronic pain
C 4.2		B. Analyzes societal, political, economic, legal, and ethical factors affecting management of the patient with chronic pain
A 4.1		C. Takes a position on issues related to care of the patient with chronic pain
C 4.2		D. Evaluates the role of the nurse as a significant health team member in the research and practice domains that address pain management
C 4.2		E. Identifies the responsibility of nursing to generate knowledge pertinent to nursing actions in helping the patient with chronic pain meet self-care demands
A 4.1		F. Declares a position on nursing's ethical and moral responsibilities in the various pain management methods used in practice

[a]The C before the behavior indicates the cognitive domain, the A indicates the affective domain, and the P indicates the psychomotor domain.

TABLE 22B. MODEL FOR A UNIT OF CLINICAL COURSE

Objectives[b]	Content	Class		Clinical	
		Teaching Method[c]	Learning Activity	Teaching Method	Learning Activity
II.M,N	I. Pain: A legitimate concern of nursing A. Definition	Two hours Lecture/discussion	Assignment: To be read prior to class 1. Unit objectives 2. Text, "Dealing with Chronic Pain", pp. 40–50	Plan with students for clinical assignment. Explain protocol for keeping a log of activities	
III.B,C,G	1. A subjective phenomenon	Transparency: Definition of pain	Participate in discussion View transparency and raise questions		
IV.B	2. Not a single entity				
VI.D	a. Multiple factors influencing response				
	3. Perception/threshold/tolerance				
	4. Chronic vs. acute				
	B. Pain: A primary reason for entry into health care system				
	C. Impact of pain 1. Patient's perception	Read letter from patient with chronic pain	Analyze message in letter		

Content	Teaching aids	Learning activities	Evaluation

D. Nursing's unique contribution
  1. Pain: A human response as a focus for nursing intervention
  2. Nurse's availability during pain experience
  3. Nurse's responsibility in planning pain management
  4. Liaison/advocate role
E. Patient's rights
  1. Decision making
  2. Mutual goal setting
F. Necessity for theoretical basis for pain management
II. Pain: Psychosocial factors
A. Coping with pain
  1. Factors affecting pain perception
B. Psychologic factors affecting pain perception and response
  1. Emotionally traumatic life experiences
	Transparency: Nursing's Role in Pain Management
	
	Film: "Coping with Pain" (25 minutes)
	What are some psychologic factors affecting pain perception and response?
	Record on transparency
		View transparency and discuss
		
		View film. Identify factors affecting pain perception
			Clinical assignment Log
			
			Select a patient with chronic pain in the clinical setting. Identify psychologic factors affecting patient's pain perception and response and evaluate their implications. Record in log

I,B,C,D

II.B–E, F

III.D

265

TABLE 22B. (Continued)

		Class		Clinical	
Objectives[b]	Content	Teaching Method[c]	Learning Activity	Teaching Method	Learning Activity
	2. Secondary gains of the patient's complaint of pain				
	3. Personal past experience with pain				
	4. Knowledge level				
	5. Developmental level	What are the effects of developmental level on response to pain?			Identify patient's developmental level and related tasks.
	a. Influence of stage of development on ability to cope with pain				Analyze effects of pain on development.
	b. Effects of pain on developmental level				Record in log
	(1) Regression to earlier stage				
	(2) Inability to meet stage-specific tasks				
	6. Powerlessness				
	7. Presence, attitudes, and feelings of others				

266

Content	Transparency/Media	Activity	Assignment/Method
8. Threat to life situation 9. Perceptual dominance of pain 10. Previous coping strategies			
C. Cultural influences affecting patient's behavioral responses and pain sensations	Transparency: Cultural influences on responses to pain	View transparency and raise questions	Clinical assignment (in or out of clinical setting) Log
1. Membership in a particular sociocultural group 2. Age and sex 3. Religion a. Source of strength or source of despair 4. Body part involved in pain 5. Meaning of pain 6. Cultural ways of coping with pain	How many religious beliefs influence ability to cope with pain?		Interview one person from a culture other than your own. Inquire regarding: —person's view of pain —how pain is handled within cultural group —cultural folk remedies —when health care is elicited. Analyze data in terms of theory about culture and identify implications for pain management. Record in log
D. Family factors influencing pain perception and response 1. Family reaction to chronic pain	Transparency: Family Factors Influencing Pain Perception and Response	View transparency and discuss one's own experiences with family when pain was present	

(Continued)

267

TABLE 22B. (Continued)

	Class		Clinical	
Objectives[b]	Content	Teaching Method[c]	Learning Activity	Teaching Method	Learning Activity
	a. Ability to function as open system			Clinical assignment Log	Select a patient with chronic pain in the clinical setting. Assess family role in terms of health leader role and role changes.
	b. Integrity of family structure				
	(1) Interdependence				
	(2) Boundaries, systems, roles				
	2. Significance of role development for family member with pain				Identify implications for care.
	a. "Health leader" role				Record in log
	(1) Prime educator and decision maker of family				
	(2) Reluctance to assume sick role				
	(3) Usually wife/mother				
	b. Role changes secondary to chronic illness				

      (1) Ability to carry on usual role varies

      (2) Centrality of role vacated

      (3) Role strain occurs until family equilibrium achieved

      (4) Member with chronic pain must be integrated into family structure

E. Environmental factors influencing pain perception and response
1. Milieu
2. Time of day

F. Other factors affecting patient's pain perception and response
1. Social isolation and loneliness
2. Anger
3. Burden of care

Transparency: Environmental Factors Influencing Pain Perception and Response

View transparency

TABLE 22B. *(Continued)*

Objectives[b]	Content	Class		Clinical	
		Teaching Method[c]	*Learning Activity*	*Teaching Method*	*Learning Activity*

	4. Reintegration into society
	  a. Normalizing
	  b. Renormalizing
	  c. Balancing options
			Assignment: Read chapters on pain theories and traditional pain management techniques in text prior to class		

I.A,E,G	III. Pain theories
	A. Pattern/summation theory
	  1. Goldscheider, 1895
	  2. Coding of impulses at periphery
	  3. Modulation of impulses by central nervous system
	  4. Limitations of theory
		One hour
		Lecture/discussion
		What is the pattern/summation theory of pain?
		Record on transparency
			Participate in discussion		

	B. Specificity theory
	  1. VonFrey, 1894
	  2. Purely anatomical basis for pain perception
		What is the specificity theory of pain?
		Record on transparency			

a. Specific peripheral pain receptors
b. Transported via spinothalamic tract in spinal cord
c. Pain center in brain
d. Rationale for many surgical interventions

3. Limitations of theory

C. Gate control theory
1. Melzack and Wall, 1965
2. Attempts to integrate physiologic and psychologic aspects of pain
3. Widely accepted today
4. Based on interaction of systems
   a. Stimulation of large diameter fibers "closes" gate to pain
   b. Stimulation of small diameter fibers "opens" gate to pain

Handout: Gate Control Theory

What is the scientific rationale underlying the gate control theory of pain?

Read handout and raise questions

Participate in discussion

(Continued)

TABLE 22B. (Continued)

Objectives[b]	Content	Class		Clinical	
		Teaching Method[c]	Learning Activity	Teaching Method	Learning Activity
	c. "Gate" located in substantia gelatinosa of spinal cord				
	d. Presence of a central descending control mechanism				
	5. Implications	What are implications of gate control theory of pain?	Discuss implications for practice	Clinical conference: Application of gate control theory in practice (one hour)	Describe patient's pain and management strategies in terms of gate control theory
	a. Pharmacologic control of pain				
	b. Sensory control of pain				
	(1) Enhancement of large-diameter nerve fibers leads to closure of pain gate				
	(2) Rationale for hypnosis, suggestion, and distraction techniques				
	6. Limitations of theory				

7. Relationship to self-management of pain

D. Endogenous opiates
   1. Location
      a. Midbrain
      b. Thalamus and hypothalamus
      c. Substantia gelatinosa in dorsal horn of spinal cord
   2. Physiologic role in pain perception
      a. Distribution
      b. Research findings
   3. Implications
      a. Central control mechanism for gate control theory
      b. Rationale for hypnosis, acupuncture, and placebos
      c. Possible use in treatment of pain

Transparency: Endogenous Opiates

Handout: Implications for Pain Management

View transparency and raise questions

Read handout and discuss

(Continued)

273

TABLE 22B. (Continued)

Objectives[b]	Content	Class		Clinical	
		Teaching Method[c]	Learning Activity	Teaching Method	Learning Activity

I.E,G
 	
II.M,O, Q,R
III.A
V.B,E
	IV. Traditional methods of chronic pain relief
	A. Surgical intervention
	B. Pain medications
	1. Utilized alone or with other treatments
	2. Choice of medication and route dependent on many factors
	  a. Diagnosis
	  b. Defect in normal physiology
	  c. Length of time treatment to be pursued
	  d. Normal vs. shortened life expectancy
	  e. Potential complications
	  f. Patient perceptions regarding definition of pain relief and desired level of control
		Lecture/discussion
		
		Handout: Pain Medications
		What factors influence the choice of medication and route in the treatment of chronic pain? Record on transparency
			Participate in discussion
			
			Read handout and raise questions
				Clinical assignment
				Log
					Choose a patient with chronic pain in the clinical setting. Review the medical record. Identify pain medications, drug classification of each, and rationale for use. Describe other methods of pain management. Record in log

3. Classifications
   a. Narcotics—including actions, analgesia, risks, and therapeutic applications
   b. Nonnarcotics—including actions, analgesia, risks, and therapeutic applications
   c. Placebos
      (1) Definition
      (2) Myths vs. facts
      (3) Use vs. misuse
      (4) Legal and ethical considerations
4. Considerations in medication administration
   a. Need for ongoing assessment and adjustments
   b. Scheduling: ATC vs. PRN
   c. Patient rights

What is a placebo?

Self-paced module: "Medications for Pain"

Complete module in learning laboratory

Clinical conference: Incident process: Issues associated with placebos (one hour)

Analyze incident in clinical conference

(Continued)

TABLE 22B. (Continued)

Objectives[b]	Content	Class		Clinical	
		Teaching Method[c]	Learning Activity	Teaching Method	Learning Activity
I,E,F,G	V. Nontraditional pain management techniques	Three hours Lecture/discussion	Assignment: Read text and references from bibliography on non-traditional pain management techniques prior to next class		
II,M,O, Q,S	A. Hypnosis 1. General effects of hypnosis	What are the effects of hypnosis in relation to pain control?	Participate in discussion		
III,A	a. Decreased awareness of pain	Record on transparency			
V,B,E	b. Substitution of other feelings for pain				
	c. Movement of pain to other body areas				
	d. Altered meaning of pain				
	e. Dissociation of body from patient's awareness				
	2. Advantages of hypnosis techniques	Transparency: Advantages of Hypnosis in Pain Management	View transparency and raise questions		

Content Outline	Media/Materials	Learning Activities
a. Minimal unpleasant side effects		
b. Maintenance of physical, mental functioning		
c. Creation of life-enhancing attitudes		
3. Limiting factors of hypnosis	Transparency: Disadvantages of Hypnosis in Pain Management	View transparency and discuss
a. Mechanism of action unknown		
b. Association with myths, entertainment		
c. Concern about practicality in relation to training	Videotape of hypnosis of client with chronic pain (20 minutes)	View videotape and discuss
d. Majority of people unhypnotizable		
B. Distraction		
1. Characteristics of distraction	Transparency: Characteristics of Distraction	View transparency
a. Focus of attention on alternate stimulus		
b. Sensory shielding effect		
c. Use of existing objective or physical stimuli		

(Continued)

TABLE 22B. *(Continued)*

Objectives[b]	Content	Class		Clinical	
		Teaching Method[c]	Learning Activity	Teaching Method	Learning Activity

	2. Distraction guidelines
	  a. Assessment of previously used or familiar distraction techniques
	  b. Provision of information regarding limitations
	  c. Use of several sensory modalities
	  d. Emphasis on rhythm
	  e. Emphasis on breathing techniques
		What are the essential features that will enhance the effectiveness of distraction techniques?
		Record on transparency			

	3. Specific distraction techniques
	  a. Visual concentration and rhythmic massage
	  b. Slow rhythmic breathing
	  c. Sing and tap rhythm
		What are examples of distraction techniques?
		Handout: Distraction Techniques
		
		Has anyone ever used distraction techniques?
			Read handout and discuss
			
			Share with class previous experiences with use of distraction techniques
				Demonstration	Following demonstration of distraction techniques, choose a partner and practice techniques presented.
					Demonstrate techniques to peers

Content	Teaching methods/materials	Learning activities

d. Auditory stimulation via earphone
4. Major advantages of distraction
  a. Simple to use and teach
  b. Practical for use in clinical setting
		Clinical assignment
		Clinical conference: Use of distraction (30 minutes)

		Select a patient with chronic pain in the clinical setting. Teach patient and/or family one or several of the distraction techniques. Discuss experience in conference

5. Problems related to distraction techniques
  a. Limited effectiveness
  b. Limited attention span of patient
  c. Inconsistent effectiveness with repeated use
  d. Hyperventilation/dry mouth
	Transparency: Problems with Use of Distraction	View transparency.
		Discuss problems with use of distraction

C. Relaxation 1. Definition/conceptualization of relaxation a. relaxation vs. "common concepts" of relaxation		

(Continued)

TABLE 22B. (Continued)

Objectives[b]	Content	Class		Clinical	
		Teaching Method[c]	Learning Activity	Teaching Method	Learning Activity
	b. Relaxation therapy vs. relaxation techniques				
	c. Interruption of stress–tension pain cycle				
	2. Overview of relaxation techniques a. Meditation b. Yoga c. Zen d. Progressive muscle relaxation e. Autogenic training f. Biofeedback	Transparency: Overview of Relaxation Techniques	View transparency		
	3. Effects of relaxation a. Reduction of stress b. Reduction of anxiety c. Distraction from pain d. Alleviation of muscle tension or contraction	What are the effects of relaxation techniques? List on transparency			

Content	Questions / Materials	Learner Activities	Teaching Methods	Objectives

e. Creation of increased suggestibility
f. Reduction of fatigue
g. Enhancement of other pain relief measures
4. Specific relaxation techniques
  a. Deep breath—clench fists—yawn
  b. Heartbeat breathing
  c. Music for relaxation
  d. Slow, rhythmic breathing
  e. Progressive relaxation of muscle groups
	What are some specific examples of relaxation techniques?
	Handout: Relaxation Techniques
	Tape recording of relaxation method for pain control: "Conditioned Relaxation" (10 minutes)
		Read handout and discuss
		Listen to tape and discuss
			Demonstration	Following demonstration of relaxation techniques, select a partner and practice techniques using handout as guide.
				Demonstrate techniques to peers

5. Potential problems of relaxation techniques
  a. Withdrawal from life
  b. Insomnia
  c. Hallucinations
  d. Enhancement of body sensations including pain
	What are problems and limitations associated with relaxation techniques?
	Record on transparency
			Clinical assignment
			Clinical conference: Use of Relaxation (30 minutes)
				Select a patient with chronic pain in the clinical setting.
				Teach the patient and/or family one of the pain relaxation techniques.
				Discuss experience in conference

(Continued)

TABLE 22B. (Continued)

Objectives[b]	Content	Class Teaching Method[c]	Class Learning Activity	Clinical Teaching Method	Clinical Learning Activity
	e. Enhancement of existing physical problems				
	D. Guided imagery				
	1. Definition of guided imagery				
	a. Use as a therapeutic tool				
	b. Guided imagery vs. distraction				
	2. Effects of imagery	What are the effects of guided imagery in relation to pain control? Record on transparency			
	a. Reduction in pain intensity				
	b. Elimination of pain				
	c. Promotion of muscle relaxation				
	d. Reduction of anxiety				
	e. Reduction of feelings of confinement				
	f. Physiologic changes				

(Continued)

3. Specific imagery techniques
a. Images in conversation
b. Standardized images
  (1) Breathing out pain
  (2) Ball of healing energy
  (3) Healthy body
  (4) Beach scene
	Handout: Imagery Techniques	Read handout and raise questions	

	Assignment: Read text and refereces from bibliography on nursing process with patient with chronic pain and issues related to pain management. Review McGill-Melzack assessment tool		Observation Log	Observe in pain clinic. Identify patients' methods for managing pain and analyze patient responses. Describe methods in terms of underlying theory. Record in log

TABLE 22B. (Continued)

Objectives[b]	Content	Class		Clinical	
		Teaching Method[c]	Learning Activity	Teaching Method	Learning Activity
II.A to E F,G to AA	VI. Nursing process A. Assessment of patient with chronic pain 1. Assessment categories a. Universal self-care requisites	Two hours Lecture/discussion What areas need to be included in the assessment of the patient with chronic pain? Record on transparency	Participate in discussion	Nursing rounds Role play	Participate in rounds. Two students to role play and others observe. Analyze using assessment criteria presented in class
III.B,C, D,f					

IV.A,B–E	b. Developmental self-care requisites
	  (1) Individual developmental level
	  (2) Family developmental level				

V.B,E,F	c. Health deviation self-care requisites: pain assessment
	  (1) Impact of pain on life style
	  (2) Patient's previous coping strategies
	d. Conditioning factors
		Transparency: Conditioning Factors	View transparency		

Content		Learning activities	Evaluation
(1) Biopsychosocial factors			
(2) Cultural factors			
(3) Support systems			
(4) Health state			
2. Self-care agency of patient with chronic pain			
a. Knowledge			
b. Skills			
c. Motivation			
3. Self-care deficit of patient with chronic pain	Case study: Assessment of patient with chronic pain	Divide in groups of six. Analyze case and identify nursing diagnoses	Clinical assignment Written assignment: Assessment
a. Nature of self-care deficit			Select a patient with chronic pain in the clinical setting. Assess patient and identify nursing diagnoses.
b. Reason for existence			Complete assessment tool and submit
4. Influence of nurse's values and biases			
5. Formulation of nursing diagnoses			
6. Assessment tool for client with chronic pain: McGill-Melzack (Modified)	Handout: McGill-Melzack Pain Questionnaire	Discuss handout	
B. Planning care for patient with chronic pain			
1. Establishment of mutual goals			

(Continued)

TABLE 22B. (Continued)

		Class		Clinical	
Objectives[b]	Content	Teaching Method[c]	Learning Activity	Teaching Method	Learning Activity

	2. Patient role in decision making
	3. Design of nursing system to meet goals
	  a. Selection of methods of helping
	  b. Selection of pain management methods: traditional and nontraditional
	  c. Determination of type of nursing system
	  d. Identification of appropriate resources				

	4. Planning nursing system
	  a. Time
	  b. Place
	  c. Environmental conditions
	  d. Equipment and supplies
		What elements are included in the nursing system plan?		Clinical assignment	Using same patient for assessment, establish goals to be achieved and plan to meet goals. Include elements of time, place, environment, and needed equipment

Content				

C. Intervention for patient with chronic pain
1. Regulatory nursing systems
  a. Interaction of nurse and patient
    (1) Meeting of patient's self-care deficits
    (2) Development of self-care agency
2. Comfort measures for patient with chronic pain
3. Traditional and/or nontraditional interventions for patient
4. Development of therapeutic relationship
5. Initiation of referrals
  a. To appropriate health care providers
6. Role as liaison
7. Role as clarifier of information
8. Documentation
	What actions characterize the intervention phase of the nursing process?
	Computer simulation: "Mrs. Shilkraut: An Uncomfortable, Terminal Patient"
	Learning laboratory
		Discuss in terms of pain management
		Complete computer simulation in learning laboratory or home
			Clinical assignment	Using same patient as for assessment and planning phase, implement plan including at least one nontraditional pain management technique

(Continued)

TABLE 22B. (Continued)

Objectives[b]	Content	Class		Clinical	
		Teaching Method[c]	Learning Activity	Teaching Method	Learning Activity

	D. Evaluation of care
	1. Ongoing process
	2. Communication with health care personnel
	3. Consistency with professional standards
	4. Evaluation criteria
	  a. Meeting of self-care deficits
	  b. Enhancement of self-care agency in relation to pain management
	5. Evaluation of outcome
	  a. Achieved outcome vs. stated goals
	  b. Adequacy of plan
	6. Modification of plan
		What actions characterize the evaluation process?		Clinical assignment
				Peer review conference: Evaluation of management plan (30 minutes per student)
					Using same patient as in assessment, planning, and implementation; evaluate effectiveness of care and suggest modifications in management plan.
					Present patient and management plan in conference for peer review

	Content	Teaching Method/Time	Learning Activities	

II.Z
III.A,B
C,E,G
IV.C
V.A,C,**D**
VI.**A**,B,
C,**F**
	VII. Personal and professional issues related to pain management
	A. Standards of care as basis of pain management
	B. Relation of personal philosophy to care of patients with chronic pain
	  1. Mind–body interrelatedness
	  2. Beliefs about health, illness, and self-care
	  3. Holistic approach to pain management
	  4. Humanistic application of scientific knowledge
		One hour
		Lecture/discussion
		Handout: Use of Nursing Standards in Pain Management
			Participate in discussion
			Read handout and raise questions
				Complete self-exploration exercise on beliefs and values associated with pain and pain management

	C. Responsibility for pain management
	  1. Patient's responsibility
	  2. Nurse's responsibility
	  3. Responsibility of other health team members
	
	Who is responsible for managing pain?
		Discuss responsibilities	Log	Analyze care provided to patient in terms of (a) relationship of personal philosophy to care and (b) responsibilities of patient and health care providers for care.
				Record in log

	D. Nurse's role as change agent
	  1. Risk taking
	  2. Role modeling
	
	How can nurses initiate change that will result in more effective pain management for the client?			

(Continued)

289

TABLE 22B. (Continued)

Objectives[b]	Content	Class		Clinical	
		Teaching Method[c]	Learning Activity	Teaching Method	Learning Activity
	E. Nurse's role as advocate			Issue conference: Patient rights in pain management (one hour)	Read vignette on patient rights. Analyze situation and discuss in conference
	F. Patient's rights				
	1. Refusal of treatment				
	2. Access to information				
	3. Privacy and confidentiality				
	4. Quality care				
	5. Termination of provider–patient relationship				
	6. Self-determination				
	G. Codes for nurses: Ethical concepts				
	H. Ethical dilemmas in chronic pain management	Decision-making situation on ethical dilemma	Divide into groups of six. Analyze decision-making situation and discuss in small groups		
	1. Evaluation of available data base				
	2. General questions				
	3. Determination of underlying values of people involved				

| 4. Patient trust and informed consent
5. Ethical and moral responsibilities in pain management
I. Accountability in chronic pain management
  1. Precautions against contributing to patient's pain
  2. Consideration of more than technical aspects
  3. Societal, political, and economic issues
  4. Ability to cope with problematic patients
  5. Recognition of different pain philosophies
    a. Nursing vs. medicine
    b. Patient's perception of own pain management
  6. Quackery
    a. Nurse's role in informing public | Multidisciplinary conference
Log | Attend multidisciplinary conference on patient with chronic pain.
Record observations in log |

(Continued)

TABLE 22B. (Continued)

Objectives[b]	Content	Class		Clinical	
		Teaching Method[c]	Learning Activity	Teaching Method	Learning Activity
	b. Patient's perception of own pain management				
	J. Need for continued learning in relation to pain management				
	1. Resources for learning				
	2. Continued development of skill				
V,B,E,**F** VI.D,E	VIII. Future directions in chronic pain management	Lecture/discussion	Participate in discussion		
	A. Transforming research into clinically useful information				
	B. Nursing research and pain management	Written assignment: Critique of research	Read one article describing nursing research in area of pain management. Critique research and identify implications for clinical practice.		
	1. Significance to nursing				
	2. Significance to other disciplines				

Submit

C. CURN project
   1. Deliberative nurs-
      ing—Bochnak
   2. Exploratory study
      of nursing ap-
      proach—McBride
D. Future directions
   for nursing
   research
IX. Summary of unit

[b] *Objectives are numbered according to the list of unit objectives and behaviors. Objectives to be attained in class are in roman type, clinical in boldface type, and class and clinical in italics.*

[c] *Questions included with Class: Teaching Method are to be asked by the teacher to initiate discussion of related content.*

(The information in this table has been adapted from course work completed by Barbara E. Banfield, Lula B. Lester, Joyce C. Miller, Judi Schneider and Katherine M. Zimnicki for the unit plan on pain management developed as part of the requirements for NUR 772's Curriculum Theory Development in Nursing at Wayne State University, Detroit, Michigan, with permission.)

A significant factor must be noted in viewing this model. In the classroom setting, the time frame for each class is designated. No time frame is noted for the clinical experiences because of the variability of the clinical environment. The intent is to demonstrate that the clinical experiences as noted will occur within the time allocated to the unit.

SUMMARY

A curriculum in nursing includes a conceptual framework of nursing, a philosophy, a statement of purpose, program and level objectives, and a sequence of courses. Not all courses in the nursing program have a clinical component, although clinical practice is required for those courses reflecting use of theories in practice. Each clinical nursing course includes objectives for clinical practice and a systematic plan for related learning in the field. Rather than representing separate competencies to be achieved in the field, clinical objectives are those course objectives and behaviors for which clinical practice is associated. Some course objectives and behaviors are accomplished in the classroom setting. Others are achieved in the clinical field, and still others are identified for attainment in both the class and clinical settings. The objectives for clinical practice provide the framework for teaching in the field since they specify the learning outcomes to be achieved there and give direction to faculty in choosing teaching methods and learning activities.

Content for a course is extrapolated from the objectives and organized in a logical sequence. Some content is addressed in the classroom and further developed in the clinical setting; other content is taught only in the classroom or in clinical practice.

Development of the plan for learning in the field involves the selection of teaching methods and learning activities to promote attainment of the clinical objectives and meet individual learner needs. Planning for the field practice experience occurs concurrently with the classroom experience since the theory and practice components of a clinical course are viewed as a whole. The model included in this chapter illustrates the relationship of the clinical component to the overall course and demonstrates the process of planning for learning in the field within the total course structure.

REFERENCES

Beauchamp, G. A. (1975). *Curriculum theory* (3rd ed.). Wilmette, Ill.: Kagg Press.
Bevis, E. O. (1978). *Curriculum building in nursing: A process* (2nd ed.). St. Louis: C. V. Mosby.
Dewey, J. (1944). *Democracy and education*. New York: Macmillan.

Reilly, D. E. (1975). Why a conceptual framework? *Nursing Outlook, 23,* 566–69.
Reilly, D. E. (1980). *Behavioral objectives—Evaluation in nursing* (2nd ed.). New York: Appleton-Century-Crofts.
Santora, D. (1980). *Conceptual frameworks used in baccalaureate and master's degree curricula.* (Pub. No. 15-1828). New York: National League for Nursing.
Torres, G., & Stanton, M. (1982). *Curriculum process in nursing: A guide to curriculum development.* Englewood Cliffs, N.J.: Prentice-Hall.

BIBLIOGRAPHY

Bloom, B. S. (Ed.). (1956). *Taxonomy of educational objectives: Handbook I: Cognitive domain.* New York: D. McKay.
Conrad, C. F., & Pratt, A. M. (1983). Making decisions about the curriculum. *Journal of Higher Education, 54,* 16–30.
Goodlad, J. H., & Associates. (1979). *Curriculum inquiry: The study of curriculum practice.* New York: McGraw-Hill.
Hunkins, F. P. (1980). *Curriculum development: Program improvement.* Columbus, Ohio: Chas E. Merrill.
Johnson, M. (1967). Definitions and models in curriculum theory. *Educational Theory, 17,* 127–40.
Krathwohl, D. R., Bloom, B. S., & Masia, B. B. (1964). *Taxonomy of educational objectives: Handbook II: Affective domain.* New York: D. McKay.
Lawrence, S. A., & Lawrence, R. M. (1983). Curriculum development: Philosophy, objectives, and conceptual framework. *Nursing Outlook, 31,* 160–63.
National League for Nursing. (1978). *Curriculum process for developing or revising baccalaureate nursing programs* (Pub. No. 15-1700). New York: National League for Nursing.
Olivia, P. F. (1982). *Developing the curriculum.* Boston: Little, Brown.
Reilly, D. E. (Ed.). (1978). *Teaching and evaluating the affective domain in nursing programs.* Thorofare, N.J.: Charles B. Slack.
Smith, C. E. (1984). Process curriculum in nursing contrasted to product orientation. *Journal of Nursing Education, 23,* 167–69.
Torres, G. (1975). Learning experiences within and outside the classroom. In *Faculty–curriculum development part IV: Curriculum revision in baccalaureate nursing education* (Pub. No. 15-1576). New York: National League for Nursing.
Torres, G., & Yura, H. (1975). The conceptual framework and its influence on learning experiences. In *Faculty–curriculum development part III: Conceptual framework—its meaning and function* (Pub. No. 15-1558). New York: National League for Nursing.
Tyler, R. W. (1949). *Basic principles of curriculum and instruction.* Chicago: University of Chicago Press.

10

Clinical Evaluation

Clinical evaluation is the process of obtaining information for making judgments about the learner's performance in the clinical field. Formative evaluation represents feedback to the learner regarding progress toward meeting the objectives for clinical practice, whereas summative evaluation provides information on the extent to which the objectives have been attained. This distinction between formative and summative evaluation is important in teaching in the field.

Middleton and Holcomb (1978) describe the elements in designing an evaluation protocol for a clinical program. They include:

1. Statement of the purposes and rationale for the program.
2. Analysis of the instructional sequence and identification of the specific clinical objectives.
3. Selection of evaluation methods which will provide the quality and quantity of data desired.
4. Evaluation of the evaluation design. (pp. 14–15)

The design must account for both formative and summative evaluation and provide direction as to when to evaluate and as to the how and what of evaluation.

The climate in which the clinical evaluation takes place is a critical determinant of the way the learner perceives the process. A supportive climate with mutual trust and respect between teacher and learner is essential for evaluation to be viewed as a means for growth and to be valued by the learner.

The nature of nursing practice and varying competencies to be achieved in the field require multiple methods for judging student learning. Evaluation methods are classified as: observation, written communication, oral communication, simulation, and self-evaluation. The teacher chooses evaluation strategies based on the objectives for clinical practice, individual learner needs, and other variables associated with the field practice experience.

CONCEPT OF EVALUATION

Evaluation is the process of obtaining information for making judgments about learners. Bloom, Hastings, and Madaus (1971) define evaluation as "the systematic collection of evidence to determine whether in fact certain changes are taking place in the learners as well as to determine the amount or degree of change in individual students" (p. 8). The educational process results in changes in learners; evaluation provides the means through which these changes are assessed.

Evaluation serves three major purposes: (1) selection of students for a given nursing program; (2) assessment of student learning in varied settings—classroom, learning laboratory, and clinical field; and (3) program revision and determination of program success. The focus of this chapter is the second purpose; i.e., evaluation of student learning, although faculty teaching in any nursing program should also be knowledgeable regarding the assessment of students for entry into the program and the processes of program and curriculum evaluation.

Evaluation is a dynamic, continuous process interwoven with the teaching–learning process. This view of evaluation emphasizes its relationship to growth of the learner; for the judgments made facilitate the learners' own further development of knowledge, skills, and potential essential for professional practice. Evaluation carried out properly in an environment of trust and respect between teacher and learner aids both the teacher in the instructional process and the student in the learning process. Feedback to the learner, obtained through evaluation, is essential for improvement in learning.

Through a review of the literature and after consultation with professional faculty teaching in the clinical field, Irby, Evans, and Larson (1978) identified nine trends concerning evaluation of clinical skills:

1. Greater emphasis on relating objectives to evaluation.
2. More focus on student learning as the function of clinical evaluation.
3. Increased attention to the clinical evaluation process as a vehicle for instructional improvement.
4. More involvement of students in clinical evaluation.
5. Provision for observer training to improve reliability among faculty evaluators.
6. Increased use of simulation techniques.
7. Use of patient records as instruments for clinical evaluation.
8. Renewed efforts toward dealing effectively with the issue of grades and clinical evaluation.
9. Combined clinical evaluation methods for more comprehensive evaluation. (p. 20)

There are two major types of evaluative processes: formative and summative. Formative evaluation represents feedback to the learner regarding the learner's progress in meeting the objectives. Occurring throughout the instructional process, formative evaluation is diagnostic in nature, providing information to assist in correcting learning deficiencies and promoting demonstrated abilities. Evaluation that is formative enables the teacher and student to identify areas in which further learning is needed and plan relevant learning experiences. The focus of such evaluation is on assisting the student in meeting the clinical objectives. Formative evaluation "intervenes during the formation of the student, not when the process is thought to be completed" (Bloom, Hastings, & Madaus, 1971, p. 20). Airasian (1971) writes, "The aim [of formative evaluation] is to foster learning mastery by providing data which can direct subsequent or corrective teaching and learning. Thus formative evaluation is an integral part of the instructional process" (p. 79). With its diagnostic focus, data obtained through formative evaluation are not subjected to the grading process.

Summative evaluation, end of instruction evaluation, provides information as to the extent to which the learner has achieved the behavioral objectives. Such evaluation occurs at the end of a unit or course and is used to determine the grade for the clinical practice experience. Summative evaluation is "final," stating what has been accomplished rather than what can be. It is concerned with how students have changed as a result of the instruction.

Evaluation that is summative in nature "occur[s] infrequently, typically covering relatively large blocks of instructional material" (Airasian, 1971, p. 78). Airasian further emphasizes that "summative evaluation is ill-suited to perform the [first] evaluative role of providing on-going evidence during the instruction, or to identify learning weaknesses to be corrected prior to grading" (p. 79). Summative evaluation, while informing the teacher and student at the conclusion of an instructional period as to the degree of attainment of objectives, is not intended to identify learning deficiencies nor the appropriate experiences to assist in overcoming them. Further, with summative evaluation, objectives not mastered are often identified too late in the instructional process for students to have an opportunity to meet them.

The distinction between formative and summative evaluation is important in teaching in the field for it is formative evaluation that, as an integral part of the teaching–learning process, provides information to the learner as to knowledge and skills which have been attained and those for which further learning is needed; it also guides the teacher in planning relevant activities to assist the student in this process. Morgan, Luke, and Herbert (1979) write that "without this distinction faculty put students in a double-bind situation. While they often tell students that the practice setting is for learning, they may later use observations made during the learning time to determine the students' grades" (p. 540). Reilly (1980) emphasizes that "the concept of formative evaluation is generally accepted in principle by many teachers, but a gap exists between expressed belief and action" (p. 97). While faculty espouse the value of such evaluation, in practice it is often not an integral part of the instructional process. A commitment to formative evaluation requires that a systematic approach be developed and feedback to learners be given on a continuous basis, not for use in grading but for facilitating learner growth and development. Effective clinical evaluation also requires summative evaluation that is conducted periodically.

Types of Evaluation

The distinction between norm- and criterion-referenced evaluation is important in planning for evaluation in the clinical field. Norm-referenced evaluation is designed to compare a student's performance with that of a group of students. Such an interpretation demonstrates that a student has more or less knowledge, skill, or ability than others in the group. The learner's performance is thus *referenced* to that of the *norm* group. Rating the achievement of students in field practice in relation to other students in the clinical group represents an example of this approach to clinical evaluation.

In contrast, criterion-referenced evaluation compares students not in relationship to others but in terms of some performance standards. The basic intent of this type of evaluation is to measure the performance of students in relation to these standards. With criterion-referenced evaluation, the criteria to be met are established by faculty and known to learners in advance of any evaluation. The behavioral objectives of a unit or course identify the behaviors to be achieved, which must be based on acceptable standards. Instead of indicating that the student in the clinical field is "average," representing a normative judgment, criterion-referenced evaluation using standards indicates the learner's attainment of the clinical objectives. Mehrens and Lehmann (1978) state: "If we can specify important objectives in behavioral terms, then, many would argue, the important consideration is to ascertain whether a student obtained those objectives rather than his position relative to other students" (p. 52). Criterion-referenced evaluation is the approach most relevant to clinical evaluation within a nursing program since competency in terms of specific knowledges, skills, and values is a critical outcome. Certain actions must be carried out in nursing. These actions must be executed skillfully for safe and efficient practice to occur. Criterion-referenced evaluation addresses this notion. The existence of goal-free evaluation, however, must be acknowledged and recognized in the evaluation summary. Coincidental learning does occur and is significant.

NATURE OF CLINICAL EVALUATION PROCESS

Clinical evaluation is a judgmental process, reflecting the values and beliefs of the participants. Value is part of the word and since values are personally chosen, there is a subjective involvement in all aspects of the process.

E | V A L U | A T I O N

It is apparent, then, that there is no such process as "objective evaluation," which is an act of rendering judgments about performance in terms of criteria that are totally external to the evaluator. Evaluation is always subjective for it involves human beings with their own set of values that influence the process. Schweer and Gebbie (1976) write: "The very nature of evaluating clinical nursing performance means that the evaluators, the students, and the setting in which the evaluation occurs deal with human beings. As such, one can hardly eliminate subjectivity in evaluation" (p. 170).

This value component of evaluation makes it critical for faculty to examine their values, attitudes, beliefs, biases, and prejudices about the process itself and the matter being evaluated, for these influence the judgments made of students in the field. Values affect the teacher's observations and interpretations of their meaning; the learner's values influence his or her own perception of performance in clinical practice and interpretation of the evaluative statements made by others in regard to the performance.

Quality of Fairness in Clinical Evaluation

Whereas clinical evaluation cannot be objective, it can be fair; and this quality of fairness in the evaluative process should be the goal of the faculty. Fairness has two requisites: (1) clarity of the objectives identified for the field practice experience, and (2) supportive climate within which the evaluation takes place.

Clinical Objectives. The clinical objectives communicate to the learner the expected behaviors to be developed and, in turn, the focus of evaluation. These behaviors need to be adhered to in the evaluation process so the learner is aware of the behavioral competencies to be evaluated and can direct his or her own learning toward them. The learner is thus free to learn with knowledge of the outcomes of learning to be judged. The clinical objectives also direct the teacher as to the specific behaviors to be evaluated in the field, rather than allowing the teacher's personal desires and beliefs to become the focus of the evaluation. The clinical objectives represent a contract between learner and teacher, communicating to the student the outcomes to be judged and providing structure for the teacher so that these objectives will be addressed in the evaluation.

Psychosocial Climate of Clinical Evaluation. The climate within which the evaluation takes place is a critical determinant of the way the learner perceives the evaluation process. A supportive climate denoting trust and respect between teacher and student is essential if evaluation is to be viewed by the learner as a *learning* experience, providing needed feedback for improvement in learning. Students must value feedback from the teacher and view it as an integral part of developing competence in clinical practice. A trusting relationship between teacher and learner will enable students to value feedback and seek from the teacher evaluation of performance as the learning process occurs.

Development of a supportive climate for clinical evaluation requires faculty clarification of one's own beliefs about evaluation. The teacher's concept of evaluation influences the way in which it is carried out. Evaluation treated as a means for control of the learner does not promote a climate in which evaluation is perceived by students as an integral part of the learning process. Instead, learners are forced to direct energies to surviving in the system rather than using the teacher as a resource for learning. A humanistic approach to clinical evaluation considers evaluation as a process for growth and development of the learner. In this context, clinical evaluation is viewed as a diagnostic process providing information to learners for their further development.

Learning in the clinical field is a difficult process for it places students in a vulnerable position. Learning, especially that which requires a demonstrated performance, occurs as a public event in front of the teacher, clients, and sometimes even staff and peers, often resulting in the student experiencing feelings of anxiety and stress. Clinical evaluation takes place under similar circumstances, and this vulnerability of the student must be acknowledged by faculty. Much of the data obtained for clinical evaluation is through observation of the learner. The act of being observed during performance is in itself stressful. A climate based on trust and respect serves to minimize some of the anxieties inherent in evaluation in the clinical field.

Meisenhelder (1982) emphasizes the need to remain positive and supportive in the clinical evaluation process. Learners who feel threatened by the teacher will not seek feedback nor value what is given. Placed in this situation, they are deterred from their pursuit of knowledge. Schweer and Gebbie (1976) discuss a climate for clinical evaluation "in which students are encouraged to continuously evaluate themselves and feel free to seek help and accept guidance accordingly" (p. 168).

RELATIONSHIP OF CLINICAL EVALUATION TO OBJECTIVES

Clinical evaluation is based on the objectives established for field practice, which are those course objectives and behaviors for which clinical practice is required for attainment. These objectives address competencies in the cognitive, psychomotor, and affective domains at different taxonomic levels. The level of competency at which the behaviors are evaluated is determined by the taxonomic level. Strategies for evaluation need to provide data for judging learning at the particular level addressed by the taxonomy.

Cognitive Domain

Evaluation of cognitive learning relates to the learner's acquisition of the knowledge base needed for problem solving and decision making and the ability to use these skills in practice. At the lower levels of the cognitive taxonomy, evaluation is directed toward assessment of the students' knowledge and understanding of relevant concepts and theories pertinent to cognitive skill development. The student's ability to comprehend and relate data and extrapolate meaning for action is important at these lower levels. At the application level, evaluation focuses on the learner's ability to *use* abstract and factual knowledge including concepts and theories in practice. At the analysis level, evaluation addresses the ability to problem solve and make decisions through an analytic process. Evaluation reflects skill in analyzing data, comparing different alternatives and their consequences, and assessing how concepts and theories relate to one another. Strategies for evaluation at the synthesis level focus on the learner's creativity and skill in developing new products relevant to clinical practice, such as the development of one's own conceptual framework of nursing practice. It is at the evaluation level in which ability to make judgments based on internal and external criteria, such as through research, is assessed.

Affective Domain

Evaluation of affective learning in the field relates to two aspects: the experiencing behaviors of the learner which may be evidenced in practice, and the critical thinking behaviors vital to the element of choice in value development (Reilly, 1978). It is important that evaluative data be obtained on both practice and cognition. Evaluation of the learner's behavior in the clinical field with clients and staff without cognitive evaluation does not enable the teacher to differentiate practice as value based or as a reflection of compliant or imitative behavior. Evaluation of cognitive behavior without assessment of the learner's practice only provides data on what the student *says* will be his or her own position.

The first two levels of the affective taxonomy address value indicators, where beliefs are expressed and some evidence of behavior is presented. Evaluation at these levels provides data on the student's acknowledgement of the existence of a given value or a situation, condition, or phenomenon and acting on or responding to it. At the third level, valuing, patterning of behavior becomes significant; thus, evaluative data must be acquired over a period of time from more than one clinical experience. Evaluation at this taxonomic level, therefore, requires data collected over time to ascertain *consistency* of behavior with stated values. This principle of evaluating affective behavior in practice over time applies to evaluation of learning at the upper levels of the taxonomy, where commitment to the underlying value is evident.

Psychomotor Domain

Evaluation of psychomotor performance competency relates to judgments of the learner's accuracy, coordination, and speed in performance. Judgment of psychomotor skill at the first two taxonomic levels reflects learner ability to perform actions with guidance, although lacking in coordination. Errors in performance and inability to carry out the skill within a reasonable time are to be anticipated at this level of development. At the precision level, performance is characterized by accuracy and ability to carry out the skill without use of a model. Critical elements of the skill are without error, although some errors may occur with other actions not requisite to effective performance of the skill. Evaluation at this level also involves collecting data on the learner's coordination in performance. It is at the articulation level that speed and timing become significant elements to be evaluated in judging skill performance. The student should be able to perform the act within a reasonable time. This dimension of speed is best evaluated in the clinical setting in which it is possible to judge ability to carry out the skill with clients and adapt it as needed. Evaluation of psychomotor learning at the upper level of the taxonomy is intended to ascertain the integration of the act in nursing practice. Performance should reflect a consistently high level of coordination and competence.

Multidomain Performance

Except in instances of evaluating specifics, much evaluation entails assessment of behaviors in two or three domains of learning. This is evident in performance evaluation situations where the student is involved in administering care to a client, thus requiring an assessment of the integration of cognitive, psychomotor and affective skills. In this situation, the learner is engaged in an activity requiring a direct observation of the implementation of theory in practice. Much of performance evaluation is conducted as formative evaluation and summative data are derived from these observations. Lenburg (1979) describes a more formal and definitive approach to obtaining summative data about student performance in providing care in the clinical field. A performance test is the method used; an action separate from the educational process. Criteria for assuring fairness are described by Lenburg (1979):

1. The test must be uniform and equivalent for all students and judged by the same criteria, by all of the faculty.
2. It must be administered at a designated time and place with specific and prescribed conditions that are known and accepted by both students and faculty.
3. The expected performance behaviors are clearly and explicitly stated and known in advance by students and faculty.
4. Students are responsible for learning the entire array of performance behaviors prior to the examination, but are tested on a sample of those that have been systematically derived according to stated criteria and are consistent with the program objectives. (pp. 2–3)

A clinical examination can be used for specific nursing actions or for a holistic action in providing care. If used, the faculty and students must approach it for what it is; an examination of performance, not an evaluation of performance within the rubric of learning.

METHODS OF EVALUATING CLINICAL PRACTICE

Clinical practice is complex and as such cannot be evaluated by one method. Since nursing practice encompasses behaviors in the cognitive, psychomotor, and affective domains, it requires an evaluation protocol that contains multiple strategies for appraising the learner's practice competence in all three domains as appropriate.

Reilly (1980) identifies five reasons for providing diversity in evaluation strategies:

1. Complexity of human behavior
2. Individual differences in responses to learning
3. Suitability of specific evaluation approaches to specific types of learning behavior
4. Motivational factor of evaluation
5. Creative dimension to the evaluation process (pp. 101–2)

Evaluation strategies applicable for use in the clinical field may be classified: (1) observation, (2) written communication methods, (3) oral communication methods, (4) simulation, and (5) self-evaluation.

Observation

Observation of learner performance is a major means of evaluating students in clinical practice. Through observation, judgments may be made regarding cognitive, psychomotor, and affective performance behaviors. There are two components to any observation of learner performance—the behaviors observed in the situation (data), and the inference or judgment as implied by the interpretation of these behaviors. The data reflect the actual performance without the observer's interpretation. Most observations also include statements of judgments of the behavior based on specific criteria that may be made by the teacher, learner, or both. It is important in use of observation for clinical evaluation that both teacher and learner are clear as to the data collected and the inferences made; often, different interpretations may be made of the same data.

Difficulties in the use of observation methods lie with: (1) the influence of teacher variables on the observation and the resulting judgments, (2) focus of the observation, and (3) sampling of behaviors observed which may or may not be representative of the usual level of performance of the student. Wood (1982) writes: "Human observation exhibits inherent bias and subjectivity, and is a subjective process" (p. 11). Any observation of a learner in the clinical field is influenced by the teacher's background, past experiences, values, attitudes, and biases. These teacher variables affect the actual observation; i.e., the behaviors noted in the clinical situation, and the resulting interpretations.

A second problem in use of observation of learner performance relates to the focus of the observation. In any clinical situation multiple aspects of the learner's behavior may be selected for emphasis in an observation if that observation is not directed toward predetermined behaviors. For example, in observing a student changing a dressing on a client, without identification of the exact behaviors to be evaluated the teacher could focus on any one or more of the following: (1) the dressing change procedure, (2) learner's use of nonverbal techniques, (3) relationship with the client, (4) means of preparing the client for the dressing change, and (5) other aspects of particular interest to the faculty. Faculty "see different things" in any observation. For this reason, observation should be directed toward specific clinical objectives to be evaluated, which are known to both faculty and student.

Another difficulty with use of observation relates to the need for an adequate sampling of behaviors over time, which often means data must be obtained from various sources before conclusions are made relative to the learner's typical performance in a particular area. Observations of performance are inevitably based on a sample of the learner's total experience in the field, so an adequate number of observations of behavior or data obtained through multiple means is necessary before drawing conclusions about the learner's achievement of specific clinical objectives.

Discussion of observations made during field practice with the involved learner is critical to provide for feedback and clarification and validation of perceptions and interpretation. Observations best fulfill a formative evaluation purpose if learners examine the data with faculty in terms of areas for further growth and development and instructional strategies for improving behavior.

Specific observations can rarely be recalled over time for a group of learners and, therefore, are generally recorded. Four methods for documenting behaviors observed in practice are: (1) anecdotal note, (2) critical incident, (3) rating scale, and (4) videotape.

Anecdotal Note. An anecdotal note is a narrative description of an observed behavior recorded in relation to a specified clinical objective(s). Some faculty enlarge the scope of the anecdotal note by including an interpretation of the behavior. DeMers (1978) emphasizes that the description of the observable behavior, the data, is recorded separately from the interpretation. The anecdotal note thus represents a record of the behavior observed in the clinical field. Provision should be made for learners to include their own perceptions and judgments of the behavior as recorded.

Effective use of anecdotal notes can be increased by developing a systematic approach to their collection. In determining evaluation strategies, the teacher decides on methods by which each objective is to be judged. Reilly (1980) recommends that at the time certain clinical behaviors are identified for evaluation by anecdotal notes, the number of notes to be recorded for each also be specified and the student so notified. Such a decision, however, does not limit the total number of anecdotal notes written, for the teacher can *always* obtain more data about student performance through this method than originally planned if the student is informed. Anecdotal notes are not the same as general notations a faculty might make after an observation.

In addition to identifying the behaviors to be evaluated with observation and anecdotal notes and specifying the number of notes to be written for each student, faculty can facilitate effective use of the note by limiting the information documented to a brief description of the incident. The observation and information recorded are to relate to the specific behavior being evaluated. Recording extraneous data should thus be avoided. If an interpretation of behavior is also included, it should be so indicated. In documenting behavior, faculty should also review the manner in which the description is recorded so as not to imply only deficiencies or negative behavior as worthy of notation.

An illustration demonstrates use of anecdotal notes for evaluation in the field. Anecdotal notes are most effective for formative evaluation but may also be used for summative evaluation.

Behavioral Objective
P 3.0 Demonstrates skill in administering medication using Z-track technique.

Evaluation
Two observations recorded in anecdotal notes.

Evaluation Criteria
1. Wipes skin with alcohol
2. Pulls skin laterally until taut
3. Injects needle at 90° angle
4. Aspirates
5. Injects medication slowly
6. Removes needle and immediately releases skin
7. Does *not* massage area.

Critical Incident. The critical incident technique is another means of recording information collected through observation of learner performance. Schweer and Gebbie (1976) define critical incident as ". . . a sample of observable human behavior in a given situation that clearly demonstrates either positive or negative factors contributing to the effective or ineffective completion of the activity" (p. 173). Critical incident technique differs from anecdotal notes in that the behavior is analyzed in terms of its positive or negative influence on the outcomes of the activity. Critical implies that the behavior has a significant impact on the outcome. Critical incidents are an effective strategy for formative evaluation since they include a record of observations made regarding performance in the field and allow for analysis of behavior in terms of its influence on the outcomes of the activity. Discussion of the critical incident with students provides them with information relative to their strengths and deficits in practice. Critical incidents are also appropriate for summative evaluation. An example of a critical incident follows.

Behavioral Objective
C 4.2 Uses nursing measures which facilitate the patient's ability to cope with pain.

Evaluation
Observation of learner's nursing actions which are recorded as critical incident.

Evaluation Criteria
Identification of measures used which were:

1. Effective in assisting patient in coping with pain.
2. Ineffective in assisting patient in coping with pain.

Rating Scale. Rating scales, used to a great extent for evaluation in the clinical field, provide a means of recording qualitative and quantitative judgments regarding the learner's performance in practice. The rating scale contains two major parts: (1) a set of defined clinical behaviors on which students are judged, and (2) an accompanying graduated scale to rate the degree of competence with which the behavior has been performed. Rather than listing behaviors, some rating devices include a list of traits to be evaluated.

With a rating scale, the teacher makes a judgment as to the degree of the learner's performance of each behavior. Most of the rating scales used in nursing programs represent five-point scales with descriptors, such as letters, A, B, C, D, E, or numbers, 5, 4, 3, 2, 1; qualitative labels, such as excellent, very good, good, fair, and poor; normative labels like superior, above-average, average, and below-average; and frequency labels, such as always, usually, frequently, sometimes, and never (Bondy, 1983).

One of the difficulties in using rating scales is apparent with this review of typical scale descriptors. First, these descriptors are not necessarily applicable to all of the behaviors or traits evaluated. Second, many of the descriptors are vague and allow for different interpretations by faculty, contributing to problems with reliability. What is the difference between an A and a B? Is there faculty consensus as to what constitutes excellent versus very good performance? With scales that use frequency labels, what about the learner who only has an opportunity to perform a behavior a few times? Schweer and Gebbie (1976) emphasize that ". . . there must be faculty agreement regarding the standards to be used for each rating" (p. 174).

Bondy (1983) developed a criterion-referenced set of scale labels to improve the validity and reliability of rating scales for clinical evaluation in nursing. The criteria for clinical evaluation are clustered into three areas: accuracy or acceptability of the behavior according to professional standards, qualitative aspects of performance, and the type and amount of teacher assistance or cues needed to perform the behavior being judged. According to Bondy (1983) five levels of competency: independent, supervised, assisted, marginal, and dependent are applicable to each of these three areas. Bondy (1984) reported that use of these criteria to define the scale labels contributed significantly to both the accuracy and reliability of faculty scores when using the rating scale.

If a standardized scale is used, the behaviors or other items listed may or may not be congruent with the clinical objectives for the particular unit or course upon which the clinical evaluation is to focus. Ideally, behaviors listed for evaluation should reflect those of the unit or course. DeMers (1978) clearly recommends that rating scales relate specifically to the learning objectives. Scales can be derived from the objectives/behaviors of a clinical course by designating the behaviors to be achieved in clinical practice and devising a format for judging performance of these behaviors.

Proper use of a rating scale requires the collection of sufficient data for judging each behavior in the scale. At times, faculty, in their desire to complete the rating scale, may rate behaviors without adequate evaluative data. Sources of rating error are noted by Dyer (1978):

1. Error of leniency—a higher rating for friends, well-known persons, etc.
2. Error of central tendency—hesitancy to mark end categories of scales.
3. Halo effect—judgment in terms of a global mental attitude.
4. Logical error—same rating for items that are logically related in the minds of the raters.
5. Contrast error—a bias whereby the rater judges others in the opposite direction from self on a given trait. (pp. 136–137)

Even though limitations exist with use of rating scales, they do have value in clinical evaluation. Scales provide a means of rating observed behavior over time so that a pattern emerges. This enables faculty to maintain a record of learner performance. Scales also provide a way of describing performance, suggesting areas of strength and those needing improvement, which serves an important formative evaluation purpose. Rating scales are effective strategies for compiling and presenting data regarding learner performance in terms of multiple behaviors and aspects of clinical practice, particularly when the behaviors represent the ones specified for the unit or course. Reilly (1980) recommends they not be used for grading clinical practice because of other problems associated with their use.

Videotape. One additional means of recording observation of learner performance is through videotape, followed by a session to critique the activity. Videotapes provide for visual and auditory recording of performance and have a valuable start–stop capability. Many types of performance behaviors may be videotaped in different practice settings. Videotaping is effective for formative evaluation, for the learner and the teacher or peers may then critique the performance immediately following it. Videotape also may be used for summative evaluation purposes.

Written Communication Methods

Evaluation strategies classified as written communication methods provide data on the ability of the learner to communicate in writing and on the quality of the content communicated. Through these methods, information is obtained for assessing the learner's skill in conveying ideas and thoughts on paper. Evaluation of the substance of the written material provides data relevant to the objectives. Strategies for clinical evaluation include:

1. Nursing care plan
2. Case study
3. Teaching plan
4. Process recording
5. Log
6. Nursing notes
7. Other written assignments

Nursing Care Plan. Nursing care plans are both teaching and evaluation strategies that enable the learner to analyze the client's health care problems and develop a related plan of care. The format of the care plan may represent the practice model or learning care plan developed by faculty for use as a learning strategy. Either type of care plan may be evaluated in terms of substance and clarity with which the information is communicated, use of proper terminology, conciseness of presentation, and format. An illustration of use of a nursing care plan for evaluation follows.

Behavioral Objectives

C 4.2 Derives goals of care from identified self-care deficits.

C 4.2 Develops with patient and family plan of care reflective of self-care deficits.

C 4.2 Selects appropriate nursing interventions.

C 4.2 Records plan of care.

Evaluation

In two out of three care plans, the student meets the criteria.

Evaluation Criteria

1. Identifies short- and long-term goals.
2. Develops goals based on identified self-care deficits as perceived by patient and care giver.
3. Involves patient and family/significant others in goal setting and planning of care.
4. Selects nursing interventions which address self-care deficits and ability of patient to engage in self-care.

5. Is comprehensive in planning care.
6. Uses format for recording plan of care properly.
7. Communicates information clearly, concisely, and with correct terminology.

It is advisable that a care plan devised as a learning tool be discontinued as soon as possible once the teacher is convinced, on the basis of evaluative data, that the student has met the requisite objectives. Some students may need to prepare a limited number of such plans, whereas others may need to submit a considerable number before mastery is achieved. Because nursing care plans are an integral part of nursing practice, it is advisable that the student move into the system that is operating in the setting and be evaluated accordingly. Ability to move into the practice mode is an important piece of evaluation data.

Changes in the communication of nursing care plans are already underway in some agencies and will be evident in most agencies in the near future as the computer becomes entrenched in the clinical setting. The computerization of nursing care plans will alter the behaviors to be evaluated in this element of nursing. The content of the plan as it is individualized to a patient will be of significance while the writing skill will be determined by the computer program in use. Evaluation will then address the skill in using the computer in planning care.

Case Study. Evaluation of a case study presentation is particularly appropriate for judging a student's ability to present a holistic perspective of a patient phenomenon drawing upon a related knowledge base, skill in synthesis of data, projected action and results, and the ability to communicate this information in a logically clear and concise manner. The complexity and depth of the case study is a function of the level of the behaviors to be evaluated. A study written at the comprehension level is primarily descriptive of events and relationships with a related rationale. At an analytic behavioral level, the case study would represent an analytic approach to the patient phenomenon drawing upon relevant theories and a synthesis of all the elements into a creative and substantive presentation. Case studies are often written, but they can be presented orally and be subject to peer review. Case studies that are written are effective summative evaluation strategies for they demand the use of cognitive skills and the cognitive component of affective skills in an integrative format. An example of a case study for evaluation appropriate in the senior level of the program is presented.

Behavioral Objectives

C 4.1 Analyzes the processes entailed in providing nursing care for a client from stress-adaptation theory framework.

A 4.1 Includes a defense of the right of the client and family to a participatory role in decisions in all phases of the care.

C 4.2 Relates nursing decisions in all phases of the process of care to those of other disciplines involved with the client.

C 4.2 Evaluates the processes used in terms of the ANA Standards.

Evaluation
Case study of a client from practice.

Evaluation Criteria
1. Includes complete and accurate data in terms of the client's status and the theoretical framework.
2. Reflects congruency among assessment data, plan of care, and intervention.
3. Includes nursing decisions compatible with those of other health care providers unless the reasons why these decisions are incompatible are stated and documented.
4. Provides evidence in each phase of the study of the client's and/or family's perception of events and participation in decisions regarding management of care.
5. Addresses evaluation outcomes in terms of goals and process in relation to the integrity of the plan.
6. Presents case in a scholarly prepared document which is logically organized, clearly expressed, and substantive in content.

Teaching Plan. Evaluation of a written teaching plan provides data relative to the learner's ability to use concepts of learning and teaching to meet the educational needs of clients or staff. When used in client situations, the data for determining the learning needs of the individual are obtained during the assessment phase and the plan is so noted in the total care plan. Evaluation includes the assessed data as well as the plan itself. Similar to other written communication methods, evaluation focuses on the quality of the content and skill in communicating the information in written form. An example follows.

Behavioral Objectives
C 3.0 Relates principles of learning and teaching to patient education.

C 3.0 Develops a teaching plan consistent with patient's and family's learning needs.

A 3.1 Accepts responsibility for involving patient and family in development of teaching plan.

Evaluation
Two teaching plans.

Evaluation Criteria

1. Identifies patient's and family's learning needs in terms of knowledge, skills, and values.
2. Develops behaviorally stated objectives reflecting patient's and family's learning needs.
3. Selects appropriate content for objectives.
4. Organizes content logically.
5. Chooses appropriate teaching methods and learner activities for objectives, with recognition of patient preferences and learning style.
6. Provides for patient and family involvement in development and implementation of teaching plan.
7. Selects appropriate educational materials for use in teaching.
8. Records teaching plan appropriately.

Process Recording. Process recording, when used as a teaching strategy, provides information on the learner's skill in interacting with others in the clinical field and may be subject to evaluation. It is particularly valuable for formative evaluation, especially when used in conjunction with individual conferences with learners in which the interaction is analyzed by both teacher and student and discussed in terms of further learning experiences. It may also be used in summative evaluation as data on the student's ability to grasp the various meanings which may occur in communications. The focus of evaluation of the process recording is dependent upon the objectives. An example of the use of a process recording for clinical evaluation is included.

Behavioral Objectives

C 4.2 Identifies verbal and nonverbal cues.
C 4.2 Relates nursing actions to identified client cues.
C 4.2 Analyzes own interactive behavior within a
therapeutic relationship.

Evaluation

Process recording of nurse–client interaction

Evaluation Criteria

1. Interprets accurately client verbal and nonverbal cues.
2. Identifies own verbal and nonverbal cues.
3. Selects appropriate nursing actions based on cues exhibited in communication.
4. Analyzes effect of own behavior in the relationship.
5. Identifies facilitators and blocks to communication.
6. Describes clearly own feelings during and perception of the interaction.
7. Uses format for recording interaction correctly.

Log. Learning log is another means of evaluating clinical objectives, but because of the nature of the log, it does not provide sufficient data on the learner's skill in communicating in written form. It is more of a process than an outcome evaluation strategy. Maintained concurrently with specified clinical experiences, it enables the evaluator to be a participant in the learning process through the eyes of the learner. The value of students' perceptions of experiences is often not recognized by faculty as a significant data base in the evaluation process. Use of a learning log for clinical evaluation is illustrated.

Behavioral Objectives
C 3.0 Identifies coping mechanisms used by client.
C 3.0 Assesses client system for need for planned change.

Evaluation
Log entries describing:
1. Observation of client for signs and symptoms of stress.
2. Coping mechanisms used by client.
3. Rationale for whether or not change is indicated in client system.

Evaluation Criteria
1. Identifies coping mechanisms used by client.
2. Differentiates between functional and dysfunctional adaptation.
3. Relates adaptation and change theories in determining need for planned change.
4. Assesses strengths and deficits of client system that may influence outcome of planned change.

Nursing Notes. The learner's ability to report and communicate in writing client data is an important outcome of clinical experience and another source of data for evaluation. As with other written communication methods, nursing notes may be judged in terms of their content and the learner's skill in recording. Nursing notes enable faculty to evaluate the learner's ability to collect and record relevant data about the client, identify nursing diagnoses from the data, develop and revise accordingly plans of care, and document client progress.

Criteria for evaluating the content of nursing notes include comprehensiveness and accuracy of data collected about the client, significance of interpretation of the data, and appropriateness of the plans of care and nursing interventions. Evaluation of the learner's skill in communication relates to clarity with which the information is recorded, use of proper terminology, conciseness with which presented, and order in which the information is recorded.

Evaluation of nursing notes may occur over a period of time as a longitudinal strategy or within a limited time frame for a selected number of recordings, depending on the objectives of the experience. Both approaches might be used, for the longitudinal strategy provides data about the degree of consistency with which the student documents care provided, while the incidental strategy provides the opportunity for a discrete evaluation of a particular documentation for which the student is responsible. Regardless of the structure of the evaluation, this strategy is particularly valuable for formative evaluation especially when the nursing notes are then discussed with the learner, but it may also be of value in summative evaluation.

It is recognized that the introduction of computers to the practice setting will alter considerably the process for documenting nursing care provided to the client. The process will resemble the present problem-oriented system where all disciplines involved record their data in the same place. Computer language will be determined by the computer program used, and evaluation will need to address the student's ability to use such a program. The concern for quality of the documentation will remain a significant factor in evaluation. An illustration of the use of nursing notes for evaluation is offered.

Behavioral Objectives

C 3.0 Records pertinent client data and progress of client.

C 3.0 Revises plan of care.

Evaluation

In two out of three nursing notes, records pertinent data and revises plan of care.

Evaluation Criteria

1. Documents relevant data collected from client, family, health team members, and other sources.
2. Interprets data accurately.
3. Records data indicative of progress of client.
4. Presents information clearly and concisely.
5. Revises plan of care appropriately.
6. Uses proper format for nursing notes.

Other Written Assignments. Other types of assignments appropriate for clinical evaluation include reports and papers which are descriptive of an event or an experience relevant to the goals of the field practice.

Oral Communication Methods

Ability to convey ideas verbally is an important skill in nursing, for in most settings nursing is practiced in groups where sharing of information or the formulation of decisions for action is a frequent occurrence. This activity may involve intradisciplinary groups or interdisciplinary groups.

Criteria for evaluation of oral communication skills include the ability to: (1) present ideas clearly and succinctly in group discussions, (2) assume a leadership or participant role within the group as indicated, (3) offer data and ideas or suggestions which contribute to group thinking, and (4) facilitate group process in arriving at decisions or solutions to problems. The quality of the content communicated in terms of accuracy and relevancy to the objectives of the group process are appropriate matters for evaluation.

Evaluation methods which provide data on the learner's ability to communicate verbally include:

1. Clinical conference
2. Issue conference
3. Nursing or multidisciplinary conference

Clinical Conference. Clinical conferences represent clinically focused discussions by groups in clinical practice and include such types as postconferences and peer-review conferences. Postconferences involve a group discussion or problem-solving activity in relation to experiences encountered during practice in the clinical field. Peer-review conferences provide for group critique and evaluation of the clinical decisions and actions of all or selected members. Conferences such as these are effective means for evaluating the ability of the learner to present ideas, listen to the ideas of others, critique those ideas presented, and lead or participate in group action toward the goals of the conference.

Whatever the format of the conference, evaluation is concerned with the quality of the content presented, ability to communicate verbally, and skill in use of group process. Clinical conferences may be used for evaluating one or several behavioral objectives and for either formative or summative evaluation. An example of a postconference for evaluation is presented.

Behavioral Objectives
A 2.2 Discusses willingly one's own feelings about caring for patients of varied cultural and ethnic backgrounds.

C 3.0 Examines the impact of cultural stereotypes on identification of patient needs.

Evaluation
One postconference in which student presents patient of different cultural or ethnic background than his or her own.

Evaluation Criteria
1. Describes accurately the cultural or ethnic background and behavior characteristics of the patient.
2. Identifies stereotypic attributes that she or he associates with such patients.
3. Describes one's own feelings about patients of this cultural or ethnic background.
4. Relates the influence of one's own stereotypic beliefs and feelings in assessing the patient's needs.
5. Promotes an atmosphere for sharing of ideas and feelings among individuals in the group.
6. Leads the group in exploring the significance of stereotyping of groups of patients and the care provided.

Issue Conference. Issue conferences involve group discussion of sociocultural-economic and political as well as professional issues that are not always generated by the particular clinical experience but are relevant to that experience. Various group modalities may be used. One student or a group of students may be responsible for the presentation to the larger group. Evaluation addresses the same elements as in other oral communication methods. However, in this type of conference another dimension is added in respect to the content. These conferences are directed toward enlarging the student's perspective of the events that occur in the setting by relating them to ideas, events, or actions beyond the present boundaries. It is the ability to move from a more prescribed technical perspective of an issue to see it within the greater context that is the concern of the evaluation. An illustration of a senior issue conference is presented.

Behavioral Objectives
    C 4.2 Analyzes the impact of DRGs on quality of care.
    C 4.2 Identifies the implications of DRGs for the nursing profession.

Evaluation
    One issue conference in which learner leads discussion on DRGs.

Evaluation Criteria
1. Explains the meaning and significance of DRGs.
2. Bases presentation on literature and related research.
3. Identifies aspects of health care in general and nursing care in particular affected by DRGs.
4. Leads group in examining implications of DRGs for professional nursing practice and proposing strategies for responding to changes resulting from DRGs.
5. Identifies some of the consequences of this payment system on patients and their families.

6. Encourages participation of group members in discussion.
7. Presents ideas clearly and in logical order.

Nursing and Multidisciplinary Conferences. Nursing team and multidisciplinary conferences provide another means of evaluating clinical objectives. The composition of the group varies from nursing practitioners only to a group of representatives from different health care disciplines, sometimes including a client. These conferences emphasize the process of collaborative decision making in which client problems are explored, plans for care are developed and revised, strategies for implementation are examined, and evaluation of care is completed. The nature of the learner's participation in these conferences varies, depending upon the objectives. In some conferences, learners may be involved primarily in sharing information about a client while in others the student may be responsible for group leadership. Criteria similar to other oral communication methods apply to evaluation of nursing and multidisciplinary conferences. An example of evaluation of a nursing team conference is included.

Behavioral Objective
C 3.0 Develops nursing diagnoses for a patient in conjunction with nursing colleagues.

Evaluation
One conference in which learner presents patient data for establishing nursing diagnoses.

Evaluation Criteria
1. Reports one's own observations of patient and data obtained through assessment.
2. Collects data from other team members.
3. Discusses patient's resources and preferences for meeting health care needs.
4. Leads group in analyzing data and identifying priority of self-care deficits.
5. Leads group in identifying nursing diagnoses.
6. Provides opportunity for members to participate in discussion and group decision making.

Simulations
A new method of performance testing for the cognitive, affective and psychomotor domains is simulations. Simulations are a valuable strategy for clinical evaluation, offering a readily available means

of judging performance. The complexity of the problems simulated and related nursing actions to be performed are able to be controlled in a simulation. Evaluation may focus on cognitive, psychomotor, or affective behaviors as indicated by the clinical objectives. The following four types of simulations presented previously as teaching methods are appropriate for use in clinical evaluation: (1) active case study method, (2) models, (3) simulated patients, and (4) role play. With the first type, in which information relative to a clinical situation is presented to the learner requiring some action to be taken, the simulation may be in paper and pencil, audiovisual media, or computer format.

Maatsch and Gordon (1978) identify three components of a simulation: setting, problem, and scenario. Setting includes the environment in which the simulation takes place, representative of the real-life clinical situation. The setting consists of any equipment, supplies, props, and other materials necessary for carrying out the simulation. Maatsch and Gordon recommend that "the setting should be simulated with the lowest fidelity possible for the task to be carried out by the learner" (p. 126).

The problem represents the task to be performed and evaluated. Included here is information relative to the client and other aspects of the clinical situation necessary for taking action. The problem is simulated with the highest fidelity possible to represent accurately the real clinical situation.

The third part of the simulation is the scenario that "captures the sequential unfolding of the real-world clinical problem being simulated" (p. 126). This relates to how the clinical situation and problem are introduced and the kinds of nursing decisions and actions to be performed, similar to the series of events that might occur if the same situation were encountered in clinical practice.

Creation of a simulation for evaluation thus proceeds from the real clinical situation through the development of the simulation to the actual evaluation in which the learner proceeds through the simulation and is judged on performance. Evaluation may take place through paper and pencil or computer format or the learner may actually carry out the actions under observation by the teacher. The simulation may involve a specific action or skill, such as insertion of a urinary catheter, or may represent a larger scope requiring a series of decisions to be made and related actions to be taken, such as an emergency situation. The type of simulation is dependent upon the objectives to be evaluated; criteria for evaluation relate to these behaviors. Simulations are appropriate for either formative or summative evaluation. Commercial models for simulation experiences are entering the market and merit faculty evaluation of their use in a clinical evaluation protocol.

Self-evaluation
Learner self-evaluation represents an important component of any clinical evaluation protocol. Development of this skill begins with the initial clinical nursing course and continues throughout the program. Fuhrmann and Weissburg (1978) emphasize that "just as skills in evaluation are not inherent in human beings but must be learned, so too must self-evaluation skills be learned" (p. 139). Regardless of the process, self-evaluation has greater value when implemented on a continuous basis in order for learners to examine their progress toward meeting goals. Self-evaluation should be accompanied by teacher–student discussions in which sharing of evaluation takes place and decisions are made regarding future learning experiences. For these reasons, self-evaluation is most appropriate for formative evaluation.

The focus of self-evaluation in clinical practice is determined by the objectives of the experience and individual learner goals. Various methods of recording evaluation data are possible, such as in anecdotal notes, logs, and reports of progress in the clinical field. Learners can also evaluate their own clinical assignments. Schweer and Gebbie (1976) propose the use of student self-rating scales for recording a final summary of progress made toward meeting the clinical objectives.

USE OF MULTIPLE STRATEGIES FOR CLINICAL EVALUATION

Clinical practice cannot be evaluated by one method alone. The range of behaviors to be judged in the practice setting and differences among learners require a variety of evaluation methods. An example demonstrating different evaluation strategies possible for a behavioral objective is included. The teacher can vary strategies with a group of learners or an individual learner based on needs and the clinical situation in which the evaluation takes place.

There are several significant values to the use of multiple strategies in evaluating clinical performance. In some instances, student difficulty in performance behavior for an objective may be a function of the evaluation strategy rather than the skill implied by the behavior. A written report of an interview may suggest that the student cannot perform an interview satisfactorily. A tape recording of an interview by the same student may signify that the student is indeed competent in that task. The difficulty that the student has is in writing, not interviewing, and it is that skill that the student needs to develop. The willingness to try another method when performance is not satisfactory provides a more accurate diagnosis of the student's learning needs, whether it entails the actual skill under assessment or another skill required for data collection.

Another advantage to maintaining a multistrategy approach relates to the teacher. Repetition leads to boredom, loss of interest, and lack of creativity. The use of varied strategies with a different or even the same group of students provides the diversity the teacher needs in his or her own practice of teaching. Acceptance of this diversity leads the faculty to be challenged to the development of more creative evaluation processes and adds a sense of excitement that often accompanies change. Evaluation approaches are developed by the willingness of the faculty to be daring and comfortable with new situations.

Behavioral Objective
C 3.0 Provides for instruction of the patient and family in required measures of self-care.

Possible Evaluation Methods
1. Observation in clinical field
2. Teaching plan
3. Simulation
4. Videotape recording of teaching
5. Clinical conference
6. Nursing notes

Evaluation Criteria
1. Bases teaching on identified self-care deficits and patient's abilities to perform self-care.
2. Determines priorities for teaching according to self-care deficits.
3. Involves patient and family in all phases of teaching.
4. Uses appropriate teaching strategies.
5. Evaluates effectiveness of teaching plan in terms of promoting self-care.
6. Revises teaching plan based on evaluative data.

EVALUATION PROTOCOL FOR UNIT ON CHRONIC PAIN

In developing the evaluation protocol, the teacher decides on methods for collecting information on the objectives for clinical practice and plans strategies for both formative and summative evaluation. The clinical behaviors specified for the unit on chronic pain management, in Table 21, Chapter 9, provide a means for illustrating the process of planning for clinical evaluation. Strategies are proposed for each behavior, although the teacher must keep in mind that a variety of methods are possible (Table 23).

TABLE 23. EVALUATION METHODS FOR UNIT ON CHRONIC PAIN MANAGEMENT

Clinical Behaviors	Evaluation Methods
I. Relate Orem's self-care model to nursing management of patients with chronic pain	
B. Evaluates the biopsychosocial and cultural influences on the individual's ability to manage one's own pain	Log
C. Identifies the impact of chronic pain on the developmental tasks of an individual	Log
D. Analyzes the impact of chronic pain on family relationships and dynamics	Log
F. Analyzes the various nontraditional pain management techniques in terms of the individual's and family's learning needs and self-care potential	Postconference
II. Use the nursing process in promoting self-care of patients with chronic pain *Assessment:*	
A. Carries out a systematic pain assessment of patient	Written Assignment: Assessment
B. Evaluates impact of chronic pain on patient's life style	Log
C. Identifies patient's strategies for coping with pain	Case Study
D. Appraises the impact of biopsychosocial and cultural factors on the patient's response to pain	Case Study
E. Identifies developmental level of patient and family	Log
F. Analyzes the influence of support systems on patient's ability to manage chronic pain	Case Study
G. Assumes responsibility for identifying one's own values and biases that may affect the assessment	Postconference
H. Integrates pain assessment data in calculation of therapeutic self-care demand	Written Assignment: Assessment
I. Identifies the nature and reasons for the existence of self-care deficits in relation to managing chronic pain	Case Study
J. Analyzes the learning needs of patient and family in relation to chronic pain management	Teaching Plan
K. Formulates nursing diagnoses based on identified self-care deficits	Case Study, Nursing Care Plan
Planning:	
L. Develops with patient goals of care congruent with nursing diagnoses	Nursing Care Plan
M. Plans nursing management related to self-care deficits of patient and family	Case Study, Nursing Care Plan, Peer-review Conference

(Continued)

TABLE 23. (*Continued*)

Clinical Behaviors	Evaluation Methods
N. Supports the patient in decision making relative to options for pain management	Anecdotal Notes
O. Selects appropriate traditional and nontraditional methods of pain management	Case Study, Nursing Care Plan, Peer-review Conference
P. Provides for use of appropriate resources to assist patient and family	Nursing Care Plan
Implementation:	
Q. Implements nursing interventions congruent with a scientific rationale, research, and the mutually established plan of care	Anecdotal Notes
R. Is competent in the use of traditional pain management techniques	Anecdotal Notes
S. Demonstrates skill in the use of nontraditional pain management techniques	Anecdotal Notes Simulation
T. Initiates referrals to health care providers and/or agencies essential in assisting patient to meet optimum self-care agency	Nursing Notes
U. Encourages patient in use of his or her own potential and resources in addressing self-care limitations	Critical Incident
V. Protects patient's self-care abilities as a means of preventing new self-care limitations	Anecdotal Notes
W. Documents pertinent nursing observations and interventions	Nursing Notes
Evaluation:	
X. Develops criteria for evaluating the effectiveness of the plan toward a decrease in self-care deficit and increase in self-care agency	Case Study Nursing Care Plan
Y. Uses criteria in evaluating patient and family outcomes of care in terms of stated goals	Peer-review Conference
Z. Uses professional nursing standards as a framework for evaluating the process of the delivery of nursing care	Peer-review Conference
AA. Modifies plan of care as indicated by the evaluation results	Nursing Notes
III. Formulate judgments which reflect respect for the inherent worth and dignity of the patient with chronic pain	
A. Defends the patient's right to be informed regarding traditional and nontraditional methods of chronic pain management relative to their expected outcomes and inherent risks	Anecdotal Notes Issue Conference
B. Supports the patient's choice regarding the selection of pain control methods	Anecdotal Notes
C. Is consistent in respecting the patient's expressed perception of the degree of self-care deficit	Postconference

TABLE 23. (*Continued*)

Clinical Behaviors	Evaluation Methods
D. Provides care reflective of the patient's own sociocultural preferences, psychologic needs, and health beliefs	Anecdotal Notes Case Study
E. Protects the patient's rights to privacy and confidentiality	Anecdotal Notes
F. Assumes responsibility for assessing one's own biases and values that may interfere with effective determination of the patient's self-care requisites	Log
G. Acts as advocate for patient and/or family when individuals or situations appear to impede progress toward goal attainment	Critical Incident Issue Conference
IV. Foster facilitative relationships with patients with chronic pain, families, and colleagues	
A. Analyzes one's own interactive behavior within a therapeutic or collegial relationship	Process Recording
B. Assumes a liaison role between patient and other persons who have an impact upon the health care of the individual	Postconference
C. Contributes readily to discussions and decisions that have an impact on matters concerning the patient's pain management	Nursing Team Conference
D. Serves as clarifier to patient, family, and other health team members in situations where misunderstanding or lack of knowledge is evident	Postconference
E. Maintains ongoing communication with appropriate health providers regarding the plans, implementation, and evaluation of care	Anecdotal Notes Nursing Notes
V. Assume responsibility for continued development of the knowledge base and competencies essential for promoting self-care agency in the presence of chronic pain	
A. Assumes responsibility for expanding one's own knowledge base regarding care of the patient with chronic pain	Case Study
B. Maintains knowledge of current research findings which address the phenomenon of pain and its management	Case Study
C. Examines one's own beliefs about health, illness, and an individual's potential as a self-care agent in formulating a philosophy of chronic pain management	Log
D. Is accountable for seeking out those learning experiences that enhance the development of requisite competencies	Anecdotal Notes
F. Identifies researchable patient care problems which lend themselves to exploration within nursing's body of knowledge	Postconference

(*Continued*)

TABLE 23. (*Continued*)

Clinical Behaviors	Evaluation Methods
VI. Affirm the accountability of nurses and the nursing profession to contribute to the development of a theory of practice for patients with chronic pain	
A. Takes a position on the responsibility of nurses and nursing to protect a vulnerable public against quackery and other kinds of deceptive methods purported to alleviate chronic pain	Issue Conference
E. Identifies the responsibility of nursing to generate knowledge pertinent to nursing actions in helping the patient with chronic pain meet self-care demands	Postconference
F. Declares a position on nursing's ethical and moral responsibilities in the various pain management methods used in practice	Issue Conference

SUMMARY

Evaluation in the clinical field provides data for making judgments of the learner's performance in all domains of learning. An evaluation protocol needs to include strategies for both formative and summative evaluation which are clearly differentiated. Formative evaluation represents feedback to the learner on progress in meeting the objectives for clinical practice. Evaluation that is formative enables the teacher and student to identify areas in which further learning is needed and plan relevant learning experiences. In contrast, summative evaluation, end of instruction evaluation, provides information as to the extent to which the objectives have been achieved. Summative evaluation is used to determine the grade for clinical practice.

There is no such process as objective evaluation. Evaluation is always subjective, for it is influenced by the values and beliefs of the participants. It is critical, therefore, for faculty to examine their own values, beliefs, attitudes, and biases which may affect judgments made of learners in the field. Although clinical evaluation cannot be objective, it can be fair.

Clinical practice is complex and as such, cannot be evaluated by one method alone. Multiple strategies are needed for appraising the learner's performance in practice. These methods are classified as observation, written communication, oral communication, simulation, and self-evaluation.

Observation of learner performance is a major means of evaluating students in the field. Methods for documenting observations include anecdotal notes, critical incidents, rating scales, and videotapes.

Evaluation strategies classified as written communication methods provide data on the learner's skill in writing and quality of the content communicated. Relevant evaluation strategies are nursing care plan, case study, teaching plan, process recording, log, nursing notes, and other written assignments.

Nurses must also be skillful in conveying ideas verbally and participating in a group format. Strategies for evaluating these skills in clinical practice include clinical conference, issue conference, and nursing and multidisciplinary conferences.

Simulation, presented in Chapter 5 as an instructional strategy, may also be used for evaluation of clinical objectives. Any protocol for clinical evaluation should also provide opportunity for learner self-evaluation.

A range of clinical evaluation methods is needed. Clinical practice cannot be evaluated by one method alone and instead requires a variety of methods for collecting information on the behavior to be achieved in the field and attending to individual needs of the learner. It is the faculty's responsibility to choose strategies that are appropriate for the objectives of clinical practice and carry out evaluation in an environment denoting trust and respect between teacher and learner.

Trends noted by Irby, Evans, and Larson (1978) are indeed evident as presented here. As computers and other instrumentation enter the clinical practice field, they will add new trends in clinical evaluation.

REFERENCES

Airasian, P. W. (1971). The role of evaluation in mastery learning. In J. H. Block (Ed.), *Mastery learning: Theory and practice.* New York: Holt, Rinehart & Winston.

Bloom, B. S., Hastings, J. T., & Madaus, G. F. (1971). *Handbook on formative and summative evaluation of student learning.* New York: McGraw-Hill.

Bondy, K. N. (1983). Criterion-referenced definitions for rating scales in clinical evaluation. *Journal of Nursing Education, 22,* 376–82.

Bondy, K. N. (1984). Clinical evaluation of student performance: The effects of criteria on accuracy and reliability. *Research in Nursing and Health, 7,* 25–33.

DeMers, J. L. (1978). Observational assessment of performance. In M. K. Morgan, & D. M. Irby, *Evaluating clinical competence in the health professions.* St. Louis: C. V. Mosby.

Dyer, E. D. (1978). Evaluation of clinical performance: Rating scales and checklists. In A. G. Rezler, & B. J. Stevens (Eds.), *The nurse evaluator in education and service.* New York: McGraw-Hill.

Fuhrmann, B. S., & Weissburg, M. J. (1978). Self-assessment. In M. K. Morgan, & D. M. Irby, *Evaluating clinical competence in the health professions.* St. Louis: C. V. Mosby.

Irby, D. M., Evans, J., & Larson, L. (1978). Trends in clinical evaluation. In M. K. Morgan, & D. M., Irby (Eds.), *Evaluating clinical competence in the health professions*. St. Louis: C. V. Mosby.

Lenburg, C. B. (1979). *The clinical performance examination*. New York: Appleton-Century-Crofts.

Maatsch, J. L., & Gordon, M. J. (1978). Assessment through simulations. In M. K. Morgan & D. M. Irby (Eds.), *Evaluating clinical competence in the health professions*. St. Louis: C. V. Mosby.

Mehrens, W. A., & Lehmann, I. J. (1978). *Measurement and evaluation in education and psychology* (2nd ed.). New York: Holt, Rinehart & Winston.

Meisenhelder, J. B. (1982). Clinical evaluation—An instructor's dilemma. *Nursing Outlook, 30,* 348–51.

Middleton, J. L., & Holcomb, J. D. (1978). Deciding when to evaluate. In M. K. Morgan, & D. M. Irby (Eds.), *Evaluating clinical competence in the health professions*. St. Louis: C. V. Mosby.

Morgan, B., Luke, C., & Herbert, J. (1979). Evaluating clinical proficiency. *Nursing Outlook, 27,* 540–44.

Reilly, D. E. (1978). *Teaching and evaluating the affective domain in nursing programs*. Thorofare, N.J.: Charles B. Slack.

Reilly, D. E. (1980). *Behavioral objectives—Evaluation in nursing* (2nd ed.). New York: Appleton-Century-Crofts.

Schweer, J. E., & Gebbie, K. M. (1976). *Creative teaching in clinical nursing* (3rd ed.). St. Louis: C. V. Mosby.

Wood, V. (1982). Evaluation of student nurse clinical performance—A continuing problem. *International Nursing Review, 29,* 11–18.

BIBLIOGRAPHY

Brown, B. J., & Chinn, P. L. (1982). *Nursing education: Practical methods and models*. Rockville, Md: Aspen.

Burgess, G. (1980). The self-concept of nursing undergraduate students in relation to clinical performance and selected biographical variables. *Journal of Nursing Education, 19*(3), 37–44.

Conklin, K. R. (1970). Educational evaluation and intuition. *Educational Forum, XXXIV,* 323–33.

Cronin-Stubbs, D., & Mathews, J. J. (1982). A clinical performance evaluation tool for a process-oriented nursing curriculum. *Nurse Educator, 7,* 24–29.

Dressel, P. L. (1980). Models for evaluating individual achievement. *Journal of Higher Education, 51,* 194–205.

Gage, N. L., & Giaconia, R. (1981). Teaching practices and student achievement causal connections. *New York University Education Quarterly, 12,* 2–9.

Huckabay, L. M. D. (1979). Cognitive–affective consequences of grading versus nongrading of formative evaluations. *Nursing Research, 28,* 173–78.

Johnson, D. M., & Wilhite, M. J. (1973). Reliability and validity of subjective evaluation of baccalaureate program nursing students. *Nursing Research, 22,* 257–262.

Kolb, S. E., & Shugart, E. B. (1984). Evaluation: Is simulation the answer? *Journal of Nursing Education, 23,* 84–86.

Krumme, U. S. (1975). The case for criterion-referenced measurement. *Nursing Outlook, 25,* 25–39.

Lawrence, R. M., & Lawrence, S. A. (1980). Clinical evaluation of students in nursing: A step toward quality nursing practice. *Image, 12*(2), 46–48.

Loustau, A., Lentz, M., Lee, K., et al. (1980). Evaluating students' clinical performance: Using videotape to establish rater reliability. *Journal of Nursing Education, 19*(7), 10–17.

McDowell, B. J., Nardini, D. L., Negley, S. A., & White, J. E. (1984). Evaluating clinical performance using simulated patients. *Journal of Nursing Education, 23,* 37–39.

McIntyre, H. M. (1972). A simulated clinical nursing test. *Nursing Research, 21,* 429–35.

Morgan, M. K., & Irby, D. M. (Eds.). (1978). *Evaluating clinical competence in the health professions.* St. Louis: C. V. Mosby.

Pearson, B. D. (1975). A model for clinical evaluation. *Nursing Outlook, 23,* 232–35.

Reilly, D. E. (1958). *Nursing student responses to the clinical field.* New York: Department of Nursing, Columbia University.

Rezler, A. G., & Stevens, B. J. (1978). *The nurse evaluator in education and service.* New York: McGraw-Hill.

Richards, A., Jones, A., Nichols, K., et al. (1981). Videotape as an evaluation tool. *Nursing Outlook, 29,* 35–38.

Rosen, M. L. (1983). Forecasting summative evaluation from formative evaluation: A double cross-validation study. *Psychological Reports, 49*(3), 843–48.

Schwirian, P. (1978). Evaluating the performance of nurses: A multi-dimensional approach. *Nursing Research, 27,* 347–51.

Scriven, M. (1967). The methodology of evaluation. In R. W. Tyler, R. M. Gagné, & M. Scriven, *Perspectives of curriculum evaluation.* Chicago: Rand McNally.

Sommerfeld, D. P., & Accola, K. M. (1978). Evaluating students' performance. *Nursing Outlook, 26,* 432–36.

Stecchi, J. M., Woltman, S. J., Wall-Haas, C. et al. (1983). Comprehensive approach to clinical evaluation: One teaching team's solution to clinical evaluation of students in multiple settings. *Journal of Nursing Education, 22,* 38–46.

Steele, S. (1978). *Educational evaluation in nursing.* Thorofare, N.J.: Charles Slack.

Sweeney, M. A., O'Malley, M., & Freeman, E. (1982). Development of a computer simulation to evaluate the clinical performance of nursing students. *Journal of Nursing Education, 21*(9), 28–38.

Woolley, A. (1977). The long and tortured history of clinical evaluation. *Nursing Outlook, 25,* 308–15.

11

Grading of Clinical Field Experience

Summative evaluation often leads to some type of system by which the results are "readily interpreted" and communicated. In American education, that system is usually referred to as *grading,* the process by which some symbol is designated to represent the sum total of achievement for an educational experience. Evaluation and grading are two distinct processes, although some persons use the terms interchangeably. Evaluation can occur without grading; grading should not occur without evaluation. The use of a grading symbol, whether a letter or number, to convey a complex and diverse array of competencies and attributes is reflective of a need for simple answers or responses. The meaning conveyed by the symbol is generally instantly "understood" by the viewer.

MEANING OF GRADES

What do grades mean? It is interesting that grades are identified as quantitative symbols of qualitative dimensions of behavior, even though no absolute standard is available for interpretation. As one ponders the meaning of the term *grade,* Boulding's (1971) postulation about the differentiation between the image and the message comes to mind. He postulates that a highly learned process of interpretation and acceptance influences how one receives a message. He states, ". . . What this means is that for any individual or group or organization, there are no such things as *facts*. There are only messages filtered through a changeable value system" (p. 14). Grades may well reflect the values, past experiences, and beliefs of the interpreter.

Although educational institutions may have protocols for ascribing meaning to grades, there is generally little consistency in their use. There can be marked differences among graders in any given institution as to the dimensions of the educational process that relate to the grading practice. This differentiation can be not only institution-wide, but found within departments and among faculty involved in the same course.

Grading is a system for ranking or rating an individual; i.e., categorizing the person in relation to a phenomenon called academic achievement. Academic achievement is a nebulous concept. Warren (1971) notes that academic achievement is itself defined only in terms of composites of course grades. "It has no independent definition against which the validity of course grades can be checked" (p. 2). The symbol used denotes unidimensional information and keeps concealed data about many different kinds of performances which may have been used to arrive at the grade. Thus the concept of academic achievement projects a single entity that is global in nature, when in reality it represents many interrelated components.

The meaning behind the ranking, therefore, lacks consistency among users whether the symbols used are letters of the alphabet, numbers, or descriptive words. Is an "A" an "A"? No standard exists for supporting such a contention; there are certain variables which mitigate against standardization in the meaning of a grade.

Individual Perception

One significant variable has already been referred to—the part played by the elements in the grader's life space and the value system by which the meaning of a grade is determined by the individual. Likewise, the elements in the life space of the interpreter influence the meaning of any particular grade.

Variation in Data Base

A second variable is the inconsistency in the quantity and quality of the evaluative data base; i.e., the summative evaluation used by the person assigning the grade. Data may measure only one type of performance, such as writing a paper or answering questions on an examination, regardless of whether or not the performances are the appropriate ones. On the other hand, a grade may represent data from a composite of numerous evaluation strategies that deal with many dimensions of the learning experience. A grade may represent the student's skill in handling the evaluative procedure rather than the attainment of the learning inherent in the objectives of the experience. Thus, a grade may reflect relevant competencies or may reflect the attempt to use one symbol to depict accomplishment as to varied and unrelated abilities.

Another dimension of quality relates to the consistency with which the data base really reflects the objectives. Does the grade have enough support to convey the student's progress, or have the evaluation strategies been irrelevant to the goals of the experience? As an example, do the objectives relate to skills in problem solving and decision making while the data upon which a grade is based relate to skills in information recall? Is it possible that a grade may reflect learner behavior unrelated to the objective such as, tardiness, appearance, or some personal attribute? Use of these latter criteria connotes a punitive dimension to the grading process when reflecting negative attributes.

Base Standard
A third variable is concerned with the basis for the standard in determining grades. In some instances, the standard is based on evidence of growth throughout the learning experience, the *process*; whereas in other instances, the standard is based on the degree of learner attainment of the objectives at the conclusion of the experience, the *outcome*.

In general, grading is directed toward the outcome pattern, the degree of learner attainment of the objectives. There are discrepancies in the approach used by various graders. Some teachers rely only on summative evaluation strategy results, whereas others incorporate formative evaluation results leading to the objective attainment.

As the concept of mastery of learning increasingly influences the educational process, the focus of evaluation is on learner attainment of the objectives. A system of formative and summative evaluation operates to assure the student's mastery of the task to be learned. Standards for grading are then criterion-referenced standards. These standards, usually ascertained from empirical evidence, derive from the performance desired for a given task. In the criterion-referenced approach, the teaching–learning process is closely interwoven with formative evaluation, with summative evaluation indicating if the learner has mastered the task.

Computation Method
The method of computing grades is a fourth variable which is highly individualized and mitigates against grade standardization. How are grades determined? In some situations, the normal curve is used as the basis for determining grades. The underlying assumption of the normal curve, however, is incompatible with an educational process, for it is based on a random sample. Do learners in nursing represent a random sample? A negative response is generally in order, especially in light of the selection procedures employed in many nursing programs. What is the random element? Teaching itself cannot meet this criterion, for it is a purposeful activity. Bloom, Hastings, and Madaus (1971) in their statement on mastery

learning state: "We may even insist that our educational efforts have been *unsuccessful* to the extent that the distribution of achievement approximates the normal distribution" (p. 46).

Grades derived from the normal curve show a small percentage of students with an "A," an equal percentage with a failure. The failure may be more representative of the student's rank order in a group than the student's failure to grasp the essential learning in the course of study. A skewed curve would be the expected outcome in a professional program.

The expectation of learner performance in the mastery of learning system is markedly different. Using a criterion-referenced approach, this theory posits the notion that 95 percent of the learners for any given task have the potential for mastery, meaning a grade of "A," if that symbol is used. The other 5 percent may have a special disability for the particular learning task and, thus, are not able to achieve mastery. Although the theory recognizes the potential for most students to achieve mastery, such an outcome is not guaranteed, for much of the mastery of any learning rests with the intent, commitment, and persevered effort on the part of the learner.

Another aspect of computing grades to be considered is the procedure for the weighting of different sources of data for arriving at the ultimate grade. Much variation exists in the way faculty allocate weight for items such as tests, especially final examinations; papers; nursing care studies; and conference presentations. Weighting is a function of any particular course, but the basis for such a decision even lacks a rationale that could be used as a standard.

In response to an earlier question, one can say that "an A is not an A." A possible definition of a grade as presently used could be that it is a symbol representing the learner's degree of academic achievement as defined by an individual teacher in light of competencies and attributes deemed appropriate and as arrived at by that teacher's choice of the data base to be used and the computation strategy to be followed. In spite of the poor fidelity the grade symbol has in encoding evaluative data and the lack of reliability and validity of the grade, the grading system is highly institutionalized in our society and thus is to be used in educational programs, especially those that carry some kind of credit.

USES FOR GRADES

The grade is a ubiquitous symbol, but it prevails in the American educational system and is used as a basis for decisions critical to the life of the individual. Administratively, grades are used as a basis for determining admission to and continuance in programs of study and for awarding honors, scholarships, or other special means of recognition. The use of grades as a predictive variable occurs in spite of data to the contrary. Warren (1971) confirms this question of predictability when he states: "For most students previous grades do predict later grades moderately well over relatively short time periods. Undergraduate grades predict first year grades in graduate and professional schools moderately well, but they predict advanced grades poorly, particularly in clinically oriented programs" (p. 10). This conclusion is based on studies by Bartlett (1967), Gough (1967), Gohn (1968), and Hanlon (1964). Erickson and Bluestone (1971) address the predictive value of grades: "Regardless of in-house controls and refinements, the accumulated grade record fails as a useful indicator of post graduation success" (p. 4).

Educationally, grades may be perceived as stimuli for learner motivation; although the motivation may be to meet academic demands, not to develop the competencies inherent in the learning task. Erickson and Bluestone remind faculty of the "distinction between study effort and learning benefit; between time spent at the books and material absorbed for productive application beyond the exam" (p. 2). In general, the effort a student extends is more a function of the value the student places on the course than the grade to be received. An additional consideration is the timing of the awarding of the grade, often at the conclusion of the experience or course. At this time it is too late for a student to become motivated to effect behavior change in the experience.

A third use of grades is social; to certify individuals to perform certain functions in society. The use of grades as an admission feature fosters the "gatekeeper" role of an educational program, the means by which it selects who may enter certain fields of endeavor, thus in essence, maintaining class structure and controlling access to high social and economic levels (Warren, 1971). Employers also use grades in selecting from applicants, a practice challenged by Erickson and Bluestone (1971) by the question: "Do colleges have either the responsibility or the right to provide encapsulated evaluation of student achievement to sources beyond the classroom?" (p. 6). A suggestion is made that the employing agency determine its own criteria for evaluation to which the college could respond.

TYPES OF GRADING SYSTEMS

The most frequently used system is the multidimensional system, usually representing a five-point scale of symbols from "A" to "D" and "F." Its long-time usage and accepted respectability by administrators, faculty, and some students make it the most common form in use.

A second pattern that became fairly popular in the seventies is the two-dimensional system with only two symbols. This dichotomous system could include such combinations as: (1) pass (P)–no pass (NP); (2) satisfactory (S)–Unsatisfactory (U); (3) credit (C)–noncredit (NC). The S–U system is usually an administrative decision and pertains to all students in the course; whereas, the P–NP is an individual student option. The premises underlying this pattern are: (1) students can take difficult courses without fear of lowering their grade point average, (2) students have more option to experiment with courses outside their major, (3) emphasis is on the learning process, (4) anxiety about grades is reduced, (5) students can be self-directing, and (6) less time is wasted by students and teachers in playing the "game of grades."

Responses to this approach vary among students and faculty. There is no doubt that articulation from undergraduate to graduate school is impeded because of administrative preference for the five-dimensional system. Students wishing to pursue advanced study may be jeopardized, especially if the system is used for courses in the major. Students who require structure and the five-dimensional grading system as a frame of reference for guiding their own learning may increase their anxiety with this less structured format. Others find that with the release from competition and "grade getting" learning is less of an anxiety-producing process. An interesting phenomenon has occurred. Students and many faculty do not perceive this two-dimensional system as a grading system, nor do they perceive that the letter symbols students receive are actually grades.

Some faculty find that they cannot change their grading practices. They keep two sets of records, one in five-dimensional grades and the other in two-dimensional grades. The change to the new system is then effected in translating symbols from one system to another. There seems little question that an ethical issue exists when a system of records of grades not chosen by the student is maintained.

When dual grading systems are used by students; i.e., selecting five-dimensional grading for some courses and two-dimensional for others, there is a tendency to place priority of learning on those subjects requiring the more discriminating five-dimensional system.

A study was conducted by faculty in the College of Nursing, Wayne State University to determine faculty and student responses to the use of a two-dimensional grading pattern (Reilly, 1973). Student responses were generally favorable to the two-dimensional system, while faculty, particularly graduate faculty, were less supportive. Results were similar to those found in the literature with some student polarity evident on such issues as the impact of the system on anxiety, motivation, and competition. Faculty were less supportive of the belief that in this system there is more emphasis on learning than on obtaining a grade. Many respondents expressed concern about the evaluation process that underlies the two-dimensional grading system, suggesting that poor evaluation processes could therein be hidden.

An often voiced objection to this system is the inability to distinguish between academic excellence and barely satisfactory performance. As a result, descriptive terms are added or the use of a plus (+) or minus (−) with the letter is instituted so that in reality a four- or five-dimensional grading system results.

A third grading system has had limited use. It is the descriptive grading system which uses no letters, but rather provides for a written evaluation of student performance. At Santa Cruz University, where this system was used with a pass–no pass system, comments ranged from one word euphemisms for letter grades to several paragraphs of expressive prose (Andrews, 1970). Although there is no agreement on terminology or criteria, there is a possibility that a computer could select from stored descriptions of student performance relevant aspects of a particular performance and merge them into a standardized summary. This descriptive approach presents difficulty to decision-making groups, such as admission officers. Descriptive grading is effective if used in conjunction with the other systems.

Very few educational programs today use the number system which denotes a specific quantitative value to the achievement rather than a range of measures as in systems using letters as symbols. The inexactness of the measurement component of many evaluation strategies mitigates against the use of such a specific quantitative symbol and makes the grader vulnerable to challenge. It is difficult to defend the choice of a grade of 89 over 90.

Contract grading is another system, which in reality uses the five- or two-dimensional system with clarification of the basis for determining the grade. Mind set is a significant dimension in approaching any learning situation. Contract grading fosters such a mind set in the student as the decision for the grade to be achieved is made by the student. The decision, however, may or may not be to the advantage of the student. An agreement to engage in learning experiences in accord with a "B" grade may not be the wisest use of the experience when selected by a student with potential for greater achievement. Likewise, a student may desire to achieve an "A" level but lack the resources to meet such a goal. Student counseling is essential in using this system so that the decision is congruent with student resources, potentials, and ultimate goals.

It is evident that there are deficiencies in all grading systems. In too many instances of change there has been a manipulation of the symbols and as Silberman (1970) states:

> This kind of tinkering fails to come to grips with the real problem; how to make evaluations serve the ends of education instead of being an

end in itself. . . . What is wrong with the present system is not the use of grades, per se, but the fact that the awarding of grades has been divorced from the large function of evaluation (p. 347).

Erickson and Bluestone (1971) concur with Silberman: "The crux of any system of grading is to establish criteria relevant in learning to reduce the disparity between evaluation and grading" (p. 5).

ISSUES ON GRADING CLINICAL PERFORMANCE

Clinical performance is a form of academic achievement in a professional program, and therefore the allocation of a grade on the basis of appropriate evaluation data is in order. The use of grades for denoting achievement in a clinical practice experience is often fraught with apprehension, uncertainty, and diverse beliefs as to its applicability. The solution selected to address this matter usually entails a shift from a five-dimensional grading system to a two-dimensional system. Faculty tend to perceive this action as the discontinuance of a grading system; the awarding of a symbol, a letter such as P, NP, and so on, is not acknowledged as a grading process.

Rationale for discontinuing the traditional approach is based on the premises previously stated for the two-dimensional system. Even more so, it often reflects the insecurity of faculty as the search for the impossible, *objective* evaluation and grading, is pursued. As previously indicated, grading is not *objective,* (no human judgment can be objective), but it can be *fair* if the data on which it is based address the objectives through judicious selection of evaluation strategies. In the clinical component of a course of study, there tends to be a greater reliance on one evaluative tool as a basis for grading than is true for the classroom component. The tool is usually some form of rating scale which is translated quantitatively for a grade. The scale may or may not reflect the objectives of the learning experience. The tool is often too limited to provide the data necessary, for the diversity of competencies at any point in time requires a variety of data-gathering methods.

Grading for classroom activities is perceived to be more accurate because the methods lend themselves more easily to quantification. Perhaps this notion is more myth than reality, for it is primarily the objective format tests that are readily quantifiable. Performance testing that employs such methods as problem-solving situations, papers, essay questions, and group activity generates as much uncertainty for the evaluator as do the clinical performance activities in the clinical field such as nursing care plans, process recordings, and performance of nursing actions. Strategies removed from the one-answer format depend upon the application of predetermined criteria and judgment on the part of the teacher if they are to be used wisely and fairly in determining grades whether for class or clinical experiences. They also require the openness to hear and see the "different," which signifies the creative approach from the learner. A touch of humility when evaluating leaves the teacher in a position to acknowledge the "new" from the learner.

Concern is often expressed about the inability of grades to differentiate among students who have competency in achieving classroom objectives but are unable to master the necessary clinical performance, or vice versa. It is acknowledged that a grade represents complex, diversified abilities and is unable to encode the values attached to specific abilities which are in essence a part of the grade. However, the inability to denote the differences in performance in either of the major components may be a function of the grading system used in arriving at a grade. If a policy exists which states that failure to achieve in either of the two components, regardless of the performance in one of the components, results in failure of the total course and that policy is explicit in public announcements of the school, then no further grade computation is necessary if the failure occurs in one component. Note that it is the computation that is stopped, not the evaluation. This policy has particular meaning if clinical practice is not passed because of the practice nature of the nursing discipline. When there is passing performance but marked discrepancy between that in the classroom or clinical field, the system of grade computation should make this fact evident. Perhaps one of the systems later proposed will address this matter for some individuals.

The trend toward using a two-dimensional grading system for clinical practice experience while maintaining the five-dimensional system for the classroom experience raises some critical concerns. When a two course system is used, one for classroom (theory) and one for clinical (practice), it becomes evident that the theory component represents more discriminating evaluation. What messages are conveyed to the learner? Theory may be perceived to be more valuable because its grading is more discriminating; therefore, time for studying and preparation is allocated in that direction. Clinical practice, on the other hand, may be perceived to be less valuable and only an activity experience with little cognitive input necessary.

If both class and clinical components are combined in one course, then the final grade represents only performance in regard to the classroom objectives. It is not possible to transfer a grade from a two-dimensional system to one in the five-dimensional system. A "P" is just that; it has no further meaning. In this instance is the grade that appears on the transcript for the clinical courses misleading since in reality it only represents the classroom experiences?

Regardless of the pattern of courses, in a mix of the two grading systems, it is the classroom grade that is perceived to be significant and the one that is used in determining the grade point average. The clinical performance is assumed to be satisfactory but carries no weight in the student's average for the total program. A less confusing approach would be for faculty to decide on one grading system for both components of the course. Any system will have its strengths and its limitations, requiring faculty to make the choice with full knowledge of the implications in the use of the selected system.

GRADING SYSTEMS FOR CLINICAL PRACTICE EXPERIENCE

With recognition of the significant place that the grading system occupies in the American educational system and the lack of standardization for whatever system is chosen, several systems for grading the clinical experience are proposed. Whatever system is ultimately developed by a faculty, it must be acknowledged that the field of grading is an inexact one and the professional judgment of faculty is the key factor in making decisions. Fairness is obtained in adhering to the use of evaluative data that address the objective and the weighting of items in relation to their significance in contributing to the goal of the course and to the ultimate goal of the program. Weighting must be justified and each faculty member is held responsible to peers for such a decision.

Whether one uses a two-dimensional or five-dimensional grading system, two criteria are essential:

1. Evaluation data-gathering strategies must be congruent with the stated objectives and behaviors.
2. The data base to be used must be identified and declared.

Because clinical practice requires certain specific competencies for safe and effective execution, a criterion-referenced system of evaluation and therefore a criterion-referenced system of grading are in order.

Objectives as Framework for Computation of Grades

As previously demonstrated, clinical course objectives include behaviors most appropriately achieved in the clinical field. The extrapolation of the clinical behaviors from those of the overall course provides the evaluation form for use in clinical evaluation. It is this list of objectives and behaviors that constitute the basis for a grading system. Since these objectives and behaviors are in essence a contract with the learners by which they are assured that the teaching and learning experiences will be directed toward the attainment of the objectives and that evaluation will be so directed, grading also must be in accord with the contractual statements. There is no assurance that students will indeed attain the designated behaviors, for student choice continues to be a major factor in making the required effort to achieve.

For each objective, specific behaviors are expressed that must be attained if the objective is to be met. Achievement in certain behaviors is essential while others are significant, but their full attainment may not be reached within the time allocated to a particular course or unit of study.

Faculty judgment is the basis for determining which behaviors are essential in a criterion-referenced system. Some persons call these behaviors critical elements; others refer to them as non-negotiable behaviors. The latter signifies a very definitive approach— these behaviors *must be achieved*. No bargaining is possible. Achievement of other behaviors is not a substitute. In other words, *all* of the non-negotiable behaviors must be attained if the objective is to be considered to be passed. Alterations in decisions about behaviors must be agreed upon by all faculty concerned. One faculty member cannot modify the decision to meet individual expectations. The objectives and behaviors with the non-negotiable behaviors so noted are provided to all faculty and students concerned. This action fosters fairness in grading as it communicates specifically the expectations for an acceptable performance.

Table 24 depicts the designation of non-negotiable behaviors for the unit Chronic Pain Management, which was previously presented Table 23, Chapter 10. Since this unit is developed for senior students, it can be expected that many of the behaviors would be classified as non-negotiable for they have been in development throughout much of the program. It is their interpretation within the context of the topic under discussion that is new.

Since achievement of non-negotiable behaviors is considered to be passing, the two-dimensional system uses the data as a basis for a passing grade. The five-dimensional system for grading involves further interpretation. In an undergraduate program using the five-dimensional grading system, a grade of "C" is considered passing in most professional schools; a grade of "B" is passing in a graduate program. Quantitative allocation of criteria in this system is presented in Table 25.

In institutions where there is use of plus (+) or minus (−) signs, the numbers of behaviors can be discriminated more finely. One other quantitative datum must be in place before the grading process can proceed. The weighting of the value of each objective is indicated on the basis of faculty judgment in terms of the purpose of the course or unit. Although categories of objectives are consistent in all courses, the value of each may vary according to the major emphasis of the course. Because nursing process is the methodology of practice, it can be assumed that the nursing process objective would receive the highest weighting in a clinical practice course.

342

TABLE 24. CLINICAL BEHAVIORS—UNIT OF CHRONIC PAIN MANAGEMENT

C 4.2 I. Relate Orem's self-care model to nursing management of patients with chronic pain
*   C 4.2   B. Evaluates the biopsychosocial and cultural influences on the individual's ability to manage one's own pain
*   C 4.2   C. Identifies the impact of chronic pain on the developmental tasks of an individual
*   C 4.2   D. Analyzes the impact of chronic pain on family relationships and dynamics
    C 4.2   F. Analyzes the various nontraditional pain management techniques in terms of the individual's and family's learning needs and self-care potential

C 4.2 II. Use the nursing process in promoting self-care of patients with chronic pain
Assessment:
*   C 4.2   A. Carries out a systematic pain assessment of patient
*   C 4.2   B. Evaluates impact of chronic pain on patient's life style
*   C 4.2   C. Identifies patient's strategies for coping with pain
*   C 4.2   D. Appraises the impact of biopsychosocial and cultural factors on the patient's response to pain
*   C 4.2   E. Identifies developmental level of patient and family
*   C 4.2   F. Analyzes the influence of support systems on patient's ability to manage chronic pain
    A 3.3   G. Assumes responsibility for identifying one's own values and biases that may affect the assessment
*   C 4.2   H. Integrates pain assessment data in calculation of therapeutic self-care demand
    C 4.2   I. Identifies the nature and reasons for the existence of self-care deficits in relation to managing chronic pain
*   C 4.2   J. Analyzes the learning needs of patient and family in relation to chronic pain management
*   C 4.2   K. Formulates nursing diagnoses based on identified self-care deficits
Planning:
*   C 4.2   L. Develops with patient goals of care congruent with nursing diagnoses
*   C 4.2   M. Plans nursing management related to self-care deficits of patient and family
    A 3.3   N. Supports the patient in decision making relative to options for pain management
    C 4.2   O. Selects appropriate traditional and nontraditional methods of pain management
*   C 4.2   P. Provides for use of appropriate resources to assist patient and family

Implementation:
*   C 4.2   Q. Implements nursing interventions congruent with a scientific rationale, research, and the mutually established plan of care
*   P 5.0   R. Is competent in the use of traditional pain management techniques
*   P 3.0   S. Demonstrates skill in the use of nontraditional pain management techniques
    C 4.2   T. Initiates referrals to health care providers and/or agencies essential in assisting patient to meet optimum self-care agency
    A 4.1   U. Encourages patient in use of his or her own potential and resources in addressing self-care limitations
    A 4.1   V. Protects patient's self-care abilities as a means of preventing new self-care limitations

TABLE 24. (*Continued*)

*	C 4.2	W. Documents pertinent nursing observations and interventions

Evaluation:

*	C 4.2	X. Develops criteria for evaluating the effectiveness of the plan toward a decrease in self-care deficit and increase in self-care agency
*	D 4.2	Y. Uses criteria in evaluating patient and family outcomes of care in terms of stated goals
	C 4.2	Z. Uses professional nursing standards as a framework for evaluating the process of the delivery of nursing care.
*	C 4.2	AA. Modifies plan of care as indicated by the evaluation results

A 4.1 III. Formulate judgments which reflect respect for the inherent worth and dignity of the patient with chronic pain

*	A 4.1	A. Defends the patient's right to be informed regarding traditional and nontraditional methods of chronic pain management relative to their expected outcomes and inherent risks
*	A 4.1	B. Supports the patient's choice regarding the selection of pain control methods
	A 4.1	C. Is consistent in respecting the patient's expressed perception of the degree of self-care deficit
*	C 4.1	D. Provides care reflective of the patient's own sociocultural preferences, psychologic needs, and health beliefs
*	A 4.1	E. Protects the patient's rights to privacy and confidentiality
	A 4.1	F. Assumes responsibility for assessing one's own biases and values that may interfere with effective determination of the patient's self-care requisites
	A 4.1	G. Acts as advocate for patient and/or family when individuals or situations appear to impede progress toward goal attainment

A 4.1 IV. Foster facilitative relationships with patients with chronic pain, families, and colleagues

*	C 4.2	A. Analyzes one's own interactive behavior within a therapeutic or colleagial relationship
	A 4.1	B. Assumes a liaison role between patient and other persons who have an impact upon the health care of the individual
*	A 4.1	C. Contributes readily to discussions and decisions that have an impact on matters concerning the patient's pain management
	A 4.1	D. Serves as clarifier to patient, family, and other health team members in situations where misunderstanding or lack of knowledge is evident
*	A 4.1	E. Maintains ongoing communication with appropriate health providers regarding the plans, implementation, and evaluation of care

A 4.1 V. Assume responsibility for continued development of the knowledge base and competencies essential for promoting self-care agency in the presence of chronic pain

*	A 4.1	A. Assumes responsibility for expanding one's own knowledge base regarding the care of the patient with chronic pain
	A 4.1	B. Maintains knowledge of current research findings which address the phenomenon of pain and its management
	C 4.1	C. Examines one's own beliefs about health, illness, and an individual's potential as self-care agent in formulating a philosophy of chronic pain management
*	A 4.1	D. Is accountable for seeking out those learning experiences that enhance the development of requisite competencies

(*Continued*)

TABLE 24. (Continued)

C 4.1   F. Identifies researchable patient care problems which lend themselves to exploration within nursing's body of knowledge

A 4.1 VI. Affirm the accountability of nurses and the nursing profession to contribute to the development of a theory of practice for patients with chronic pain

     A 4.1   A. Takes a position on the responsibility of nurses and nursing to protect a vulnerable public against quackery and other kinds of deceptive methods purported to alleviate chronic pain

     C 4.2   E. Identifies the responsibility of nursing to generate knowledge pertinent to nursing actions in helping the patient with chronic pain meet self-care demands

*   A 4.1   F. Declares a position on nursing's ethical and moral responsibilities in the various pain management methods used in practice.

*Denotes a non-negotiable behavior.

As an illustration, a possible weighting of the objectives for the unit on Chronic Pain Management is noted:

Weight	Objective
20%	1. Relate Orem's self-care model to nursing management of patients with chronic pain.
40%	2. Use the nursing process in promoting self-care of patients with chronic pain.
15%	3. Formulate judgments which reflect respect for the inherent worth and dignity of the patient with chronic pain.
10%	4. Foster facilitative relationships with patients with chronic pain, families, and colleagues.
10%	5. Assume responsibility for continued development of the knowledge base and competencies essential for promoting self-care agency in the presence of chronic pain.
5%	6. Affirm the accountability of nurses and the nursing profession to contribute to the development of a theory of practice for patients with chronic pain.

When the evaluation process has been completed, data are ready to be translated into the symbol designated by the grading process which the faculty selected. Each objective is accorded the grade symbol allocated to the behaviors that have been attained as specified in the system for quantifying the behaviors. An illustration of this process with the unit Chronic Pain Management is in Table 26. Because the five-dimensional grading system is most often used for classroom grading, it is the one used in the illustration.

After the grade and numerical value are determined for each objective, these data are used in accordance with the weighted value for each objective to obtain the grade for the clinical component for

TABLE 25. QUANTITATIVE ALLOCATION FOR GRADING

Undergraduate			Graduate		
Letter Grade	Numerical Equivalent	Criteria	Letter Grade	Numerical Equivalent	Criteria
A	4	All behaviors met	A	4	All behaviors met
B	3	All non-negotiable behaviors and at least half of the others met	B	3	All non-negotiable behaviors and at least half of the others met
C	2	All non-negotiable behaviors met	C	2	One half or more non-negotiable behaviors met
D	1	One half or more non-negotiable behaviors met			
F	0	All or most non-negotiable behaviors not met	F	0	All or most non-negotiable behaviors not met

the unit. In this illustration, the computation generates the grade as depicted in Table 27.

A further step is indicated in instances when one course grade representing both clinical and classroom components is the practice. Grading in this manner has the advantage of communicating to students and others that a clinical nursing course is a total entity

TABLE 26. GRADING OF CLINICAL PRACTICE

Objective	Total No. Behaviors	Total No. Non-Negotiable Behaviors	No. of Behaviors Achieved		Grade	Numerical Value
			Non-negotiable	Others		
I	4	3	3	1	A	4
II	27	17	17	6	B	3
III	7	4	4	3	A	4
IV	5	3	3	1	B	3
V	5	2	2	1	C	2
VI	3	1	0	1	F	0

TABLE 27. COMPUTATION OF THE CLINICAL GRADE

Objective	Grade	Numerical Value	Weight	Numerical Weight
I	A	4	20	4×20 = 80
II	B	3	40	3×40 = 120
III	A	4	15	4×15 = 60
IV	B	3	10	3×10 = 30
V	C	2	10	2×10 = 20
VI	F	0	5	0×5 = 0
			Total	310
			Numbered Value	3.10
			Grade	B

which entails a synthesis of theory and practice. When these two components are separated into two courses, their interrelationship is often not as apparent.

In order to combine the classroom and clinical grade, one must know the credit allocation for each component within the course. The grading process for the clinical achievement using the objectives and behavior has been developed so as to result in one grade. The same process could be used for computing the classroom grade. The weight attached to each cumulative grade is a function of the credit allocation. In the current illustration, each component represents three credits, thus the course grade is the result of averaging the cumulative grade for each component. In the instance where the distribution is not equal, the grade for the course is comprised of the averaging of the two cumulative grades as prescribed. As an example, were the unit credit allocation is designated as two credits for classroom activities and four credits for clinical activities, the course grade computation would be:

$$\begin{array}{ll} \text{Classroom grade} & \times 1 \\ \text{Clinical grade} & \times 2 \\ \text{Total} \end{array}$$

Designated Evaluation Strategies as a Basis for Grading

The grading process presented uses the objectives and behaviors directly as the data source in determining the grade to be awarded. It is noted that the word *awarded* is used instead of the word *given*. The teacher does not *give* a grade; the student earns it and the teacher awards it.

Another approach is to use the objectives and behaviors indirectly through the use of selected evaluation strategies as the major source of data. One evaluation strategy may provide data on one

TABLE 28. COMPUTATION OF CLINICAL GRADE II

Evaluation Strategy	Grade	Numerical Value	Weight	Numerical Value
Process Recording	C	2	15	2×15 = 30
Care Conference Presentation	A	4	30	4×30 = 120
Performance Rating	A	4	35	4×35 = 140
Analysis of Log	B	3	20	3×20 = 60
				Total 350
			Numbered Value	3.50
			Grade	B

behavior or numerous behaviors. If the source of data for each behavior is so designated and all behaviors are included in the evaluation process, the results on the various evaluation strategies can become the data base. It is still possible to highlight the non-negotiable behaviors for special consideration. The evaluation strategies selected and the weighted value of each are functions of faculty judgment based on the purpose of the course or unit. An illustration of this pattern of grading is presented in Table 28.

The cumulative clinical grade is then subjected to the same computation procedure for determining a course grade when it comprises both classroom and clinical components as was described for the previous grading system.

Several approaches to arriving at a clinical grade when the five-dimensional grading system is used have been described. They are not meant to be inclusive, but rather they suggest means of addressing the grading of clinical practice that are congruent with that generally found in grading the classroom performance. The systems are criterion referenced using the stated objectives and behaviors as the framework. Criterion-referenced grading is the method of choice because nursing is a practice discipline which calls for certain competencies that must be mastered. The standard used as a basis for criterion-referenced grading must be selected with care in terms of the purpose of the grading and must not be too narrow and rigidly fixed. This approach does not suggest an objective system, but it does foster a fair system.

Reliability of grades is a function of internal consistency of individual instructors. Internal consistency of a grade measures the degree to which the various observations made by a teacher to arrive at judgment about grades of students in a course reflect a common form of academic performance (Warren, 1971). Reliability of grades is a function of their dimensionability with a decrement in reliability occurring as attributes used increase unless there is a strong relationship among attributes. Warren suggests that: "The high reliability of grades across courses and instructors, for example, in spite of differences in course emphasis and methods of evaluation is probably due to the common element of verbal ability in most academic evaluation" (p. 21).

One of the significant limitations of the computation patterns presented is the tendency to foster rigidity with no room for flexibility and recognition of a transcendent quality in the student, which portends success or failure in future endeavors. Just as intuition is an important element in nursing, so too is it meaningful in teaching. The demand in present society for specific documentation for each computation precludes decisions which arise from faculty's own perceptions and judgment. There is a phenomenon known as goal-free learning which can often get lost in the measurement process.

Faculty who acknowledge this nonmeasureable attribute in grading often place themselves at risk. Students have the right to know the basis used for grading for any learning experience, but when a trusting relationship exists between the student and the teacher, the teacher is more free to interpose his or her own professional judgment in the final interpretation of the data used in grading. As an illustration, if a "C" is equal to 2.0, the teacher might feel that a particular student with a grade point average of 1.8 will succeed in the program more readily than a particular student with a 2.2 average. Could the former student receive the grade "C," while the latter student did not receive a passing grade? An analysis of the data for the grade may provide the rationale for such a decision. The latter student may have received the 2.2 average on the basis of a high grade in a group activity, sufficient to compensate for a poorer performance in self-directed activities. Likewise, the former student may evidence satisfactory performance in most activities, but the skill required for one type of activity may be deficient.

Grading is a fact of life in the American educational system and evokes many ambivalent feelings among all involved. Westland (1969) speaks of grades thusly: "Grades probably do represent something useful; we just don't know what it is" (p. 358). Warren (1971) raises the issue of our lack of knowledge as to what grades represent as indices of academic performance. He states: "When the components and structure of grades are better described, we will be able to attack not only the current, rather limited issues, but the more substantial ones that bear heavily on the entire educational enterprise" (p. 26).

SUMMARY

Grading is a process by which some symbol is used to designate some degree of academic achievement. Various systems are selected by faculty, such as the two-dimensional or five-dimensional. The symbol is arrived at through a computation system for interpreting evaluation data. Grades have different meanings and lack a universal standard due to various individual perceptions of grading and grades, variations in data base used, differences in base standard, and types of computation methods.

Many issues accompany the concept of grading the clinical practice experience, often arising out of faculty uncertainty, insecurity with the process, and the search for an "objective" grading system. Fairness, not objectivity, is the goal. When a two-dimensional grading system is used for clinical practice and a five-dimensional grading system is used for classroom activities, confusion results and it is only the five-dimensional grading system that is ultimately used in determining the grade point average of the total program of study for a student. The five-dimensional system is often perceived to be more discriminating, thus suggesting greater value for the activities involved than is noted with the two-dimensional system.

The grading processes that are criterion referenced are: (1) the use of objectives and behaviors of a course which are to be achieved in the clinical field with certain ones designated as non-negotiable, and (2) the use of evaluation strategies which imply indirectly the objectives and behaviors. Both of these approaches lend themselves to either the two- or five-dimensional system of grading.

Grading is an integral part of the American system of education and thus cannot be dismissed. The selection of a system must reflect thoughtful consideration on the part of the faculty involved as to its strengths, limitations, and consequences.

REFERENCES

Andrews, F. C. (Ed.). (1970). *Report on grading at the University of California, Santa Cruz,* Committee on Educational Policy.

Bartlett, J. (1967). Medical school and career performance of medical students with low medical college admission test scores. *Journal of Medical Education, 42,* 231–37.

Bloom, B. S., Hastings, J. T., & Madaus, G. F. (1971). *Handbook on formative and summative evaluation of student learning.* New York: McGraw-Hill.

Boulding, K. E. (1971). *The image.* Ann Arbor, Mich.: The University of Michigan Press.

Erickson, S. C., & Bluestone, Z. (1971). *Grading and evaluation: Memo to faculty,* No 46. Ann Arbor, Mich.: Center for Research in Learning and Teaching, University of Michigan.

Gohn, L. A. (1968). An investigation of the selection techniques of veterinary science and medical students at Purdue. *University Abstracts* 28A, 446.

Gough, H. C. (1967). Non-intellective factors in the selection and evaluation of medical students. *Journal of Medical Education, 42,* 642–50.

Hanlon, L. (1964). College grades and admission to medical schools. *Journal of Higher Education, 35,* 93–96.

Reilly, D. E. (Ed.). (1973). *Report of ad hoc committee to study grading.* Unpublished manuscript. Wayne State University, College of Nursing, Detroit, Mich.

Silberman, C. E. (1970). *Crisis in the classroom: The remaking of American education.* New York: Random House.

Warren, J. R. (1971). *College grading practices: An overview, Report 7.* Washington, D.C.: ERIC Clearinghouse on Higher Education.

Westland, G. (1969). The philosophy of student assessment. *Universities Quarterly, 23,* 350–60.

BIBLIOGRAPHY

Beyer, F. J. (1983). Setting passing scores. *Nursing & Health Care, 4,* 518–22.

Hales, L. W., Bain, P. T., & Rand, L. P. (1973). The pass–fail option: The congruence between the rationale for and student reasons in electing. *Journal of Educational Research, 66,* 295–98.

Hills, J. R., & Gladney, M. B. (1968). Factors influencing college grading standards. *Journal of Educational Measurement, 5,* 31–39.

Huckabay, L. M. (1979). Cognitive–affective consequences of grading versus nongrading of formative evaluations. *Nursing Research, 28,* 173–78.

Kelly, S. P., & Thompson, R. (1968). Grading and the nature of the discipline. *Journal of Higher Education, 39,* 517–18.

Kramer, M., Sr., & Coules, J. T. (1974). Weighting and distributing course grades. *Nursing Outlook, 22,* 176–79.

Lenburg, C. B. (1979). *The clinical performance examination.* New York: Appleton-Century-Crofts.

McFarland, M. B. (1983). Contract grading. *Nurse Educator, 8*(4), 3–6.

Morgan, M. K., & Irby, D. M. (Eds.). (1978). *Evaluating clinical competence in the health professions.* St. Louis: C. V. Mosby.

Perry, L. B. (1968). College grading: A case study and its aftermath. *Educational Record, 49*(4), 78–84.

Reijai, R., & Stopak, R. (1972). On grades: Their function in academia. *The American Psychologist, 27,* 166–67.

Rezler, A. G., & Stevens, B. J. (Eds.). (1978). *The nurse evaluator in education and service.* New York: McGraw-Hill.

Sgan, M. R. (1970). Letter grade achievement in pass–fail courses. *Journal of Higher Education, 40,* 638–44.

Stallings, W. M., Smock, H. R., & Leslie, E. K. (1968). The pass–fail grading option. *School and Society, 96,* 179–80.

Wolfe, D. (1968). Are grades necessary? *Science, 161,* 1203.

12

A Future Perspective:
The Clinical Field

A familiar adage cites the need for nurse educators in preparatory programs to prepare nurses not only for today, but also for tomorrow. Likewise, staff educators are charged not only with keeping practicing nurses up to date with current knowledge and practice, but they must prepare them for tomorrow. But tomorrow is today. The seeds of tomorrow are already evidenced today. What does today suggest tomorrow will be like in nursing practice, and therefore what will teaching in the clinical field be like at that time?

Loye (1984) makes note of the fragile nature of future forecasts.

> All forecasts for the future upon which we rely for personal and national survival . . . are warped and distorted by the personality and ideology of the forecaster and because these personal differences are hidden, from us and indeed generally from the forecaster themselves, we walk on quicksand in viewing the future. (p. 66)

With some risk, the future of nursing practice is forecasted and the resultant implications for teaching this practice are examined and addressed. It is essential that faculty explore the potential directions of the future and search for their meanings, for the way nursing practice responds to these directions, the roles and responsibilities attributed to nurses, and the very actions the nurses undertake are all part of the substance of today's nursing education.

Caution in examining the future is suggested by Bolles (1983) when he states that the future has two parts: *change* and *constancy*. He sees both parts as essential, with change representing "challenge risk taking, adventure and at its height, a kind of magic and enhancement lent to our life while constancy represents familiarity, safety, comfort and security" (p. 7). A view of the future that stresses only change provokes a state of anxiety, fear, uncertainty, and powerlessness. Likewise, a future perceived as constant with an aura of nostalgia provokes a state of boredom and inertia, as well as emotional, mental, and spiritual stagnation. It is both elements, the constant and the change, which must be incorporated in the faculty's perception of the future as it pertains to teaching in the clinical field.

Nursing practice is not an island unto itself. It has its own microworld with its own boundaries and delineated actions, but it is part of the macroworld, which constantly moves, threatens, and even permeates the boundaries. It functions within an ever-expanding knowledge generation and within a rapidly evolving information society characterized by high technology and marked demands on all resources. As with other disciplines, nursing's rapidly developing knowledge base is demanding efficient means of organizing that knowledge so that it can be readily available for use. This new knowledge is altering for the better the capabilities of nursing in intervening both qualitatively and quantitatively in health matters, while modifying its roles, responsibilities, and activities. Its constancy rests in the certain goal of assisting clients in meeting their health care needs toward fulfilling their maximum potential.

The information society with its concomitant high technology provides for intervention in physiologic or anatomic aberrations to a remarkable degree but at such cost that it threatens financial resources for all health care in the society and poses moral and ethical questions relative to the "rightness" of the intervention and the eligibility of the recipient. In an effort to address the dislocation of health care dollars, regulation of the health care delivery system through cost effective measures is undertaken in the public and private sector. One effect of these measures is a marked change in both of these settings. Changes in clinical practice for the future are concerned both with the practice settings and the characteristics of the activities within those settings, while constancy is maintained through the affirmation of the helping role with the client as the primary focus. Many nursing functions will be basically constant, but they may seem different because of the changes in their execution.

THE INFORMATION SOCIETY

Naisbitt (1982) states that our society is ". . . drowning in information, but starved for knowledge" (p. 17). Information is perceived to be high in quantity but low in usability in its present disorganized and uncontrollable state. Nurses are only too aware of Naisbitt's observation as they seek to deal with the extraordinary influx of information generated not only by their own discipline, but also by disciplines whose knowledge bears directly or indirectly on nursing practice. Knowledge will continue to evolve with increased momentum and must be harnessed so that it can be a directed force used to improve the health care in the society. Ownership of knowledge cannot be a private preserve for the health professional; knowledge must be used for the benefit of others within the context of professional practice.

Technology
The fact that technology permeates the lives of all, at least in the western world, is well acknowledged. The fact that its intrusion is occurring at such a rapid rate so that in many instances there is not enough time to react to its presence is not as readily realized until it threatens some way of life. Some technology improves life for individuals; some causes disequilibrium in the balance of an individual's life, while some may threaten the very existence of life.

The health care field is in the center of much new technology: some of it has been proven essential for forward movement; some of it has yet to attest to its value; and some of it may address one problem but create new ones. The use of technology in health care has occurred in two major areas; the instrumentation of care and cure and the computerization of data into information systems.

Instrumentation. Technology is a significant part of the cure component of health care. Assessment instrumentation has moved far beyond the glass thermometer and the stethoscope and in time these tools will become obsolete as newer devices are developed to monitor vital signs more efficiently and accurately. Monitoring can now occur even when geographic distances separate the client from the health care provider. Technology provides for continuous observation of many body functions as is evidenced in intensive care units. New technology, such as scanners and their successors, permit more accurate assessment of body structures and functions not easily accessible with the usual assessment techniques.

Technology has altered significantly the instrumentation aspect of intervention so that many aberrations in body structure or function previously unperceived or untreatable are now addressed with reasonable assurance of improvement in the quality of life for the individual. Some technology is making older intervention strategies obsolete. The advent of laser surgery portends the obsolescence of some currently used surgical procedures. Technology has permitted life processes to be maintained when the body's own mechanism fails; an action which may be important for a prescribed period of time, but which possesses the potential of extending beyond the need, resulting in feelings of anxiety and guilt on the part of the families and care givers when the purpose is no longer relevant and cessation of the process should be undertaken.

It is beyond the purview of this book to identify the various types of instrumentation currently used in practice or on the drawing board for future implementation. Suffice it to say, the assessment of and intervention in body dysfunction is becoming increasingly technologic. This is a significant factor in preparation of practitioners.

Computerization. The reference to "information society" causes an immediate association with the word computer. The computer is one means for bringing order to the vast array of available information and making it more accessible for use. Naisbitt (1982) sees the computer as liberating, particularly in its ability to manage complexity of data.

Hospitals, community health agencies, and other facilities are rapidly developing information systems which incorporate the essential data relative to their purposes and functions and provide for demonstration of their interrelationships as needed. This communication network organizes the multitude of data pertinent to agency functioning and readily yields data necessary for meeting a designated problem or situation. It is obvious that employees in these agencies who have any decision-making responsibility will be required to be functional in the use of a computer.

Information systems are appearing in nursing departments in many health care settings and are becoming an integral part of nursing practice. Ball and Hannah (1983) refer to two computer programs for recording observations of clients. One program contains a library of frequently used phrases to assist nurses in reporting observations. The other program provides for a branching questionnaire which leads the nurse through a series of questions in an effort to make more precise observations. Ball and Hannah suggest several significant results of this computer programming:

> . . . (a) increased number of observations as a result of forced recall, (b) increased accuracy and reliability of observations, (c) shorter time required than when writing nursing notes, and (d) readily available statistical data for various nursing purposes. (pp. 134–35)

Efforts to computerize nursing diagnoses are reported in the literature, (Romano, McCormick, & McNeely, 1982; Simmons & Ryan, 1984). Simmons and Ryan see a computerized system of diagnoses as a means of providing a logical structure that guides the nurse in the thinking process entailed when considering a patient problem. Simmons and Ryan raised four questions following their effort to implement a computer program for nursing in their agency:

1. Is there adequate conceptual knowledge related to diagnostic categories?
2. Are the clinical reasoning skills of nurses in the agency lacking, underdeveloped, unrewarded?

3. Are there inherent intuitive conclusions nurses make that relate to certain populations?
4. Is there a diagnostic formulation that is not documented? (p. 282)

The present state of the art in the development of nursing diagnoses, their describing characteristics, and the underlying phenomena of nursing concern as well as the present limited use of nursing diagnoses by nurses in practice suggest that the use of computers for nursing diagnosis is not operational on a wide scale. At the Sixth Conference on Nursing Diagnosis held in St. Louis in 1984, reports were given that action in coding and computerizing diagnoses with the goal of eventually providing a national data base was in process. Such a data base will be in the future of nursing.

Nursing care plans have been computer programmed. As a rule, the program includes a master plan which can be modified for each client. Ball and Hannah (1983) indicate possible advantages to the use of plan stored in a computer memory: ". . . (a) accountability is identified through a print-out of the plan, (b) errors and omissions are decreased, (c) more consistent care is possible, especially among nurses in the different shifts, and (d) time for planning is greatly decreased" (p. 137).

The role of computers in concert with technology is presently in use for monitoring the many physiologic processes of vital functions of clients. The addition of the computer provides an important dimension, for it lessens the demand for the nurse to "monitor the machine." The computer also interprets the findings and provides the protocol for action when any findings suggest body system dysfunction.

The role of the computer in nursing care will become increasingly prominent in the information age. Its ability to provide a record system, not only for a particular client but also for retrieval of clinical data, will greatly facilitate the development of a knowledge base of practice and the precision of nursing decision making as well as raising research questions. Protocols of care for various client problems which are retrievable from the computer minimize the time required for planning and enable the establishment of more accurate and inclusive patient care management systems. It has particular value in providing for nursing audit of care through the design of its program and the retrieval of the data. The validity of the contribution of nursing practice to health care management can also be ascertained as a basis for determining the costing out of the economic value of nursing and other purposes.

Influence of Technology on Hospital Care

Donley (1984) refers to hospitals as "temples of technology" (p. 4). Technology is well integrated into all systems of hospitals with evidence that this trend will continue in the future. High technology is associated primarily with acuity of illness. This factor accounts for hospitals becoming centers of acute care requiring sophisticated technologic instrumentation used by highly trained technical practitioners. McClure and Nelson (1982) note that the acuity issue has fostered an increased specialization phenomenon relative to medical and nursing care and concomitantly to specialization or segregation of particular areas of the hospital. Although this costly technologic specialization occurs predominantly in medical centers, even small community hospitals are required to have intensive care units to provide for immediate service to their communities.

A significant factor about high technology in health care to consider is the difference of its impact on the health care system from what one finds in industry. In the latter, technology often reduces the cost for labor, causing a shift of the cost to capital which can be spread out over a period of time. Curtin (1984) notes that in the health care system, the introduction of cybernetics increases capital costs without the concomitant decrease in labor costs, for in practice it actually increases the need for employment. Two results of using high technology in the delivery of health services are cited by Curtin:

1. Sicker people now can survive, but their care consumes more human and material services.
2. The resultant increase in population ultimately increases demand for services. (p. 70)

She concludes, "In short, mortality rates still come one to a person, only now people tend to die of long-term, chronic or debilitating diseases that require increasingly sophisticated interventions over longer periods of time" (p. 70).

Technology, rather than contributing to a reduction in costs of health care, in essence accounts for much of its increase. Its effect is found in its ability to prolong life, with or without improvement in its quality. Value questions arise in addressing cost in relation to life. Health care dollars are not finite, hard choices lie ahead in their control and allocation.

Because of the high cost of technology, patient days in the hospital are restricted to the time necessary for the use of the technology, not to the time necessary for the patient to be prepared to manage self-care outside the hospital. This means that hospital stays for patients will be shorter, patient turnover will be more rapid, and hospitals will be centers of intensity and complexity with high stress for all a complicating factor. Naisbitt (1982) refers to the effects of technology in changing the care aspect in the hospital: "The more high technology we put into our hospitals, the less we are being born there, dying there . . . and avoiding them in between" (p. 38).

Hospital care as previously known is in transition, if not in revolution. Birthing centers for new life, hospices for the dying, chronic hospitals as step-down centers for persons discharged from high-tech centers, ambulatory centers for general surgery and medical therapies, and organized home care services will be the pattern for delivery of health care in those matters previously tended to within the hospital domain. The decrease in the dependence on hospitals will foster the self-care movement in which individuals will place more emphasis on staying well and learning how to meet their own health needs except in acute situations or those which impede their usual activities.

Changes in Role and Responsibilities of Nursing

The technology diffusion in health care settings has altered the responsibilities of nursing. Donley (1984), using Toffler's notion of societal waves, considers the mechanical technologic nursing seen today as reflective of a second-wave society with some evidence of a third-wave society in the use of some sophisticated technology. To a lesser degree, hands-on care, characteristic of the first wave continues. In a mechanical technologic setting, nursing responsibilities entail clinical knowledge for rapid decision making and technologic expertise. Naisbitt (1982), however, sees high technology creating dissonance in life patterns of many persons resulting in resistance to the dehumanizing effects of such mechanisms.

Nurses working in high-tech hospital settings, although challenged by the "wonder machine," must develop skills in "high touch"; a process of sensitivity to the humanity of the client and to those who share love and concern for the client. High-touch skills are most vulnerable in a highly charged environment where client stay is short, negating a long-term relationship and where client response level is diminished by the nature of the pathologic processes and the therapies being used to ameliorate these processes.

Nurses need to participate in decisions as to what advances in technology are acceptable in the setting. Questions as to technology's value, its effect on the value system of individuals and the society, and its effect on the health care delivery system are in order.

The high-tech environment in hospitals includes computerization of the data relative to assessment of patient physiologic responses and protocols for patient management or treatment for deviations in response. Many clinical judgments are thus preprogrammed, with the major decisions related to the selection of the appropriate protocols for the particular problem involved.

A group of nurse practitioners responding to the Delphi technique for identifying the major direction nursing in hospitals will take specified two relevant trends as described by Hill (1984):

1. Use of computers by all nursing staff members for autonomous decision making concerning patient care.

2. Use of skilled technical nursing for all direct nursing care of hospitalized patient. (p. 8)

There is some concern in the minds of some nursing leaders relative to the possibility of nursing autonomy, legitimate control over nurses' own work, becoming reality in hospital settings (Donley, 1984; Jacox, 1982; Rosenow, 1983). Although nurses have the ability to make clinical judgments, their actions are limited by role definition in a bureaucratic system. Rosenow notes: ". . . the authority for nursing actions comes from physicians through orders or from the hospital through rule and specified routines" (p. 35). In describing the intensive care situation with its high technology, she identifies the activities of the triad: administration, physician, and nurse; the administration assures the availability of essential resources, the doctor determines the services to be offered and the nurse executes and monitors the delivery of services. The nurse in this setting does not have professional autonomy; rather, the nurse functions in a supportive role carrying out tasks delegated by a member of another profession. To have professional autonomy, Freidson (1971) cites two significant criteria: ". . . (a) the professional must have control over an area of work separate from that of a dominant profession; (b) the practice must occur without routine contact or dependence on the dominant profession" (p. 79).

The question is posed as to whether or not hospitals will require professional nurses if activities are delegated by another profession and most protocols of care are computerized. Some efforts are underway to seek more control of nursing by nursing. Clifford (1982) reported on her effort to move in this direction in the institution where she is director. A significant action was the decentralization of decision making nearer the locus of action. In the study of magnet hospitals (American Academy of Nurses, 1983) the decentralization of decision making was a major factor in attracting and maintaining nurses because it enabled nurses at the unit level to have a sense of control over the immediate work environment.

The decentralization of decision making is an essential concept of the networking system which affords authority to those who know, not to those who hold a designated position in a hierarchy. Networking as an organizational framework has not appeared at this time in hospitals to any significant degree in the mid-eighties, but its acceptance in other major organizations will influence the processes in hospitals. Three reasons are cited by Naisbitt (1982), for the emergence of a network system:

1. Dearth of traditional structures.
2. Din of information overload.
3. Past failures of hierarchies. (p. 220)

Differences between a hierarchical system and a networking system are identified by McInnes (1984):

1. Authority tends to be decentralized, residing in individuals with pertinent information rather than in those who occupy an assigned position.
2. Policies and boundaries tend to be fluid rather than fixed.
3. Personnel tend to relate among themselves and with others as equals rather than as subordinate or superior.
4. Procedures tend to be people centered.
5. Style tends to be sociable rather than officious.
6. Structure tends to be polycentric rather than monocentric. (p. 9)

Present trends in some nursing departments suggest that in the future, nursing will move into a networking system which provides for information linkages horizontally, vertically, and multidirectionally. This system change will result as more highly educated and prepared nurses enter the practice setting with professional knowledge and the expectation to be active participants in the decision-making process with control over their own practice. Because of nurses' need to manage large quantities of information in a short space of time, nurses will see validity to Naisbitt's concept of networking as a "structure for transmitting information in an organization that is quick, more high touch and more energy efficient" (p. 215).

Alterations in locus of decision making relative to patient care have potential for fostering a networking organizational system in hospitals. Jacox (1982) notes the internal authority conflict occurring in hospitals as outside forces exert control over patient care decisions, formerly the primary responsibility of the physician. The cost-effective measure, prospective payment for health care provided for Medicare patients, places the administration with the support of government in a decision-making position relative to patient discharge, a practice rarely occurring in the past. The change in power of the physicians in the hospital and their movement toward becoming salaried employees of hospitals and other health care groups, as well as the affirmation of nursing's knowledge domain, provide an opportunity for nursing to consolidate its domain of practice over which it has autonomy. With the recognition and acceptance of the expertise of each group working within the hospital and the allocation of responsibility and authority accordingly, a networking- rather than a power-oriented management system is a real potential for the hospital of tomorrow. The increasing complexity of decisions is no longer the domain of any one group; decisions require the synthesis of expertise of all involved.

PROSPECTIVE PAYMENT: IMPACT ON HEALTH CARE SETTINGS

A direct outgrowth of the diffusion of high technology into the health care system is the changing nature of the hospital as a health care agency and the shift of many of its former activities to other agencies in the community. Although this shift has been underway for some time in response to high cost and impersonality in a mechanized environment; e.g., development of birthing centers, hospices, and self-care movements, the major change came about in 1984 when government-sponsored reimbursement for hospitalized patients receiving Medicare became prospective rather than retrospective.

In a retrospective reimbursement system the hospital was paid at the conclusion of services rendered including a per diem for routine and special care as well as ancillary services such as diagnostic and therapeutic tests at a cost specified by the hospital. With few restrictions on costs to health care providers, individuals, and agencies, there was no sense of urgency to provide cost-efficient care. The inflation of health care costs at a higher rate than was evident for other aspects of society prompted the government to develop a system of payment with built-in cost controls, which are in effect expenditure controls.

Prospective Method of Case Mix Reimbursement
Since the 1960s, efforts have been made to develop a means of determining realistic costs for treating patients in hospitals. The prevailing system in most hospitals uses an approach which costed out such factors as per diem, treatment modalities, services, and meals, all directed toward the utilization of hospital resources but not addressing illness and demographic data which cause variations in resource utilization. Plomann and Shaffer (1983) cite nine different prospective case mix plans that were in evidence:

1. ICD 9 CM, list A—international classification of diseases adopted—9th revision clinical modification.
2. DRG—diagnostic related groups.
3. MD–DADO—physician discharge abstract data optional.
4. AS Score—appropriations of hospital length of stay.
5. VA MLL—Veterans Administration multilevel care.
6. Patient management categories—reason for admission.
7. Disease staging—similar conditions.
8. Severity of illness index.
9. Generic algorithms—purpose of classification dictates group formation. (p. 493)

Diagnostic Related Group Case Mix Reimbursement System
On April 20, 1983, the Social Security Amendments of 1983, law H.R. 1900 (Pl 98-21), passed by Congress, was signed by President Reagan. This law authorized the use of a prospective payment system based on DRG (diagnostic-related categories) for all hospitals serving Medicare. This system was developed by the Yale Center for

Health Studies and Yale, New Haven Hospital. The primary objective of the system is to define types of cases that would be expected to be similar in the amount of usage of hospital services, with the length of stay as a measure of hospital services (Plomann & Shaffer, 1983). The length of stay is a significant factor, for experience suggests that ancillary services, such as diagnostic tests and treatments, increase proportionally to the time the patient stays in the hospital.

The categories selected are based on patient diagnosis, age, treatment procedures (inclusive of surgery), discharge status, and sex. This classification system reinforces the already established disease orientation of the hospital, in contrast to nursing's health orientation. The original DRG classification included 383 groups, but it became evident that too many illness factors in patients could not be accommodated. The current system, based on ICD-9-CM Diagnostic and Procedure Code, includes 467 groups. Lichlig (1982) cites two critical criteria in developing such a classification system:

1. Statistically coherent—statistically significant so that patients in a DRG tend to consume similar amounts of hospital resources.
2. Medically meaningful—patients in a DRG have similar clinical conditions and treatment regimes. (p. 14)

Hospital reimbursement for Medicare patients occurs in terms of rates set in advance according to a formula which also takes into account the regional and national rates and for each hospital, the 1982 cost experience updated for inflation, The rate is fixed for a year with adjustment anticipated as cost data become more precise and care costs alter with such factors as new technology and new care regimes. A three-year time span is planned before a national system is in place. It can be anticipated that states will adopt a similar system for their Medicaid recipients and that the private sector will respond in similar ways to control costs.

As this book goes to press, the DRG mixed-case reimbursement system is in the initial phase; the results are projected to be most effective in controlling costs and insuring quality care. The reality of these expectations awaits further experience with the system and a critical analysis of the data generated. Serious questions are raised as to the applicability of the system in accommodating illnesses which do not fit neatly into the current classifications; the viability of such a system in small hospitals where numbers of clients in any one group are too limited to be meaningful; and the adaptability of the system in accounting for advances in technology, diagnostic measures, and treatment modalities as well as the differences among hospitals in resources which ultimately may affect the patterns of care provided and the length of stay of patients. The present development is evolutionary and it may well be subject to drastic change as experience grows with usage. It can be assured, however, that cost containment will be a constant in health care delivery services, whether through the DRG prospective reimbursement system or some other one. Financing in health care in the future will most likely be responsive to the protection of the public purse rather than to the quality of care.

Influence of a Case Mix Prospective Reimbursement System
As the system becomes institutionalized, several observations are noted. Shaffer (1983) recognizes that the system provides "a means of exerting more external influences over hospital activities and plans as a means of building cost containment constraints or incentives into hospital payments" (p. 388). Since length of hospital stay is a critical variable in the use of hospital resources, each category in the system is designated a time frame called *trim point*. Patients falling outside this time range are called *outliers* (Joel, 1983). If patients are discharged before the designated length of time, the hospital keeps the surplus; if the patient extends the stay beyond the trim point, the hospital does not get full reimbursement for the extension.

In this system, the incentive is to expedite the care of the client and the movement of the individual as quickly as possible from the hospital. This action presupposes a vast network of community health care services, hospitals for chronic care, long-term care facilities, nursing homes, and home health services which provide care after the acute episode is over.

The incentive in the system which enables hospitals to keep surplus money if patient discharge occurs early can be taken advantage of if quality controls are not maintained. The Health Care Financing Administration according to Davis (1984) has two processes in place to prevent abuse of the system:

1. Extension of system of admission pattern monitoring to prospective payment.
2. Use of Professional Review Organization (PRO) to validate diagnoses, monitor appropriateness of admission, and review outlier cases. (p. 20)

A significant change resulting from this prospective reimbursement system will be in the types of information systems developed in hospitals. Fedorowicz (1983) comments on the present hospital management philosophy which provides for two organizations:

1. Administration, which controls finances and resources of hospital and provides financial and utilization data for management purposes.
2. Medical, which directs volume of services offered to patient and provides data to support medical functions.

The case mix reimbursement system will require a health information system which combines medical and financial data providing for on-line entry and retrieval of all data related to hospital patient.

The delivery of health care in this country is undergoing a marked shift, with the end result difficult to project. Changes in philosophy, values, and meaning of health care; alterations in loci of decision making and control; modifications in classifications, roles, and responsibilities of health care providers; shifts in dollar allocations for health care; and continued examination and alteration in purposes and functions of health care agencies all portend a very different health care system. The use of the health care dollar has emphasized the cure aspect, but the realization of the high cost of cure is causing some individuals and groups to accept the value of money spent on prevention and maintenance of people in a healthy state. Governmental efforts to reduce environmental factors which are etiologic agents in illness, the development of education programs (especially in the mass media) which promote healthful living, and the monitoring of occupational practices for elimination of health hazards are directions which support the notion of health promotion and prevention of illness.

The hospital will no longer serve as the main source of publicly or privately remunerated health care. Except for a limited number of highly skilled technically prepared individuals, many health care providers will be employed in the various health care agencies in the community. Some types of health care workers will be eliminated as their work becomes obsolete; others will decrease in numbers as demand for their service is lessened due to lack of need or technology, while other health care workers will need to develop new knowledge and skills to meet new demands. It is clear that all health care workers will need to be knowledgeable about the prospective case mix reimbursement system and about cost containment factors in the health care system. The constant variable for these individuals is their ultimate purpose to minister to the health care needs of persons; the change variable will be evidenced in the manner the ministrations are carried out, the settings where they occur, and the characteristics of their roles and responsibilities.

Change in Nursing Roles and Responsibilities in a Prospective Case Mix Reimbursement System

What will nursing be like under the new system? The literature about the system relative to its evolution and present state is negligible as far as the nursing component is concerned. It is only in nursing literature that the new system of reimbursement is examined in relation to nursing's role and responsibility. In general, nursing, a major health care resource, is classified as a nonmedical entity in the systems.

An opportune moment for a group to make a significant change is when the larger system of which it is a part is also undergoing a change. How will nursing respond, for its future is being determined now? One direction of response continues nursing in its "supportive" and "doing" role, obtaining functional knowledge of the new system and all it involves toward cost containment, while still accepting directions from other groups in the system and supporting the expressed values of the organization. The other direction sees nursing seizing the opportunity to assert itself, declare its parameters based on its own knowledge over which it will have professional autonomy, and through an appropriate data base, determine nursing intensity required for each DRG classification as a basis for costing out the use of nursing resource. It is the latter direction that speaks to professional nursing.

Since the stimulus for change is the need to develop a reimbursement system directed toward cost containment, nursing has an immediate need to ascertain the cost of the utilization of the nursing resource. Such an effort must be in accord with the system used by the larger body as it addresses the use of all resources. This delineation of costs must not only pertain to nursing care delivered in the hospital, but also that provided in community health agencies and home care. Formulas for approaching costs in hospitals are available with some modification; there is little available for cost determination outside the hospital. One significant question is how does one put a monetary value on resource use for health promotion?

The costing of resource utilization requires quantification of nursing care but must answer to questions of quality. Such questions relate to the kind of nursing resource consumed, frequency and duration of its use, quality of care required by the severity of illness, and appropriate staff mix. Johns Hopkins Hospital began a study in 1983 on the cost of nursing care by developing a Nursing Intensity Index, which looks not only at acuity of nursing care but also provides a description of the overall nursing needs of patients. These data should be helpful in not only predicting staff needs, but also nursing resources required for a particular patient (Horn, 1984). Research questions need to be raised and explored if nursing is to cost-out its care incorporating the values it deems to be significant. Hegyvary (1984) raises three pertinent questions in relation to the prospective reimbursement:

1. What does the patient receive for a given cost?
2. What does a hospital or patient receive in quality for a given level of payment toward cost?
3. What decisions do hospital managers make about quality when costs increasingly overrun reimbursement? (p. 51)

The relationship of the use of nursing resources to these questions is critical. The tendency to equate money spent with quality is often detrimental to the actual quality component of care. The action of management to lay off higher salaried professionally prepared nurses to decrease cost may in reality increase costs if staff is not prepared to meet demands. More staff at a lower salary may be needed, and their inability to meet clients' needs may result in the development of complications or recidivism, both of which increase health care costs. Cost containment can entail using the best prepared professionals capable of providing the expertise required. The institution of the primary nursing modality in health care settings is one endeavor to provide the quality and expertise needed.

The emergence of the information society places demands on nursing to hone up its information system so that data are readily retrievable. Clarity, accuracy, and comprehensiveness in documentation are increasingly significant since documentation is used by a medical recorder, not a member of the writer's profession, to determine DRGs and the ultimate cost reimbursement. Donaho (1984) stresses the need for documenting the use of nursing resource in a retrievable form so that it can be linked to the system-wide parameters (p. 37). This action requires linkage between nursing data and clinical data, which suggests that nursing terminology must be accepted by all and be compatible with that used by others. Donaho stresses the need for national uniformity as she notes that the present trend of each institution in setting up its own standards using its own measures for quality makes nurses very vulnerable. Uniformity of standards derived from research is very much in order.

The shortened hospital stay greatly increases the need for nursing research in discharge planning for the patient, for this activity is primarily under the direction of nursing. Clifford (1984) poses the critical questions:

- What is the impact of early discharge on community health agencies?
- What are post hospital care requirements?

The latter question needs also to be addressed by research, for the intensity of the question is new within the present system of reimbursement. Wagner (1984) raises additional questions relative to the early hospital discharge process. Aware of the limitations of many communities to provide services, her questions are:

- What nursing services will be available in the community?
- What nursing services are appropriate to be provided in the community?
- What nursing services will be acceptable to client and at what cost?

The movement of more health care into the community signifies a different client–health care provider relationship than one encounters in the hospital. In the latter, the client is "captive" with relatively little say about services provided. Tests are done, routines are followed, standard meals are served, and each group's territory is specified. In the community, however, the health caregiver is on the client's turf and the client is more free to decide whether or not to follow the prescribed regime of care, or indeed to accept any care. Some of the decisions will be based on clients' priority for expenditure of their own money, for there is less reimbursement money for diagnostic and therapeutic measures when carried out outside the hospital domain. Care of clients within their own cultural milieu represents a different source of power in health care decisions than when caring for a client within the hospital culture.

The early discharge of patients means a change in the nature and amount of nursing that will be required in the home. Some patients will move into chronic hospitals as a transition from the acute care hospital to home. Others, however, will be discharged directly to their homes, often needing care and the use of technical equipment, once thought to be available only in the hospitals. Teaching of patients, families, and even volunteers will become a major focus of nursing action in the maintenance of a therapeutic regimen within the community settings. Because the early discharged patient still needs monitoring and care, Schraff (1984) recognizes that the planning for these patients involves more than the types of professional services needed; planning will need to consider client needs over a 24-hour period. Interagency planning, flexibility of community agencies with time schedules determined by need for services, and a networking system designed so that client and family have access for whatever care is needed are essential if continuity of care is to be provided.

Other activities, formerly conducted in the hospital, will be incorporated into community health care. The high cost of acute hospital care means that the time as a patient in that setting must be maximized and focused directly on the resolution of the health problem. The practice of admitting patients for preoperative preparation, both diagnostically and educationally, can become obsolete as practice increasingly occurs in the community prior to hospital admission.

All of these changes in practice occur with a shift in population groups needing care. The increasing age level of the public is documented in the literature and brings with it increased demand for use of health care resources and dollars; for illness, especially chronic, is more frequent in the older age group. Care emphasis will shift from custodial to the maximizing of the social potential of these elderly individuals so that they can assume greater responsibility for self-care. Another goal of this change is to minimize the cost of their care.

At the opposite end of the age spectrum are the very young who need the essential care to assure a healthful life. Neglect at this age often dooms the individual to a life of health problems which puts increased demand on health care resources. Prevention, early correction of deviations, and health promotion and teaching are the foci of health care dollar expenditure for this young group. Although these two groups of the population place the highest demands on health dollars and resources, other age groups have specific health needs which must also be addressed.

Nursing practice will change. Nursing knowledge will change. Nursing administration will change with more involvement of nurses in decision making. What knowledge will the future nurse need? A Delphi study carried out to determine knowledges and skills nurses will need in the future indicated computer language, computer skills, information skills, information systems, program analysis, nursing knowledge, and coping with organizational complexity (Hill, 1984). Other areas to suggest are leadership, costing strategies, technology, and teaching.

Donley (1984) sees dimensions of knowledge needed as a "gestalt of technical, humanistic and ethical knowledge" (p. 6). She elaborates on each of these dimensions. Super-technical knowledge refers to the professional who has established parameters of assessment and use of information to make clinical decisions. Humanistic knowledge enables nurses to address the philosophical meaning of health, illness, life, and death. Ethical knowledge enables the nurse to ascertain the goodness or badness of both clinical decisions and social policies which influence public decisions about resource allocation.

Harriman (1984) believes that in any rapidly changing world, ". . . innovative skills will be increasingly sought and implemented as more and more competing new challenges appear because it will be practical to do so" (p. 104). The ability to move within a changing system requires problem-solving skills that do not rely on past solutions but rather call upon the formulation of new ideas. This requires the ability to connect seemingly irrelevant data to a problem without the demand for assurance of fit but with the willingness to risk to think differently. Change is not linear; neither is problem solving. Nurses will need skills far removed from a routine, principled, or procedural approach to seek answers to obstacles or novel problems which will characterize the future of health care. The report of the study of medical education by a panel of the Association of Medical Colleges endorses this notion in speaking of the need for medical students to ". . . become critical, original thinkers who are constructively skeptical" (Conclusions, 1984, p. 17).

THE USE OF THE CLINICAL FIELD IN THE FUTURE

Change in the present presages the directions that will be found in the future. Health care, delivery of health care, and nursing practice are all enmeshed in a radical change that alters the foreseeable future. Nursing education, likewise, is an integral part of this change. The current directions influence nursing practice in the future and thus will influence the character of learning knowledge and skills in the clinical field. Two significant changes in the use of the clinical field are apparent: change in the settings and change in the types of learning in these settings.

Change in Setting

The prospective reimbursement system will have a marked impact on the settings where students learn to practice as professionals. Cost-containment measures in the system do not include educational costs for students using hospitals as a practice field. Although in some instances, nursing service is charging a fee for use of the setting as a student affiliation, this practice was not supported by four nursing directors discussing the future of nursing (Nursing & Health Care, 1984). Walker, responded to this trend thusly: "I think it is absolutely ridiculous for nursing directors to get into this mentality, because then we are cutting off our nose to spite our face" (p. 314). Another director, Sr. Michael noted a disadvantage to interfering with the system of clinical affiliation, especially in chronic care hospitals. Positive experience as a student is an important factor in the recruitment of graduate nurses. It is also recognized that the presence of students in a practice setting positively influences the quality of care provided, for they serve as an incentive to the staff to improve care and reevaluate the care they are providing. The future possibility of charging for clinical affiliation remains to be decided, but such a decision is critical relative to its possible impact on both nursing service and nursing education.

Although the nursing literature in recent years has referred to the emphasis on wellness through prevention and health promotion as a primary focus in professional nursing preparation, there has been little evidence of this fact in many nursing curriculums. In most instances, the majority of clinical experiences, indeed even the first such experience for a student, occur in the hospital, where emphasis is on cure. The pattern continues in spite of the increasing complexity of patient needs while hospitalized. If the development of professional competencies proceeds from simple to complex, practice fields must be selected that provide for the orderly process to occur. Movements to the community and its agencies, other than acute hospitals, for learning experiences is in the future, with hospitals providing experience in acute nursing care at an appropriate time in the program when students have the requisite entry competencies for practicing in such a setting.

Community as a Practice Field

The reference to the community as a practice field must recognize its diversity in purpose, clientele, and services within the system of health care delivery. Its chronic care hospitals, long-term facilities, and nursing homes provide experience which is generally continuous, not subject to radical changes in patient health status, and is opportune for learning to establish a nurse–patient relationship and to use the nursing process in practice. Emphasis can be on prevention, health promotion, and cure, which brings persons to optimum health status. The experience is available for such learning but may need to be selective with the arrival of more acutely ill patients coming from an early discharge from the hospital.

Ambulatory care facilities will increase and provide experience in monitoring health status, participation with diagnostic and therapeutic measures, and fostering self-help capacities of clients and their families. The facilities will also be the locus for preparation of people for hospital admission, which includes preoperative and pretherapeutic teaching, thus enabling the student to gain experience in addressing the informational and emotional needs of clients prior to hospitalization. The nurse–patient relationship is episodic and may or may not recur. In this field, the student learns to maximize time with the client and develop precision with assessment and intervention skills, particularly teaching and counseling competencies. Students also learn to accommodate their own notions of health care to the culture of clients in terms of their practices, life styles, values, and priorities.

Home care as a field of practice brings the student in direct contact with the client's culture where client acceptance or rejection of care and counsel may be related to the nurse's sensitivity to the multiple forces that affect health care decisions. Nursing experience in a home care setting ranges from simple to complex and often entails a continuing nurse–patient relationship. Experiences are selected on the basis of the student's readiness to participate. In some situations monitoring and teaching are the primary activities. In situations where the patient is discharged from the hospital early and requires considerable technologic intervention, students must be reasonably competent in their own practice to become involved. Whereas many of these interventions are carried out in a regular regime in the hospital and in the home, the patient, family, or others must be prepared to follow the regime beyond the nurse's professional visit. A network for patients' use summoning for assistance whenever needed is a critical component of care. The high nursing intensity required by these patients is the proper concern of the more advanced student.

The illustrations of different types of community agencies and some of the learning experiences available have been identified. The illustrations are not inclusive but suggestive of the experiences which faculty can choose as the curriculum is developed. Knowledge of and skill in computer usage within an information system will be required for all students in community settings, for linkages will be established and data from patients will be computerized. Many of the agencies are multidiscipline organizations, with each discipline submitting data for synthesis on a client's record. Simmons (1984) describes a computer system for ambulatory care used in a visiting nurses association which uses the patient's clinical record as a source of data for payroll, other financial purposes, personnel needs, demographics, medical diagnosis, and patient's problems (p. 19). To these data, nursing diagnoses must be added.

Greater use of the community as a field of practice demands that students be more informed about various community resources to assist client health needs. Often the nurse serves as the coordinator of care and needs to have a functioning knowledge of appropriate resources to which the client must be referred as well as the systems by which they operate, the procedures for entry, and costs and financial arrangements required.

Hospital as a Practice Field
The role of the hospital in preparing nurses will be altered as the result of the system of health care which is evolving. The acuity of patient needs and problems and the intensity of nursing demands in a high-stress environment will be a practice field for more experienced students who have mastered skill in making clinical judgments, using the nursing process and using technical skills, and who are comfortable with themselves in a patient care milieu. The experiences provided include opportunity to participate in care where decisions are apt to be made rapidly and where patient–nurse–family relationships occur under highly stressful situations. The use of information systems by which care data and therapeutic prescriptions are computerized gives significant meaning to "Hi-Tech–Hi-Touch" care. Sharing in the decision-making process not only with nurses, but with members of other disciplines provides a broad perspective of the various perceptions of individuals involved in patient care. Skills in moral reasoning become particularly developed when decisions as to who receives care, who pays for the care, and what care is appropriate become of concern.

Discharge planning skills of the student will be fostered as patients are sent from the hospital with a lesser degree of recovery than previously. Many institutions will develop a computerized discharge planning model which assures a systematic approach to providing continuity of care. A multidisciplinary discharge planning model using the Computerized Medical Information System

(MIS) has been developed at the Clinical Center, National Institute of Health and is reported in the literature (Romano, 1984). New knowledge is needed relative to discharge planning which addresses the needs of early discharged patients and the use of community resources, often limited, to meet these needs.

Implications of Setting Change for Faculty

The change in emphasis on setting and the inherent nursing activities will place new demands on the preparation of faculty so as to use effectively the various fields available for experience. Most faculty preparation dichotomizes nursing faculty roles into those prepared to teach within hospitals and those prepared to teach in the community. Another type of faculty is required: one who has the competencies to function in both settings and can facilitate involvement of students in the patient's transition from home to hospital and then to another community agency or home. The essence of continuity will become a critical factor in teaching, for the transfer of patients to various health care settings poses a real danger of the patient becoming "lost" in the process.

Many faculty teaching in hospitals today will not have the high technological knowledge and expertise necessary for patient care and for teaching that care to students. This factor will require these faculty to further their education in the competencies required or to be retrained to function within a community setting. It is in the latter where the need for faculty will be greatest in the future and where there is the greatest deficit currently. These faculty must be expert in home or long-term care and in coordination of health care resources, and comfortable with the values, practices, and life styles of various cultural groups. There will also be a need for coordination between faculty associated with acute episodic care in the hospital and those involved with long-term needs in the community so that the student experience provides for a holistic perspective of the client's needs for health care. Changes in health care patterns and delivery affect markedly the preparation of nursing faculty and support the need for faculty to maintain their practice competencies. Increasingly, faculty practice plans will become commonplace in nursing education institutions.

Research in nursing education is a critical need in the future, especially as it explores the new knowledge and skill demands and their incorporation in a teaching modality which is most cost effective. Cost factors in educating future students relative to the new patterns of care must be identified through research for they are critical variables in determining programs. A teacher–student ratio appropriate for a geographical field reasonably circumscribed may not be sufficient for one with more diffuse boundaries as characteristic of nursing in the community.

New uses of information processing teaching modalities, preceptors in practice settings as models, and new knowledges derived from research in the learning process must be explored and instituted into the teaching program. Delineation of the *essential* knowledges and skills which are within the purview of any particular preparatory program is needed. Trivial pursuits and vested interests of faculty or others cannot with impunity dominate program decisions. Quality and quantity of the substance of learning, cost-effective teaching strategies, and the most expeditious use of faculty and clinical experts in the field are all matters for specific renewed exploration. The future demands precision in nursing education with quality of experience provided by those with expertise in their domain of nursing practice and teaching practice.

EFFECT OF CHANGE ON PURPOSES
FOR USE OF CLINICAL FIELD
FOR PREPARATION OF PRACTITIONERS

The caution that any view of the future must incorporate both change and constancy was stipulated by Bolles (1983). The change component has received the bulk of the attention in this chapter, but some explicit and implicit references were made to the constancy in the goal of nursing which is providing health services to clients in such a way as to contribute to the quality of their lives. Does any other constancy exist for the future which is significant for faculty?

This book began with suggestions for use of the clinical field in professional education as proposed by Argyris and Schön, which are: learning how to learn, handling ambiguity, thinking like professionals, and developing personal causation. Although the general notion of the goal of applying theory to practice is acknowledged, the other purposes denote a broader concept of this application more fitting for a professional so that the *how to do* does not become an end in itself.

Is there evidence of constancy in these four purposes, in spite of all the changes that are affecting nursing and nursing education? A review of their intent suggests that they are even more relevant today and for the future. They are most important outcomes in a field whose students will enter a society dominated by change.

The first outcome stated is *learning how to learn*. Facts and "how to do" are not sufficient subject matters for the clinical field experience, for both are consistently subject to questioning and are often altered as new knowledge is developed. Students must learn the facts and the *how to do* acceptable at any point in time, but they must equally be prepared to accept the probability of their transiency. Ever alert to the advent of new knowledge, the student will need to acquire the cognitive skills of rational and creative thinking, problem solving that provides for innovation as indicated, and decision making within a humanistic context. These skills enable the student to adopt the present state of knowledge, yet maintain the flexibility to accommodate to the new. Learning how to learn means the rigidity of knowledge ownership is inappropriate. It means the development of the posture of a continuous learner, the mainte-nance of a scholarly approach to developing knowledge, and a read-iness to examine decisions and actions critically. The projection of the future of nursing includes the potential instability of much of its current knowledge and practices and affirms that *learning how to learn* is still an important purpose for clinical experience.

The second purpose stated is *handling ambiguity*. Nursing, like other health disciplines has many ambiguities in its practice. In particular, the delivery of health care services lacks a rationale which assures the delivery of the right care to the right client at the right time with the right intensity. The ambiguity of many actions in the entire health field becomes even more evident with the intro-duction of cost effectiveness as a major priority in the delivery of services. The health care provider who is a dualist thinker needing the *right and only answer* will be at a great disadvantage in the world of future nursing. Studies cited earlier showing that nursing programs are remiss in moving students from dualistic to rela-tivistic thinking and ultimately to commitment is a cause of great concern. The future of nursing requires practitioners who can han-dle ambiguity and not rely on absolutism, but are self-confident in making decisions with use of the best of present knowledge, even when the outcome is not certain. Uncertainty, not certainty, will characterize nursing in the future, thus supporting the purpose, *dealing with* ambiguity as a legitimate one for use of the clinical field in nursing education.

The third purpose stated is *thinking like professionals*. The evo-lution of a theory of nursing practice is ongoing and will become increasingly obvious. Professional nurses base their practice not from a task orientation, but rather from a questioning and explora-tory posture which seeks answers to the *why* and *what if* of nursing actions. Each professional practitioner is expected to develop an individual theory of practice that includes a systematic self-exam-ination of decisions and actions. An action is not a *fait accompli*—it demands an analysis based on theories of nursing and other rele-vant disciplines in terms of its potential contribution to nursing practice knowledge.

Professionals also examine their own practice, beliefs, and modalities as they interface with the sociopolitical and economic forces of the larger society. Practice is not perceived from the posi-tion of personal territory; it is recognized as a part of a larger system which is influenced by that system but must also contribute to the system. Nursing in the future will be involved intimately with that larger system of health care, which in turn will be involved with the greater society—locally, regionally, and nationally.

Thinking like a professional means that the students in the future have a large view of their practice, develop as a scholar and contributor to nursing knowledge, and assume an active role in helping nursing to meet health needs of individuals in a complex world. If nursing is to take its rightful place in that endeavor, practice experience needs to move the student from a self-interest posture to one that is enlightened by the values and behaviors of the professional in a world society. The purpose of the clinical experience to help students learn to *think like professionals* is basic for the attainable future for the profession.

The fourth purpose is *developing personal causation.* Accountability for one's actions is an essential criterion for any member of a society, but is required of those who are licensed by society to practice nursing. Developing information systems in health care settings will monitor the actions of nurses and others in the delivery of their services and more specifically identify the issues of accountability. The complexity of health care and the varied settings in which it occurs place demands on the nurses, not only for what they do, but also for the possession of requisite knowledge and skills for engaging in these actions. Accountability for knowing and doing in a future world of rapid knowledge generation will be a particular charge to the nurse.

Students need to develop this quality of personal causation early in their clinical experience as it pertains to their accountability for their own knowledge and skills for the actions in which they participate. The emphasis, however, must accommodate the expectation that learners make mistakes in the process of learning and can learn from their mistakes. Accountability for preparation for clinical assignments, recognizing areas of knowledge and knowledge deficits as they pertain to the involved activities, and careful documentation of actions help students to recognize professional accountability as a legitimate value of a professional. The purpose *personal causation* development will become a critical outcome of nursing education as the student prepares to enter a field characterized by ambiguity with some uncertainty of its areas of autonomy which is involved in a society capable of declaring its expectations and issuing sanctions if its expectations are not realized.

A constancy in the future of nursing education's use of the clinical field has been identified. Although the substance of the practice and settings where it occurs will be subject to alteration, its purposes remain constant. The charge to nursing educators is to accept the constancy of the purposes while interpreting them within the context of change, a characteristic of the future.

SUMMARY

The future of nursing and thus the future of nursing education is already evident today. The current developing practices need to be examined in relation to their predictive value for the future.

The change is resulting from many strong movements in society which are altering patterns for delivery of health care. The entrenchment of technology into the health field is evident in many diagnostic and therapeutic modalities and in the computerization of much data resulting in the introduction of new information processing systems. Technology in the health field has brought about marked increase in health care costs.

Increases in health care costs occurring within a limited financial resource has resulted in the federal government's initiation of the prospective case mix reimbursement system as a basis for payment of services provided for hospitalized Medicare patients. The issue of cost containment will be paramount in all health care services for the future. Patterns of health care delivery are already being altered, so that hospital care which is the most costly, will be reserved for the acutely ill requiring high technology intervention. Hospitals will foster early discharge of patients, thus placing a much greater burden of health care on the community agencies.

The changes influence the delivery of nursing care by making the hospital the setting for high intensity acute care requiring nursing competencies reflected in a well-developed knowledge base, skill in technology with a high-touch component, and the requisite knowledge and skills for making clinical judgments in a rapidly changing, high-stress environment. The community agencies will require many more nurses equipped not only with the requisite knowledge of a professional practitioner, but also the knowledge and skills essential for coordination of patient care over a 24-hour period with use of multiple community resources. Nurses will be carrying out many activities of care previously carried out only by nurses practicing in the hospital, such as preparation of patient for hospital admission, assisting with surgical procedures in ambulatory centers, and carrying out many more complex technical interventions in client's homes, clinics, or other settings.

A third major force in the change process is the increasing age of the population which will put greater demand on the use of health care resources. Technology is now permitting life to many individuals who in earlier days would have died. Now with lengthening life spans, the need for continuous monitoring of health status requires increased health care dollars.

The clinical field for nursing experience of students will be more prominent in the community with the hospital designated as the field for the more experienced student who is able to cope with and learn in a highly technical, stressful environment. The shift to more use of practice fields in the community will raise questions as to the appropriateness of the present preparation of faculty, costs entailed in using the fields which are less geographically circumscribed, and the identification of the knowledge and skills essential for a professional practitioner.

Change in the future relates to where students will have their practice experience and the knowledge and competencies they will need to practice in the future. Constancy in the future rests with the intent of the preparation—to provide nursing care to clients in order to facilitate the best possible health. For the educators, the source of constancy remains in the purposes for the use of the clinical field in preparation of tomorrow's nurses; learning how to learn, dealing with ambiguity, thinking like professionals, and developing personal causation. Both constancy and change are in the future of nursing education.

The past is recollected in the present. The future is anticipated in the present. In a sense, the "past" is gone; the "future" never comes. Now is the time to move with the future.

REFERENCES

American Academy of Nursing. (1983). *Magnet hospitals: Attraction and retention of professional nurses.* Kansas City, Mo.: American Nurses Association.

Ball, M. J., & Hannah, L. J. (1983). *Using computers in nursing.* Reston, Va.: Reston.

Bolles, P. N. (1983). Life/work planning: Change and constancy in the world of work. *The Futurist, 12*(6), 7–11.

Clifford, J. C. (1982). Professional nursing practice in a hospital setting. In L. H. Aiken (Ed.), *Nursing in the 1980's: Crises, opportunities, challenges.* Philadelphia: Lippincott.

Clifford, J. C. (1984). *Discussion.* In American Academy of Nursing. *Nursing research and formation of policy. The case for prospective payment.* Kansas City, Mo.: American Nurses Association.

Conclusions and recommendations of panel on medical student education. (1984, Sept. 26). *Chronicle of Higher Education,* pp. 15–20.

Curtin, L. L. (1984). Prospective payment: Winners and losers. In American Academy of Nursing, *Nursing research and policy formation: The case of prospective payment.* Kansas City, Mo.: American Nurses Association.

Davis, C. K. (1984). The status of the reinbursement policy and future directions. In American Academy of Nursing, *Nursing research and policy formation: The case for prospective payment.* Kansas City, Mo.: American Nurses Association.

Donaho, B. A. (1984). Prospective payment: Focus on nursing administration. In American Academy of Nursing, *Nursing research and policy formation: The case for prospective payment.* Kansas City, Mo.: American Nurses Association.

Donley, R., Sr. (1984). Nursing: 2,000, an essay. *Image, 16*(1), 4–6.

Fedorowicz, J. (1983). Will your computer meet your case-mix information? *Nursing & Health Care, 4,* 493–97.

Freidson, E. (1971). *The profession of medicine: A study of the sociology of applied knowledge.* New York: Dodd, Mead.

Harriman, R. (1984). Creativity: Moving beyond creativity. *The Futurist, 18*(4), 17–20.

Hegyvary, S. T. (1984). Prospective payment: Focus on quality of care. In American Academy of Nursing, *Nursing research and policy formation: The case for reimbursement.* Kansas City, Mo.: American Nurses Association.

Hill, D. A. (1984). A delphi application health care, practice, education and educator, administrator; Circa 1992. *Image, 16*(1), 6–8.

Horn, S. D. (1984). Overview of current models for prospective payment. In American Academy of Nursing, *Nursing research and policy formation: The case for prospective payment.* Kansas City, Mo.: American Nurses Association.

Jacox, A. J. (1982). Role restructuring in hospital nursing. In L. H. Aiken (Ed.), *Nursing in the 1980's: Crises, opportunities, challenges.* Philadelphia: Lippincott.

Joel, L. A. (1983). DRG's: The state of the art of reimbursement for nursing services. *Nursing & Health Care, 43,* 560–63.

Lichlig, L. K. (1982). Data systems for case-mix. *Topics in Health Care Financing,* 13–19.

Loye, D. (1984). The forecasting brain: How we see the future. *The Futurist, 18*(1), 63–68.

McClure, M. L., & Nelson, M. J. (1982). Trends in hospital nursing. In L. H. Aiken (Ed.), *Nursing in the 1980's: Crises, opportunities, challenges.* Philadelphia: Lippincott.

McInnes, N. (1984). Networking: A way to manage our changing world? *The Futurist, 18*(3), 9–10.

Naisbitt, J. (1982). *Megatrends.* New York: Warner Books.

Nursing service in transition: Four perspectives. (1984). *Nursing & Health Care, 5,* 312–16.

Plomann, M. P., & Shaffer, F. A. (1983). DRG's as one of nine approaches to case-mix in transition. *Nursing & Health Care, 5,* 438–43.

Romano, C. (1984). A computerized multidisciplinary discharge care planning model: NIH model. In *Computer Technology: 2nd National Conference.* Monograph of National Institute of Health.

Romano, C., McCormick, R. A., & McNeely, L. D. (1982). Nursing documentation: A computerized data base. *Advances in Nursing Science, 4,* 43–56.

Rosenow, A. M. (1983). Professional nursing practice in the beaurocratic hospital-revisited. *Nursing Outlook, 31*(1), 34–39.

Schraff, S. H. (1984) as quoted in Nursing service in transition: Four perspectives. *Nursing & Health Care, 5,* 312–16.

Shaffer, F. A. (1983). DRG's history and overview. *Nursing & Health Care, 4,* 388–96.

Simmons, A. (1984). Computer implementation in ambulatory care: A community health model. In *Computer Technology: 2nd National Conference.* Monograph of National Institute of Health.

Simmons, S., & Ryan, L. (1984). The implementation of nursing diagnosis using a computerized information system. In M. J. Kim, G. K. Mac-

Farland, & A. M. McLane, (Eds.), *Classification of nursing diagnosis: Proceedings of Fifth National Conference.* St. Louis: C. V. Mosby.
Wagner, D. (1984). Discussion. In American Academy of Nursing. *Nursing research and formation of policy: The case for prospective payment.* Kansas City, Mo.: American Nurses Association.

BIBLIOGRAPHY

Adams, E. (1983). Frontiers of nursing in 21st century: Development of models and theories in concepts of nursing. *Journal of Nursing Administration, 8*(1), 41–45.
Aiken, L. H. (1982). *Nursing in the 1980's: Crises, opportunities, challenges.* Philadelphia: Lippincott.
Anderson, R., Pierce, I., & Rengal, K. (1983). Networking: A method of retaining nursing staff. *Journal of Nursing Administration, 13*(1), 26–28.
Barnett, G. O. (1984). Application of computer-based medical record systems in ambulatory practice. *New England Journal of Medicine, 310*(25), 1643–50.
Computer Technology and Nursing: 2nd National Conference. (1984). Monograph of the National Institute of Health.
Computerized nursing information system: An urgent need: Report of study group in nursing information systems. (1983). *Research in Nursing and Health, 3,* 101–105.
Curtin, L. (1983). Determining costs of nursing service per DRG. *Nursing Management, 14*(4), 11–20.
Davidson, R. A., & Louver, D. (1984). Nurse practitioner and physician roles: Delineation and complementarity of practice. *Research in Nursing and Health, 7,* 3–9.
Davis, C. K. (1983). The federal role in changing health care financing: Prospective payment and its impact on nursing, part 2. *Nursing Economics, 1*(2), 98–104, 146.
Deiman, P. A., Noble, E., & Russell, M. (1984). Achieving a professional practice model: How primary nursing can help. *Journal of Nursing Education, 14*(7,8), 16–22.
Edmunds, L. (1983). Hospital information system—the need for a nursing subsystem. *Computer Nursing, 1*(1), 1–3.
Edmunds, L. (1983). Computer assisted quality assurance model. *Journal of Nursing Administration, 13*(3), 36–43.
Gaynor, J. M., Kant, D. A., & Mills, E. M. (1984). DRG's regulatory and budgetary adjustment. *Nursing & Health Care, 14,* 275–79.
Grayson, C. J., Jr. (1984). Networking by computer. *The Futurist. 18*(3), 14–17.
Grimaldi, P. L., & Micheletti, J. A. (1982). *DRG's: A practitioner guide.* Chicago: Pluribus Press.
Hamilton, J. M. (1984). Nursing and DRG's: Proactive response to prospective reimbursement. *Nursing & Health Care, 5,* 155–59.
Hassett, M. R. (1984). Computers and nursing education in 1980's. *Nursing Outlook, 32*(1), 34–36.
Horn, S. D., & Shumacher, D. N. (1979). An analysis of case-mix complexity using information theory and DRG. *Medical Care, 17*(4), 382–89.
Jacox, A. J. (1984). Prospective payment: Focus on clinical research. In

American Academy of Nursing, *Nursing research and policy formation: The case for prospective payment.* Kansas City, Mo.: American Nurses Association.

Lagona, T. G., & Stritzel, M. M. (1984). Nursing care requirement as measurement by DRG. *Journal of Nursing Administration, 11,* 15–18.

Long-Term Care in Perspective, Past, Present and Future Directions for Nursing. (1973). Monograph of the American Academy of Nursing. Kansas City, Mo.: American Nursing Association.

Marran, G. (1976). The comparative costs of operating a team and primary nursing unit. *Journal of Nursing Administration, 6*(4), 21–24.

McCormick, K. A. (1983). Preparing nurses for the technologic future. *Nursing & Health Care, 4,* 379–82.

McCormick, K. A. (1984). Nursing in the computer revolution. *Computer Nurse, 2*(2), 4, 30.

Mikan, K. J. (1984). Computer integration, a challenge for nursing education. *Nursing Outlook, 32*(1), 6.

Models for Health Care Delivery: Now and for the Future. (1974). Monograph of the Academy of Nursing. Kansas City, Mo.: American Nurses Association.

Munschauer, R. J. (1983). Decentralized management—Moving authority and accountability closer to the operational level. *Nursing Management, 14*(4), 21–22.

Nursing Research and Policy Formation: The Case for Prospective Payment. (1984). Monograph of the American Academy of Nursing. Kansas City, Mo.: American Nurses Association.

Piper, L. A. (1983). Accounting for nursing functions in DRG's. *Nursing Management, 14*(11), 46–48.

Rosenour, J., Stanford, D., Morgan, W., & Curtin, R. (1984). Prescribing behaviors of primary nurse practitioners. *American Journal of Public Health, 74*(1), 10–13.

Saba, V. K. (1982). The computer in public health, today and tomorrow. *Nursing Outlook, 30*(9), 510–14.

Shaffer, F. A. (1984). A nursing perspective of DRG, Part 1. *Nursing & Health Care, 5,* 48–51.

Smith, M. J. (1984). Transformation: A key to shaping nursing. *Image, 16*(1), 28–30.

Stegman, C. B., & Dison, C. C. (1984). Changing service-education relationships: The impact of primary nursing. *Journal of Nursing Education, 14*(3), 26–29.

Toffler, A. (1980). *The third wave.* New York: Bantam Books.

Toth, R. M. (1984). DRG's: Imperative strategies for nursing service administration. *Nursing & Health Care, 5,* 196–203.

Vanderzee, H., & Glusko, G. (1984). DRG's, variable pricing and budgeting for nursing service. *Journal of Nursing Administration, 14*(5), 11–14.

Walker, D. D. (1983). The cost of nursing care in hospitals. *Journal of Nursing Administration, 13*(3), 13–18.

Washington focus: DRG's, the new pulse of health policy. *Nursing & Health Care, 4,* 208–9.

Zielstorff, R. D. (1984). Why aren't there more significant automated nursing information systems? *Journal of Nursing Administration, 14*(1), 7–10.

Index

Italicized page numbers represent figures and tables.